MEDICAL MANAGEMENT OF TYPE 2 DIABETES

EIGHTH EDITION

Edited by
Luigi F. Meneghini, MD, MBA

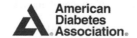

American Diabetes Association

Associate Publisher, Books, Abe Ogden; *Director, Book Operations,* Victor Van Beuren; *Managing Editor, Books,* John Clark; *Associate Director, Book Marketing,* Annette Reape; *Acquisitions Editor,* Jaclyn Konich; *Senior Manager, Book Editing,* Lauren Wilson; *Editor,* Absolute Services; *Composition,* Cenveo; *Cover Design,* Jody Billert; *Printer,* Lightning Source.

Printed in the United States of America
1 3 5 7 9 10 8 6 4 2

The suggestions and information contained in this publication are generally consistent with the *Standards of Medical Care in Diabetes* and other policies of the American Diabetes Association, but they do not represent the policy or position of the Association or any of its boards or committees. Reasonable steps have been taken to ensure the accuracy of the information presented. However, the American Diabetes Association cannot ensure the safety or efficacy of any product or service described in this publication. Individuals are advised to consult a physician or other appropriate health care professional before undertaking any diet or exercise program or taking any medication referred to in this publication. Professionals must use and apply their own professional judgment, experience, and training and should not rely solely on the information contained in this publication before prescribing any diet, exercise, or medication. The American Diabetes Association—its officers, directors, employees, volunteers, and members—assumes no responsibility or liability for personal or other injury, loss, or damage that may result from the suggestions or information in this publication.

Barry Ginsberg, MD, PhD, conducted the internal review of this book to ensure that it meets American Diabetes Association guidelines.

♾ The paper in this publication meets the requirements of the ANSI Standard Z39.48-1992 (permanence of paper).

ADA titles may be purchased for business or promotional use or for special sales. To purchase more than 50 copies of this book at a discount, or for custom editions of this book with your logo, contact the American Diabetes Association at the address below or at booksales@diabetes.org.

American Diabetes Association
2451 Crystal Drive, Suite 900
Arlington, VA 22202

DOI: 10.2337/9781580406314

Library of Congress Cataloging-in-Publication Data

Names: Meneghini, Luigi, MD, editor. | American Diabetes Association, issuing body.
Title: Medical management of type 2 diabetes / edited by Luigi Meneghini.
Other titles: Medical management of type two diabetes
Description: Eighth edition. | Arlington, VA : American Diabetes Association, [2020] | Includes bibliographical references and index.
Identifiers: LCCN 2020011341 (print) | LCCN 2020011342 (ebook) | ISBN 9781580406314 (paperback ; alk. paper) | ISBN 9781580406970 (ebook)
Subjects: MESH: Diabetes Mellitus, Type 2
Classification: LCC RC660.4 (print) | LCC RC660.4 (ebook) | NLM WK 810 | DDC 616.4/62--dc23
LC record available at https://lccn.loc.gov/2020011341
LC ebook record available at https://lccn.loc.gov/2020011342

Contents

Detection and Treatment of Chronic Complications   215

Diabetes Self-Management Education and Behavior Change 303

A Word About This Guide

Type 2 diabetes is a worldwide epidemic fueled by the increasing prevalence of obesity, sedentary lifestyles, and poor nutrition. We now predict that one in three American children born in 2000 will develop type 2 diabetes with the attendant risks of early morbidity and mortality. In the U.S. in 2017, annual expenditures for people with diabetes approximated $327 billion, taking an increasing portion of expenditures for healthcare (1 in 7 healthcare dollars), making this disease a problem for both society and the individual. Reversing these trends will take a concerted effort in public education directed toward developing better eating and lifestyle habits, as well as sustainable behavior change.

Although prevention of type 2 diabetes is a necessary key to addressing the epidemic, for the foreseeable future clinicians will be caring for an increasing number of individuals with diabetes. Since the last edition of this guide, there has been a significant increase in our knowledge of the pathogenesis of type 2 diabetes, its complications, and the options for treatment. Numerous studies have shown that lifestyle changes and pharmacological interventions make a significant impact on the well-being of the patient. Several cardiovascular and renovascular intervention trials have demonstrated the benefits of novel classes of anti-hyperglycemic medications such as GLP-1 receptor agonists and SGLT2 inhibitors in reducing the progression and complications of this disease, and in some cases reducing cardiovascular mortality. The aggressive intervention with medications to control blood pressure and lipids, smoking cessation, and antiplatelet therapy have been shown to prevent cardiovascular events in people with type 2 diabetes. When diabetes requires pharmacologic intervention, multiple drugs can and should be used in combination to control hyperglycemia in a timely fashion in order to avoid therapeutic inertia and prevent long-term complications. The introduction of medications that have unique mechanisms, such as the long-acting (once-daily and once-weekly) GLP-1RA, have changed our approach to the patient needing to transition to injectable therapy to improve glycemic control. These agents are recommended before insulin therapy is considered, unless hyperglycemia is very symptomatic. New insulin analogs and improved delivery devices can facilitate insulin administration for patients, which should improve treatment acceptance and adherence. Using available behavioral, educational, and therapeutic tools in the context of a multidisciplinary team approach to care for individuals with type 2 diabetes should translate into reduced diabetes-related complications and comorbidities.

This edition of *Medical Management of Type 2 Diabetes* has been updated to provide state-of-the-art information on these issues by a select group of experts. It also reflects the most recent *Standards of Medical Care in Diabetes* from the American Diabetes Association. This book, along with other American Diabetes Association publications, including *Medical Management of Type 1 Diabetes, Therapy for Diabetes Mellitus and Related Disorders, Intensive Diabetes Management,* and *Medical Management of Pregnancy Complicated by Diabetes*, were designed to provide healthcare professionals with the comprehensive information needed to give the best possible medical care to patients with diabetes mellitus.

The American Diabetes Association believes that you will find this book as useful as previous editions, with timely and valuable updates based on published evidence. We hope that it will encourage you to add other American Diabetes Association publications to your library and, in so doing, continue to optimize your approach and management for people with diabetes.

LUIGI F. MENEGHINI, MD, MBA
Editor

Contributors to the Eighth Edition

EDITOR

Luigi F. Meneghini, MD, MBA
Department of Internal Medicine,
   Division of Endocrinology
University of Texas Southwestern
   Medical Center
Parkland Health & Hospital System
Dallas, Texas

CONTRIBUTORS

Marconi Abreu, MD
Department of Internal Medicine,
   Division of Endocrinology
University of Texas Southwestern
   Medical Center
Global Diabetes Program
Parkland Health & Hospital System
Dallas, Texas

Sadia Ali, MD
Department of Internal Medicine,
   Division of Endocrinology
University of Texas Southwestern
   Medical Center
Dallas, Texas

Perry E. Bickel, MD
Department of Internal Medicine,
   Division of Endocrinology
University of Texas Southwestern
   Medical Center
Dallas, Texas

Abha Choudhary, MD
Department of Pediatrics
University of Texas Southwestern
   Medical Center
Dallas, Texas

**Nancy Drobycki, RN, MSN,
   CDCES**
Department of Internal Medicine,
   Division of Endocrinology
University of Texas Southwestern
   Medical Center
Dallas, Texas

Fredrick Dunn, MD
Division of Nutrition and Metabolic
   Diseases
University of Texas Southwestern
   Medical Center
Dallas, Texas

Uma Gunasekaran, MD
Department of Internal Medicine,
   Division of Endocrinology
University of Texas Southwestern
   Medical Center
Parkland Health & Hospital System
Dallas, Texas

Olga Gupta, MD
Department of Pediatrics
University of Texas Southwestern
   Medical Center
Dallas, Texas

Iram Hussain, MD
Department of Internal Medicine,
Division of Endocrinology
University of Texas Southwestern
Medical Center
Dallas, Texas

**Nisha Jacob, DNP, FNP-C,
CDCES, MBA**
Department of Internal Medicine,
Division of Endocrinology
University of Texas Southwestern
Medical Center
Dallas, Texas

Asra Kermani, MD
Department of Internal Medicine,
Division of Endocrinology
University of Texas Southwestern
Medical Center
Southwestern Health Resources
Dallas, Texas

Ildiko Lingvay, MD, MPH
Global Diabetes Program
Parkland Health & Hospital System
Dallas, Texas

**Anitha Litty, DNP, FNP-C,
CDCES**
Department of Internal Medicine,
Division of Endocrinology
University of Texas Southwestern
Medical Center
Dallas, Texas

**Janice MacLeod, MA, RDN, LD,
CDE, FAADE**
Head of Clinical Advocacy
Companion Medical
Columbia, Maryland

**Jacqueline Nicole McNulty,
PharmD, BCACP**
Global Diabetes Program
Parkland Health & Hospital System,
Dallas, Texas

Sasan Mirfakhraee, MD
Department of Internal Medicine,
Division of Endocrinology
University of Texas Southwestern
Medical Center
Dallas, Texas

**Kellie Rodriguez, RN, MSN,
CDCES**
Global Diabetes Program
Parkland Health & Hospital System
Dallas, Texas

Kyaw Soe, MD
Department of Internal Medicine,
Division of Endocrinology
University of Texas Southwestern
Medical Center
Dallas VA Medical Center
Dallas, Texas

Acknowledgments

The American Diabetes Association gratefully acknowledges the contributions of the following healthcare professionals and members of the Association's Professional Section to previous editions of this work:

Robert M. Anderson, EdD; Christine A. Beebe, MS, RD, CDE; John B. Buse, MD, PhD; Nathaniel G. Clark, MD, MS, RD; Komel Benjamin Craig, MPH, RD, LDN; Mayer B. Davidson, MD; Martha M. Funnell, MS, RN, CDCES, FADCES, FAAN; Roma Gianchandani, MD; William Herman, MD, MPH; Harold E. Lebovitz, MD; David Nathan, MD; Robin B. Nwankwo, MPH, RD, CDE; Rodica Pop-Busui, MD, PhD; Philip Raskin, MD; Matthew C. Riddle, MD; Harold Rifkin, MD; Robert A. Rizza, MD; F. John Service, MD, PhD; Robert Sherwin, MD; Martin Stevens, MD; Jennifer Wyckoff, MD; and Bruce R. Zimmerman, MD.

The Association also gratefully acknowledges the editors of the seventh edition of this work: Charles F. Burant, MD, PhD, and Laura A. Young, MD, PhD, and the review of this edition by Susan Braithwaite, MD, Sacha Uelmen, RDN, CDE, and Barry Ginsberg, MD, PhD.

Diagnosis and Classification

Highlights
Diagnosis and Classification

■ Diabetes is diagnosed by one of the following, confirmed by repeat testing in the absence of unequivocal hyperglycemia:

- Hemoglobin A_{1c} (A1C) ≥6.5% (48 mmol/mol) by laboratory method; point-of-care A1C assays are not sufficiently accurate to use for diagnostic purposes
- Fasting plasma glucose (FPG) ≥126 mg/dL (7.0 mmol/L)
- 2-h plasma glucose ≥200 mg/dL (11.1 mmol/L) during a 75-g oral glucose tolerance test (OGTT)
- Random plasma glucose ≥200 mg/dL (11.1 mmol/L) in a patient with classic symptoms of hyperglycemia (polydipsia, polyuria, unintentional weight loss) or hyperglycemic crisis.

■ The two most common types of diabetes are type 1 diabetes, which has absolute insulin deficiency and propensity to develop ketoacidosis, and type 2 diabetes, which has relative insulin deficiency combined with defects in insulin action. Type 2 diabetes accounts for 90%–95% of the incidence of the disease in Western societies and is most often (but not always) associated with obesity.

■ Prediabetes describes individuals with plasma glucose or A1C levels higher than normal but lower than those diagnostic of diabetes. Such individuals are at higher risk for both progression to type 2 diabetes and cardiovascular disease. Diagnostic criteria for prediabetes include:

- A1C 5.7%–6.4% (39–46 mmol/mol)
- FPG 100 mg/dL (5.6 mmol/L) to 125 mg/dL (6.9 mmol/L), also known as impaired fasting glucose (IFG)
- 2-h plasma glucose during the 75-g OGTT 140 mg/dL (7.8 mmol/L) to 199 mg/dL (11.0 mmol/L), also known as impaired glucose tolerance (IGT).

■ Gestational diabetes mellitus (GDM) is defined as hyperglycemia diagnosed during the second or third trimesters of pregnancy. It affects approximately 6% of all pregnancies in the U.S. As many as 50% of women with GDM later develop type 2 diabetes. If diabetes is diagnosed at the initial prenatal visit within the first trimester, using standard criteria for diabetes, it should be classified as "diabetes complicating pregnancy."

■ Screening for GDM is recommended between the 24th and 28th week of pregnancy for all women who are not known to have diabetes. The two approaches used in the U.S. include the following:

- "One-step approach" with 75-g OGTT with plasma glucose measurement of fasting at 1 h and 2 h. GDM is diagnosed if
  - FPG ≥92 mg/dL (≥5.1 mmol/L), or
  - 1-h plasma glucose ≥180 mg/dL (≥10.0 mmol/L), or
  - 2-h plasma glucose ≥153 mg/dL (≥8.5 mmol/L).

- "Two-step approach" with a 50-g nonfasting screen, which if abnormal is followed by 100-g OGTT.

■ All women diagnosed with GDM should be screened at 4–12 weeks postpartum for diabetes or prediabetes using usual nongestational glycemic criteria and rescreened periodically (at least every 3 years) thereafter.

Diagnosis and Classification

Sadia Ali, MD

DEFINITION OF DIABETES

- Diabetes is a group of chronic metabolic diseases characterized by hyperglycemia resulting from defects in insulin secretion, insulin action, or both. These defects result in abnormalities in carbohydrate, protein, and fat metabolism from deficient action of insulin on target tissues.[1]
- Chronic, sustained exposure to hyperglycemia is associated with long-term damage, dysfunction, and failure of various organs leading to microvascular complications (e.g., retinopathy, nephropathy, and neuropathy), as well as macrovascular complications (e.g., stroke, myocardial infarction, and peripheral arterial disease).[2,3]
- Symptoms of marked hyperglycemia include polyuria, polydipsia, weight loss, sometimes polyphagia, and blurred vision. Acute, life-threatening consequences of uncontrolled diabetes are hyperglycemia with ketoacidosis or hyperglycemia hyperosmolar nonketotic syndrome.

Because the syndrome of diabetes encompasses many disorders that differ in pathogenesis, natural history, and responses to treatment, it is important that clinicians and researchers use commonly accepted terminology as well as standardized classification and diagnostic criteria when categorizing patients with glucose intolerance.

Following the findings of the Diabetes Prevention Program, recognition of degrees of carbohydrate intolerance led to the description of categories of increased risk for diabetes as well as cardiovascular disease (prediabetes). The designation encompasses the previously described impaired fasting glucose (IFG), impaired glucose tolerance (IGT), and individuals with A1C of 5.7%–6.4% (39–46 mmol/mol). Identification of such individuals should facilitate efforts to intervene early and reduce the incidence of diabetes and cardiovascular disease.

The Hyperglycemia and Adverse Pregnancy Outcomes Study (HAPO)[4] demonstrated an increased risk of adverse maternal, fetal, and neonatal outcomes of pregnancy as a function of maternal glycemia at 24–28 weeks' gestation even within ranges previously considered normal for pregnancy. As a result the American Diabetes Association developed revised criteria for the diagnosis of gestational diabetes mellitus (GDM), which will significantly increase the prevalence of GDM, but with appropriate treatment, should optimize gestational outcomes for women and their babies.

DIAGNOSIS OF DIABETES

According to current American Diabetes Association criteria, diabetes may be diagnosed based on fasting plasma glucose (FPG) ≥126 mg/dL (≥7.0 mmol/L), a 2-h oral glucose tolerance test (OGTT) ≥200 mg/dl (≥11.1 mmol/L), or A1C ≥6.5% (≥48 mmol/mol) (Table 1.1).[1] Except for patients in hyperglycemic crisis or with classic hyperglycemia symptoms associated with a random plasma glucose ≥200 mg/dL (≥11.1 mmol/L), diagnosis requires a second test for confirmation of diabetes[5]; this could be two different tests from the same sample (i.e., A1C and FPG) or a repeat test on a different day (same or different lab test). In patients where diabetes is diagnosed on the basis of symptoms and a random glucose ≥200 mg/dL, a confirmatory A1C adds additional value in terms of initial treatment options.

When comparing different tests, the A1C has several advantages over OGTT and FPG, including greater convenience as the patient does not need to fast, less day-to-day variation, and greater pre-analytic stability. Relative disadvantages include lower sensitivity of A1C at the designated cut point, greater cost, limited availability of A1C testing in certain regions of the developing world, and the imperfect correlation between A1C and average glucose in certain individuals.[6] National Health and Nutrition Examination Survey (NHANES) data indicate that an A1C cut point of ≥6.5% (≥48 mmol/mol) identifies a prevalence of undiagnosed diabetes that is one-third of that using glucose criteria.[7]

In addition, A1C may not accurately reflect glycemic exposure in patients with certain hemoglobinopathies, thalassemia syndromes, states of increased red cell turnover—including those related to hemolysis, cytotoxic chemotherapy, erythropoietin therapy, or transfusion—and in patients with iron deficiency. Uremia and hyperbilirubinemia may also interfere with some assays. In such patients, the diagnosis of diabetes must employ other glycemic criteria.

Table 1.1–Criteria for the Diagnosis of Diabetes

1. A1C ≥6.5% (≥48 mmol/mol). The test should be performed in a laboratory using a method that is National Glycohemoglobin Standardization Program certified and standardized to the Diabetes Control and Complications Trial assay.

   OR

2. FPG ≥126 mg/dL (≥7.0 mmol/L). Fasting is defined as no caloric intake for ≥8 h.

   OR

3. 2-h plasma glucose ≥200 mg/dL (≥11.1 mmol/L) during OGTT. The test should be performed as described by the World Health Organization (WHO), using a glucose load containing the equivalent of 75 g anhydrous glucose dissolved in water.

   OR

4. In a patient with classic symptoms of hyperglycemia (polydipsia, polyuria, unintentional weight loss) or hyperglycemic crisis, a random plasma glucose ≥200 mg/dL (≥11.1 mmol/L).

The FPG and the 2-h OGTT are the other two tests that may be used to diagnose diabetes. The FPG and 2-h OGTT tests do not always match in diagnosing diabetes; the same is true of the A1C test and either glucose-based test (FPG or OGTT). Numerous studies have confirmed that compared with FPG and A1C cut points, the 2-h OGTT value is more sensitive and diagnoses more people with diabetes.[8] Therefore, OGTT could be considered in patients with elevated but nondiagnostic A1C or FPG in whom there is a high index of suspicion for diabetes (e.g., in patients with evidence of cardiovascular disease or microvascular complications). The OGTT is not required for patients with symptoms and concurrent random glucose levels ≥200 mg/dL (≥11.1 mmol/L), A1C ≥6.5% (≥48 mmol/mol), or fasting glucose level ≥126 mg/dL (≥7.0 mmol/L).

CLASSIFICATION OF DIABETES

Having established a diagnosis of diabetes, the next task is to classify the type. The purpose of classification is to differentiate and identify the various forms of the disease, as the treatment approach will vary for different types of diabetes. Of note, a number of individuals do not fit into a single class at time of diagnosis.[1]

The first generally accepted classification system was developed by the National Diabetes Data Group (NDDG) and published in 1979.[9] The World Health Organization (WHO) Study Group on Diabetes Mellitus endorsed the substantive recommendations of the NDDG in 1980 and 1985.[10] These groups recognized two major forms of diabetes, which they termed insulin-dependent diabetes mellitus (IDDM, type I diabetes) and non–insulin-dependent diabetes mellitus (NIDDM, type II diabetes). In 1997, the American Diabetes Association Expert Committee on the Diagnosis and Classification of Diabetes Mellitus recommended modifications to this classification system. The revised classification scheme was designed to reduce some of the confusion created by the previous scheme and to reflect both etiology and stage of disease. The terms insulin-dependent diabetes mellitus (IDDM) and non–insulin-dependent diabetes mellitus (NIDDM) and their acronyms were eliminated, as they frequently resulted in classifying patients based on treatment rather than etiology, and substituted with the terms type 1 diabetes and type 2 diabetes, respectively.

Diabetes is now generally classified into the following categories (see Table 1.2):

1. Type 1 diabetes (due to destruction of pancreatic β-cells, usually leading to absolute insulin deficiency).
2. Type 2 diabetes (due to a combination of loss of β-cell insulin secretion and insulin resistance).
3. GDM (diabetes diagnosed in the second and third trimester of pregnancy in a woman without a prior diagnosis of diabetes).
4. Other specific types of diabetes from various causes, e.g., monogenic diabetes syndromes (from genetic defects of β cell function and defects in insulin action), diseases of the exocrine pancreas (e.g., cystic fibrosis and pancreatitis), and drug- or chemical-induced diabetes (from glucocorticoid use, HIV/AIDS treatment, or after organ transplantation).[1]

—

Table 1.2–Etiologic Classification of Diabetes

I. Type 1 diabetes* (β-cell destruction, usually leading to absolute insulin deficiency)

  A. Immune mediated

  B. Idiopathic

II. Type 2 diabetes* (may range from predominantly insulin resistant with relative insulin deficiency to a predominantly secretory defect with insulin resistance)

III. Other specific types

  A. Genetic defects of β-cell function
    1. Chromosome 12, hepatic nuclear factor HNF-1α (formerly MODY3)
    2. Chromosome 7, glucokinase (formerly MODY2)
    3. Chromosome 20, HNF-4α (formerly MODY1)
    4. Chromosome 13, insulin promoter factor-1 (IPF-1; MODY4)
    5. Chromosome 17, HNF-1β (MODY5)
    6. Chromosome 2, *NeuroD1* or BETA2 (formerly MODY6)
    7. Mitochondrial DNA
    8. Others

  B. Genetic defects in insulin action
    1. Type A insulin resistance
    2. Leprechaunism
    3. Rabson-Mendenhall syndrome
    4. Lipoatrophic diabetes
    5. Others

  C. Diseases of the exocrine pancreas
    1. Pancreatitis
    2. Trauma/pancreatectomy
    3. Neoplasia
    4. Cystic fibrosis
    5. Hemochromatosis
    6. Fibrocalculous pancreatopathy
    7. Others

  D. Endocrinopathies
    1. Acromegaly
    2. Cushing syndrome
    3. Glucagonoma
    4. Pheochromocytoma
    5. Hyperthyroidism
    6. Somatostatinoma
    7. Aldosteronoma
    8. Others

  E. Drug or chemical induced
    1. Vacor
    2. Pentamidine
    3. Nicotinic acid
    4. Glucocorticoids
    5. Thyroid hormone
    6. Diazoxide
    7. β-Adrenergic agonists
    8. Thiazides
    9. Dilantin
    10. Atypical antipsychotics
    11. Antidepressants associated with weight gain (such as tricyclic antidepressants, selective serotonin reuptake inhibitors, and monoamine oxidase inhibitors)
    12. HIV/AIDS medications
    13. α-Interferon
    14. Immune checkpoint inhibitors
    15. Others

  F. Infections
    1. Congenital rubella
    2. Cytomegalovirus
    3. Others

  G. Uncommon forms of immune-mediated diabetes
    1. "Stiff-man" syndrome
    2. Anti-insulin receptor antibodies
    3. Immune checkpoint mediator-induced diabetes
    4. Others

  H. Other genetic syndromes sometimes associated with diabetes
    1. Down syndrome
    2. Klinefelter syndrome
    3. Turner syndrome
    4. Wolfram syndrome
    5. Friedreich ataxia
    6. Huntington chorea
    7. Lawrence Moon Beidel syndrome
    8. Myotonic dystrophy
    9. Porphyria
    10. Prader-Willi syndrome
    11. Others

IV. Gestational diabetes mellitus

*Patients with any form of diabetes may require insulin treatment at some stage of their disease. Use of insulin does not, of itself, classify the patient.[11–18]

Type 1 diabetes and type 2 diabetes are heterogeneous diseases in which clinical presentation and disease progression may vary considerably. Classification is important in determining therapy, but some individuals cannot be clearly classified as having type 1 or type 2 at the time of diagnosis. The traditional paradigms of type 1 occurring only in children and type 2 occurring only in adults are no longer accurate, as both diseases occur in any age group.

TYPE 1 DIABETES

Type 1 diabetes accounts for 5%–10% of all diabetes and results from cell-mediated destruction of pancreatic β-cells, leading to absolute insulin deficiency. These individuals are prone to develop ketoacidosis. This form includes cases resulting from both autoimmune process (type 1A) and those for which an etiology is unknown (type 1B, idiopathic). Autoimmune markers of this process include islet cell autoantibodies, autoantibodies to insulin, autoantibodies to glutamic acid decarboxylase (GAD), the tyrosine phosphatases IA-2 and IA-2B, and zinc transporter (ZnT8).[19] One or more autoantibodies is present in ≤90% of individuals with type 1 immune-mediated diabetes at diagnosis. Patients with type 1 immune-mediated diabetes are prone to other autoimmune disorders, including autoimmune thyroid disease, celiac disease, Addison disease, autoimmune gastritis, and vitiligo. In these patients, the prevalence of positive antithyroid antibodies can be ≤20%, hypothyroidism 2%–5%, and hyperthyroidism <1%.[20–27] For other autoimmune disorders, the prevalence of positive anti-endomysial or tissue transglutaminase is ≤10%, biopsy proven celiac disease 5%,[28–31] autoimmune gastritis 5%–10%, pernicious anemia 2%–4%,[32–34] Addison disease <1%, and positive 21-hydroxylase antibodies ≤2%.[35]

In addition, this type of diabetes has strong HLA associations, which can be either predisposing (DR3/DR4) or protective.[1] Type 1A (autoimmune) diabetes is currently classified into three stages that reflect the onset of autoimmunity, the development of dysglycemia (IGT or IFG), and eventually the progression to symptomatic hyperglycemia (see Table 1.3).[36,37]

Immune-mediated type 1 diabetes commonly occurs in childhood and adolescence but can occur at any age. The rate of β-cell destruction is quite variable. In general, it is more rapid in children and slower in adults. This may explain why children present with ketoacidosis as the first manifestation of disease, and adults may retain sufficient β-cell function to prevent ketoacidosis for many years. Although patients are often not obese when they present with type 1 diabetes, the presence of obesity is not incompatible with the diagnosis, especially given the increased prevalence of obesity in the general population. In the late stages of type 1 immune-mediated diabetes, there is little or no insulin secretion as manifested by low or undetectable levels of plasma C-peptide in the setting of hyperglycemia.

Patients that present with ketoacidosis and have no evidence of autoimmunity and no clear etiology are classified as having idiopathic type 1 diabetes; other terms include type 1B or 1.5 diabetes, atypical diabetes, Flatbush diabetes, or ketosis-prone type 2 diabetes. These patients are insulinopenic and are prone to episodic ketoacidosis. This form of diabetes is thought to account for 25%–50% of new diabetic ketoacidosis presentations in African American and Hispanic individuals and has also been described in Asian populations.[38] While it is not HLA associated,

Table 1.3–Staging of Type 1 Diabetes

	Stage 1	Stage 2	Stage 3
Characteristics	■ Autoimmunity ■ Normoglycemia ■ Presymptomatic	■ Autoimmunity ■ Dysglycemia ■ Presymptomatic	■ New-onset hyperglycemia ■ Symptomatic
Diagnostic criteria	■ Multiple autoantibodies ■ No IGT or IFG	■ Multiple autoantibodies ■ Dysglycemia: IFG and/or IGT ■ FPG 100–125 mg/dL (5.6–6.9 mmol/L) ■ 2-h PG 140–199 mg/dL (7.8–11.0 mmol/L) ■ A1C 5.7%–6.4% (39–47 mmol/mol) or ≥10% increase in A1C	■ Clinical symptoms ■ Diabetes by standard criteria

Source: Imsel[36] and Skyler. [37]

the majority of patients have a family history of type 2 diabetes and are overweight or obese. Individuals with this form of diabetes suffer from episodic ketoacidosis and exhibit varying degrees of insulin deficiency between episodes. An absolute requirement for insulin replacement therapy in affected patients may come and go. Fasting C-peptide levels >0.33 nmol/L collected 1 week after resolution of ketoacidosis or >0.5 nmol/L at 6–8 weeks following the acute event are predictive of remission to near-normal glycemia.[38]

TYPE 2 DIABETES

Type 2 diabetes accounts for 90%–95% of all diabetes diagnosed in adults and is characterized by both impairment of insulin secretion and defects in insulin action. Although patients with this type of diabetes may have insulin levels that appear normal or elevated, insulin levels are low relative to the ambient hyperglycemia. Thus, insulin secretion is defective in these patients and insufficient to compensate for the degree of insulin resistance. Although the specific etiology of type 2 diabetes is unknown, autoimmune destruction of β-cells does not occur. Type 2 diabetes is often associated with a strong genetic predisposition; however, the genetics of this form of diabetes are complex and not clearly defined.

The risk of type 2 diabetes increases with age, obesity, and physical inactivity. Although type 1 diabetes remains the most common type of diabetes in children and adolescents, type 2 diabetes now accounts for one-quarter to one-third of diabetes in adolescents, particularly in racial and ethnic minority populations. Patients with type 2 diabetes who are not obese by traditional weight criteria (e.g., Asian populations) may have an increased percentage of body fat distributed predominantly in the intra-abdominal region.[39,40] Type 2 diabetes occurs more frequently in women with prior gestational diabetes and in individuals with hypertension and dyslipidemia. Its frequency varies in different racial and ethnic groups. Diabetic ketoacidosis seldom occurs spontaneously in type 2 diabetes, but it can be seen in association with the stress of another illness such as infection or use of certain other drugs (e.g., corticosteroids, atypical antipsychotics, and sodium–glucose transporter 2 inhibitors).[41,42]

GESTATIONAL DIABETES MELLITUS

GDM is defined as diabetes diagnosed in the second or third trimester of pregnancy that was not present prior to pregnancy;[1] in the past, GDM had been defined as glucose intolerance that was first recognized during pregnancy,[43] regardless of whether the condition may have predated pregnancy. Approximately 6% of pregnant women in the U.S. have GDM,[44] while global estimates of GDM vary from 10% to 25% depending on different regions, populations, and methods of diagnosis.[45]

GDM carries risks for mother and neonate. Both the size of the baby and need for a first cesarean delivery are related to the degree of maternal hyperglycemia. The HAPO study[4] demonstrated that the risk of adverse maternal, fetal, and neonatal outcomes continuously increased as a function of maternal glycemia at 24–28 weeks of gestation, even within ranges previously defined as normal. These results emphasize the importance of recognition and treatment of GDM, with a focus on glycemic control as it reduces the risk of adverse outcomes in the mother and the fetus.

Screening for diabetes is recommended for all pregnant women, starting at the first prenatal visit. Women at high risk of diabetes should be screened immediately, using standard diagnostic criteria including A1C, fasting, or post–glucose-load glucose level. Diabetes diagnosed at this stage is considered to have preceded pregnancy. Women not found to have overt diabetes at that first prenatal visit should undergo further testing to rule out GDM at 24–28 weeks' gestation. Currently there are two approaches to diagnose GDM in the U.S. (Table 1.4):[1] "one-step" 75-g OGTT or "two-step" approach with a 50-g (nonfasting) screen followed by a 100-g OGTT for those who screen positive.

Approximately 5%–10% of women with GDM are diagnosed with type 2 diabetes in the postpartum period, and ≤50%–70% develop type 2 diabetes within 15–25 years.[48] Because of this increased risk, women with GDM should be retested for diabetes or prediabetes 4–12 weeks postpartum and every 1–3 years thereafter.[1] A 2-h 75-g OGTT is recommended postpartum because A1C levels may still be impacted by increased red blood cell turnover or delivery-related blood loss; the results are interpreted using nonpregnancy criteria.[49] Thereafter, an A1C, FPG, or 2-h OGTT can be used for screening purposes. Women with a history of GDM found to have prediabetes should receive education about intensive lifestyle interventions or metformin to prevent diabetes.[1]

OTHER SPECIFIC TYPES OF DIABETES

In the current classification scheme, the class of other specific types of diabetes includes the following categories: 1) genetic defects of β-cell function; 2) genetic

Table 1.4–Screening for and Diagnosis of GDM at 24–28 Weeks' Gestation in Women Not Previously Diagnosed with Overt Diabetes

One-step approach

Perform a 75-g OGTT after an overnight fast ≥8 h.
The diagnosis of GDM is made when any of the following plasma glucose values are met or exceeded:

- Fasting: ≥92 mg/dL (5.1 mmol/L)
- 1 h: ≥180 mg/dL (10.0 mmol/L)
- 2 h: ≥153 mg/dL (8.5 mmol/L)

Two-step approach[46]

Step 1: Perform a 50-g glucose load test nonfasting, with plasma glucose measurement at 1h.

If plasma glucose level 1 h after load is ≥130 mg/dL (≥7.2 mmol/L) ,* proceed to a 100-g OGTT.

Step 2: The 100-g OGTT should be performed when the patient is fasting. The diagnosis of GDM is made when at least two of the following four plasma glucose levels (measured fasting and at 1 h, 2 h, and 3 h during OGTT) are met or exceeded (Carpenter-Coustan criteria):[47]

Fasting: 95 mg/dL (5.3 mmol/L)
1-h: 180 mg/dL (10 mmol/L)
2-h: 155 mg/dL (8.6 mmol/L)
3-h: 140 mg/dL (7.8 mmol/L)

*American College of Obstetricians and Gynecologists notes that one elevated value can be used for diagnosis.

Source: Modified from American Diabetes Association.[1]

defects in insulin action; *3)* diseases of the exocrine pancreas; *4)* endocrinopathies; *5)* drug- or chemical-induced diabetes; *6)* infections; *7)* uncommon forms of immune-mediated diabetes; and *8)* other genetic syndromes sometimes associated with diabetes. These categories may represent <5% of all people with diabetes. Nevertheless, correct identification of these patients is important because their treatment and prognosis may differ. Recognition of patients with other specific types of diabetes requires clinical alertness to identify the history or physical features that lead to the correct diagnosis.

Monogenic Diabetes Syndromes

A small number of cases of diabetes (<5%) result from monogenic defects in β-cell function. About 80%–85% cases of "neonatal" or "congenital" diabetes, which is diagnosed <6 months of age, is monogenic in cause.[50] Maturity-Onset Diabetes of the Young (MODY) is monogenic diabetes that presents with hyperglycemia at a younger age (generally <25 years, although diagnosis may occur at older age). MODY is inherited in an autosomal dominant pattern and is characterized by impaired insulin secretion with minimal or no defects in insulin action.[1] Abnormalities in ≥13 genes on different chromosomes have been identified to date, the most common of which are GCK (glucokinase gene)-MODY (MODY 2), HNF1A (hepatic nuclear factor)-MODY (MODY 3), and HNF4A-MODY (MODY 1). Rare forms of MODY include defects in PDX1(IPF1) and NEU-ROD1.[1] A diagnosis of MODY should be suspected in younger and thinner patients diagnosed with diabetes who also have multiple family members affected by the disease. Correctly diagnosing MODY can result in simplification of treatment approaches and in identification of other affected family members.[51] For example, no treatment is usually indicated for GCK-MODY, while HNF1A- and HNF4A-MODY often respond to sulfonylurea therapy.[1] These individuals should be referred for consultation to a center specializing in diabetes genetics for further evaluation, treatment, and genetic counseling.

Diseases of the Exocrine Pancreas

Any process that causes diffuse and extensive injury of pancreatic tissue can cause diabetes. Diabetes in the context of disease of the exocrine pancreas has been termed pancreoprivic diabetes.[1] Acquired causes include pancreatitis, infection, trauma, pancreatectomy, and pancreatic carcinoma. Pancreatic carcinoma at earlier stages can also cause diabetes from a mechanism different from β-cell destruction. In earlier stages of pancreatic cancer, new onset diabetes can occur from increased insulin resistance. Extensive cystic fibrosis and hemochromatosis can also cause β-cell damage and impaired insulin secretion.

Cystic Fibrosis–Related Diabetes

Diabetes is a common complication seen in patients with cystic fibrosis, mainly due to β-cell deficiency (due to destruction of pancreatic islets) and exacerbated by the insulin resistance associated with infection and inflammation common in cystic fibrosis.[52] Cystic fibrosis–related diabetes (CFRD) is the most common comorbidity in people with cystic fibrosis, with a prevalence of ~20% in adolescents and 40%–50% in adults.[53] OGTT is the recommended screening test; however, some recent publications suggest using an A1C cut point <5.4% (<5.8% in second study) would detect >90% of cases and reduce patient screening burden.[1,54,55] Screening for diabetes <10 years old can identify the risk for progression to CFRD in those with abnormal glucose tolerance.[1] Annual screening for CFRD with OGTT is recommended to start at age 10 years in all patients with cystic fibrosis not previously diagnosed with CFRD.[1] CFRD is associated with a decline in pulmonary function, poor nutritional status, and an increase in mortality.[56,57] Insulin is the recommended therapy for treatment of hyperglycemia in patients with CFRD.[58]

Endocrinopathies

Several hormones, including growth hormone, cortisol, glucagon, and epinephrine, can impair insulin action. Endocrinopathies, which lead to excessive production of these hormones (e.g., acromegaly, Cushing syndrome, glucagonoma, and pheochromocytoma), can cause diabetes. Somatostatinoma and primary hyperaldosteronism can also cause diabetes by the hypokalemia-induced inhibition of insulin secretion. Hyperglycemia is generally resolved when hormone excess is corrected.[1]

Drug- or Chemical-Induced Diabetes

Many drugs can impair insulin secretion and can lead to diabetes in individuals with underlying insulin resistance. One of the newer categories recently added includes immune checkpoint inhibitors used for cancer treatment.[59] This is a relatively new cancer treatment modality and is becoming more widely utilized as new U.S. Food and Drug Administration approval for drugs and cancer treatment indications are added. The mechanism of diabetes with these drugs is autoimmune mediated, and insulin and islet cell antibodies have been identified in individuals with new onset diabetes on immune checkpoint inhibitors. Corticosteroids are known to increase insulin resistance and can uncover underlying β-cell insufficiency or cause stress-related hyperglycemia at high doses. Atypical antipsychotics can be associated with weight gain, insulin resistance, and hyperglycemia, at times presenting as diabetic ketoacidosis.[60] Protease inhibitors used for HIV/AIDS can also be associated with hyperglycemia and diabetes.

Infections

Certain viral infections have been associated with β-cell destruction leading to certain cases of diabetes. These include rubella, coxsackie virus B, cytomegalovirus, adenovirus, and mumps.

Posttransplantation Diabetes

Patients after transplant are at an increased risk for developing diabetes.[61,62] Hyperglycemia is common in the few weeks following transplant, but in most cases stress or steroid-induced hyperglycemia resolves.[63] Patients should be screened for diabetes following organ transplantation once the patient is stable on maintenance immunosuppressive therapy.[1] While the 2-h OGTT is the gold standard to screen for diabetes following transplant, an FPG or A1C test can identify high-risk patients requiring further assessment. Several terms have been used in literature to describe post–organ transplantation diabetes, including new onset diabetes after transplantation (NODAT).[1] Currently, the term posttransplantation diabetes mellitus (PTDM) is favored[64] as it describes all diabetes diagnosed after a transplant irrespective of the time of onset of hyperglycemia (i.e., some people may have had undiagnosed diabetes prior to their transplant). Diagnosis of diabetes is made using the same diagnostic criteria as for nontransplant patients.

Risk factors for PTDM include both the traditional risk factors for diabetes (e.g., age, family history of diabetes, ethnicity, obesity) as well as transplant-specific factors, such as use of immunosuppressive agents like glucocorticoids and calcineurin inhibitors.[65]

Insulin is the agent of choice for glycemic management in the inpatient setting. In the outpatient setting, the choice of glycemic agent can be assessed based on patient condition, side effect profile of medication, and possible interaction with immunosuppressive regimen, with particular attention given to changes in glomerular filtration rate commonly seen in transplant patients.[65] Metformin was reported to be safe for use in renal transplant recipients in a small short-term pilot study, but its safety has not been studied in other types of organ transplant.[66]

Thiazolidinediones have been successfully used in people with liver and kidney transplants; however, they have been associated with side effects, including fluid retention, heart failure, and osteopenia.[67,68] Dipeptidyl peptidase-4 inhibitors have demonstrated safety in small clinical trials for transplant patients.[69,70]

STAGE OF DISEASE

In addition to reflecting etiology, the American Diabetes Association classification system attempts to describe the stage of disease in relationship to glycemic exposure.[1] A disease process may be present but may not have progressed enough to cause hyperglycemia. For example, in type 2 diabetes, there may be insulin resistance with a compensatory increase in endogenous insulin secretion and maintenance of normoglycemia. Progressive β-cell dysfunction will lead to impaired fasting glucose or impaired glucose tolerance (prediabetes), which could progress to hyperglycemia diagnostic of diabetes. For type 1 diabetes, the early stages of the disease are characterized by the presence of autoimmune antibodies in the setting of normal glucose tolerance, which might progress to the loss of first-phase insulin release and presymptomatic impaired glucose tolerance and eventually frank symptomatic hyperglycemia (see Table 1.3).[36] The degree of residual β-cell function determines the need for exogenous insulin replacement. For type 2 diabetes or GDM, this may range from no need for insulin to insulin required for adequate glycemic control; for type 1 diabetes, most patients require insulin for survival.[1] The severity of the metabolic abnormality can progress or stay the same. Thus, the degree of hyperglycemia reflects the severity of the underlying disease process more than the nature of the process itself. Thus, classification of type of diabetes can be made independent of stage.

SCREENING FOR DIABETES

Approximately one-quarter of Americans with diabetes and nearly half of Hispanic, Black non-Hispanic, and Asian non-Hispanic people with diabetes remain undiagnosed.[71] Screening for diabetes has been recommended to identify individuals with previously undiagnosed diabetes so that they may receive appropriate medical care. Support for diabetes screening is not based on randomized, controlled clinical trials, but on observational studies that have found that people diagnosed with diabetes as a result of screening have lower A1C levels and better outcomes than those presenting spontaneously with diabetes. Most organizations, including the American Diabetes Association, recommend that at-risk individuals be screened periodically for diabetes as a part of their routine medical care (opportunistic screening).[72] Few, if any, organizations recommend population screening.

Some additional factors to consider regarding testing for type 2 diabetes and prediabetes in asymptomatic individuals include age, BMI, ethnicity, and medications. Age is a major risk factor for diabetes. BMI ≥25 kg/m² is also a risk factor for diabetes; however, data suggest that the BMI cut-point should be lower for the Asian American population.[73,74] WHO data also suggest using a BMI cut-off ≥23 kg/m² to define increased risk in Asian Americans.[75] Evidence suggests that other populations may also benefit from lower BMI cut-points. A large multiethnic cohort study showed that a BMI of 30 kg/m² in non-Hispanic whites was equivalent to a BMI of 26 kg/m² in African Americans, for an equivalent incidence rate of diabetes.[76]

Criteria for testing for type 2 diabetes and prediabetes in asymptomatic adults are as follows:[1]

- Testing should be considered in individuals who are overweight or obese (BMI ≥25 kg/m² or ≥23 kg/m² in Asian Americans) and who have one or more of the following risk factors:
  - First-degree relative with diabetes
  - High-risk race/ethnicity (e.g., African American, Latino, Native American, Asian American, Pacific Islander)
  - History of cardiovascular disease
  - Hypertension (≥140/90 mmHg or on therapy for hypertension)
  - HDL cholesterol level <35 mg/dL (<0.90 mmol/L) and/or a triglyceride
  - LDL cholesterol level >250 mg/dL (>2.82 mmol/L)
  - Women with polycystic ovary syndrome
  - History of physical inactivity
  - Other clinical conditions associated with insulin resistance (e.g., severe obesity, acanthosis nigricans)
- Patients with prediabetes (A1C ≥5.7% [≥39 mmol/mol], IFG, or IGT) should be tested yearly.
- Women who were diagnosed with GDM should have lifelong testing ≤3-year intervals. For all other patients, testing for diabetes should begin at age 45 years.
- If the results are normal, testing should be repeated at ≤3-year intervals, with consideration of more frequent testing depending on initial results and risk status.

The incidence of type 2 diabetes in children and adolescents has increased dramatically in the last decade, especially in minority populations.[77] Children and youth at increased risk for the presence or the development of type 2 diabetes should be tested within the healthcare setting, and testing should be repeated every 3 years. Beginning at age 10 years or at the onset of puberty (if puberty occurs at a younger age), children who are at risk based on the following criteria should be tested for diabetes.

Risk-based screening for type 2 diabetes or prediabetes in asymptomatic children and adolescents in a clinical setting:[1]

- Testing should be considered in youth who are overweight (≥85th percentile) or obese (>95th percentile) and who have one or more additional risk factors based on strength of their association with diabetes:
  - Maternal history of diabetes or GDM during the child's gestation.
  - Family history of type 2 diabetes in first- or second-degree relative.
  - High-risk race/ethnicity (Native American, African American, Latino, Asian American, Pacific Islander).
  - Signs of insulin resistance or conditions associated with insulin resistance (acanthosis nigricans, hypertension, dyslipidemia, polycystic ovarian syndrome, or small-for-gestational-age birth weight).

CATEGORIES OF INCREASED RISK FOR DIABETES

Prediabetes includes a category of individuals who are at an increased risk for developing diabetes and have glucose levels higher than normal but lower than those diagnostic of diabetes[78] (Table 1.5). This category includes individuals with IGT and /or IFG and/or A1C 5.7%–6.4 %. IGT is diagnosed by the 2-h 75-g OGTT, where FPG is <126 mg/dL (<7.0 mmol/L) and 2-h glucose is between 140 and 199 mg/dL (97.8–11.0 mmol/L).[43] IFG is defined by fasting blood glucose between 100 mg/dL and 125 mg/dL (5.6–6.9 mmol/L).[1]

Prediabetes is associated with an increased risk for diabetes and cardiovascular disease.[1,79–81] In general, the incidence of type 2 diabetes in individuals with IGT is 5% per year, with a range from 4% to 9% per year. Risk factors for progression to diabetes include higher 2-h post–glucose load glucose levels or A1C levels and Hispanic or Native American ethnicity. For example, a systematic review showed that individuals with A1C between 5.5% and 6.0% had an increased 5-year incidence of diabetes of 9%–25%, while for those with A1C 6.0%–6.5%, the 5-year risk of progression was between 25% and 50%.[82] For all three tests, risk is continuous, extending below the lower limit of the range and becoming disproportionately greater at higher ends of the range.

Individuals with IGT have a risk of cardiovascular disease and cardiovascular mortality approximately twofold higher than individuals with normal glucose tolerance and similar to individuals with type 2 diabetes. Hence, it is important to consider testing for prediabetes in high-risk individuals. Once identified, interventions should be considered, including lifestyle modifications and metformin use for select patients, and if appropriate treat other cardiovascular risk factors.

IFG is defined as FPG between 100 mg/dL and 125 mg/dL (5.6–6.9 mmol/L) and IGT with 2-h 75-g OGTT as blood glucose between 140 mg/dL and 199 mg/dL (7.8–11.0 mmol/L).[1,43,78] It is important to note that WHO and some other diabetes organizations use the cutoff at 110 mg/dL (6.1 mmol/L) to define IFG. Some data in literature support that subjects diagnosed with IFG are different from subjects with IGT and, in general, are at lower risk for both diabetes and cardiovascular disease.[83]

METABOLIC SYNDROME

Glucose intolerance and type 2 diabetes may also be manifestations of an underlying disorder known as the metabolic syndrome. Individuals with the metabolic syndrome are at risk for type 2 diabetes and cardiovascular disease.[84–86]

Table 1.5–Categories of Increased Risk for Diabetes (Prediabetes)

- A1C 5.7%–6.4% (39–46 mmol/mol).
- FPG 100 mg/dL (5.6 mmol/L) to 125 mg/dL (6.9 mmol/L, also known as IFG).
- 2-h plasma glucose during the 75-g OGTT 140 mg/dL (7.8 mmol/L) to 199 mg/dL (11.0 mmol/L), also known as the IGT.

There is no uniform definition of the metabolic syndrome, but there are similarities between the criteria proposed by the U.S. Expert Panel on Detection, Evaluation, and Treatment of High Blood Cholesterol in Adults (Adult Treatment Panel III [ATP III])[87,88] and the WHO (Table 1.6). Data from the NHANES III, which used the ATP III criteria, found that the prevalence of the metabolic syndrome in the U.S. was ~20%–25%.[89] The prevalence of the metabolic syndrome increases with age and is highest in Hispanic populations, affecting ≤50% of adults.[90]

Controversy surrounding the metabolic syndrome has not disputed the clustering of cardiovascular risk factors, including central obesity, dyslipidemia, and hypertension, or the association of the metabolic syndrome with the risk of diabetes and cardiovascular disease. Instead, the controversy has focused on the etiology of the syndrome, how best to define it, how clinical decision making should be modified based on those definitions, and whether there are more effective ways to screen for the risk of diabetes and cardiovascular risk.

EVALUATION AND CLASSIFICATION OF PATIENTS BEFORE TREATMENT

Before therapy is initiated for diabetes, the patient should have a complete medical evaluation (see Chapter 3). The complete medical evaluation helps the physician classify the patient, detect the presence of complications and comorbidities associated with diabetes (see Chapter 5), and provide the basis for formulating a management plan. Table 3.1 (page 55) provides an outline for the initial medical evaluation.

A thorough history, physical exam, complete personal and family history, and the diagnostic test results can often lead to an initial classification of diabetes.

Table 1.6–Diagnosis of the Metabolic Syndrome

	ATP III	WHO
Criteria for diagnosis	Any three of the five criteria below	Insulin resistance or diabetes, plus two out of five criteria below
Obesity	Waist circumference >102 cm in men and >88 cm in women	Waist-to-hip ratio >0.90 in men or >0.85 in women and/or BMI >30 kg/m²
Triglycerides (TG)	TG ≥150 mg/dL (≥1.695 mmol/L) or drug treatment for elevated TG	TG concentration ≥150 mg/dL (≥1.695 mmol/L)
HDL cholesterol	HDL <40 mg/dL (<1.036 mmol/L) in men and <50 mg/dL (<1.295 mmol/L) in women	HDL <35 mg/dL (<0.9 mmol/L) in men and <39 mg/dL (<1.0 mmol/L) in women
Blood pressure (BP)	BP ≥130/85 mmHg or drug treatment for elevated BP	BP ≥160/90 mmHg
Other	FPG: ≥110 mg/dL (≥5.6 mmol/L) or drug treatment for elevated blood glucose	Urinary albumin excretion rate ≥20 µg/min or an albumin-to-creatinine ratio ≥20 mg/g

Patients should not be classified on the basis of age alone or on whether or not they are taking insulin. If the diagnosis of diabetes had been made previously, an initial evaluation should also review the previous treatment and the past and present degrees of glycemic control. Laboratory tests appropriate to the evaluation of each patient's general medical condition should be performed.

It is sometimes difficult to assign the patient to a particular type of diabetes (i.e., type 1 or type 2) despite an initial work-up. For example, the normal-weight patient with type 2 diabetes who has been taking insulin may appear to have type 1 diabetes. Some patients with type 2 diabetes require insulin for glycemic control but do not depend on insulin to prevent ketoacidosis or to sustain life. Another example is the newly diagnosed child or adolescent who is a member of a family with an autosomal dominant form of diabetes such as MODY. The family history will provide the clue to the correct diagnosis. Such a patient should not be classified as having type 1 diabetes on the basis of age alone. Other patients, particularly adults, have type 1 immune-mediated diabetes but are at a stage in which they still have β-cell function and clinically appear similar to individuals with type 2 diabetes. It usually is not necessary for clinicians to determine the presence of islet cell or other antibodies or the degree of insulin secretion, but if type 1 diabetes is suspected, these measurements may be helpful. These autoimmune markers include islet cell autoantibodies and autoantibodies to GAD, insulin, tyrosine phosphatases IA-2 and IA-2B, and ZnT8.

REFERENCES

1. American Diabetes Association. 2. Classification and Diagnosis of Diabetes: Standards of Medical Care in Diabetes 2020. *Diabetes Care*. 2020;43(Suppl 1):S14-S31. Epub 2019/12/22. doi: 10.2337/dc20-S002. PubMed PMID: 31862745

2. Nathan DM. Long-term complications of diabetes mellitus. *N Engl J Med* 1993;328(23):1676–1685. doi: 10.1056/NEJM199306103282306. Epub 1993 Jun 10. PubMed PMID: 8487827

3. Deckert T, Poulsen JE, Larsen M. Prognosis of diabetics with diabetes onset before the age of thirty-one. II. Factors influencing the prognosis. *Diabetologia* 1978;14(6):371–377. Epub 1978 Jun 1. PubMed PMID: 669101

4. Metzger BE, Lowe LP, Dyer AR, Trimble ER, Chaovarindr U, Coustan DR, et al. Hyperglycemia and adverse pregnancy outcomes. *N Engl J Med* 2008;358(19):1991–2002. doi: 10.1056/NEJMoa0707943. Epub 2008 May 9. PubMed PMID: 18463375

5. Selvin E, Wang D, Matsushita K, Grams ME, Coresh J. Prognostic implications of single-sample confirmatory testing for undiagnosed diabetes: a prospective cohort study. *Ann Intern Med* 2018;169(3):156–164. doi: 10.7326/M18-0091. Epub 2018 Jun 19. PubMed PMID: 29913486; PubMed Central PMCID: PMCPMC6082697

6. American Diabetes Association. Standards of medical care in diabetes 2018: abridged for primary care providers. *Clin Diabetes* 2018;36(1):14–37.

doi: 10.2337/cd17-0119. Epub 2018 Feb 1. PubMed PMID: 29382975; PubMed Central PMCID: PMCPMC5775000

7. Cowie CC, Rust KF, Byrd-Holt DD, Gregg EW, Ford ES, Geiss LS, et al. Prevalence of diabetes and high risk for diabetes using A1C criteria in the U.S. population in 1988–2006. *Diabetes Care* 2010;33(3):562–568. doi: 10.2337/dc09-1524. Epub 2010 Jan 14. PubMed PMID: 20067953; PubMed Central PMCID: PMCPMC2827508

8. Meijnikman AS, De Block CEM, Dirinck E, Verrijken A, Mertens I, Corthouts B, et al. Not performing an OGTT results in significant underdiagnosis of (pre)diabetes in a high risk ad151ult Caucasian population. *Int J Obes (Lond)* 2017;41(11):1615–1620. doi: 10.1038/ijo.2017.165. Epub 2017 Jul 20. PubMed PMID: 28720876

9. National Diabetes Data Group. Classification and diagnosis of diabetes mellitus and other categories of glucose intolerance. *Diabetes* 1979;28(12):1039–1057. Epub 1979 Dec 1. PubMed PMID: 510803

10. Diabetes mellitus: report of a WHO study group. *World Health Organ Tech Rep Ser* 1985;727:1–113. Epub 1985 Jan 1. PubMed PMID: 3934850

11. Johns DR. Seminars in medicine of the Beth Israel Hospital, Boston: mitochondrial DNA and disease. *N Engl J Med* 1995;333(10):638–644. doi: 10.1056/NEJM199509073331007. Epub 1995 Sep 7. PubMed PMID: 7637726

12. Yamagata K, Furuta H, Oda N, Kaisaki PJ, Menzel S, Cox NJ, et al. Mutations in the hepatocyte nuclear factor-4alpha gene in maturity-onset diabetes of the young (MODY1). *Nature* 1996;384(6608):458–460. doi: 10.1038/384458a0. Epub 1996 Dec 5. PubMed PMID: 8945471

13. Froguel P, Zouali H, Vionnet N, Velho G, Vaxillaire M, Sun F, et al. Familial hyperglycemia due to mutations in glucokinase. Definition of a subtype of diabetes mellitus. *N Engl J Med* 1993;328(10):697–702. doi: 10.1056/NEJM199303113281005. Epub 1993 Mar 11. PubMed PMID: 8433729

14. Yamagata K, Oda N, Kaisaki PJ, Menzel S, Furuta H, Vaxillaire M, et al. Mutations in the hepatocyte nuclear factor-1alpha gene in maturity-onset diabetes of the young (MODY3). *Nature* 1996;384(6608):455–458. doi: 10.1038/384455a0. Epub 1996 Dec 5. PubMed PMID: 8945470

15. Stoffers DA, Ferrer J, Clarke WL, Habener JF. Early-onset type-II diabetes mellitus (MODY4) linked to IPF1. *Nat Genet* 1997;17(2):138–139. doi: 10.1038/ng1097-138. Epub 1997 Nov 5. PubMed PMID: 9326926

16. Horikawa Y, Iwasaki N, Hara M, Furuta H, Hinokio Y, Cockburn BN, et al. Mutation in hepatocyte nuclear factor-1 beta gene (TCF2) associated with MODY. *Nat Genet* 1997;17(4):384–385. doi: 10.1038/ng1297-384. Epub 1997 Dec 17. PubMed PMID: 9398836

17. Bellanne-Chantelot C, Chauveau D, Gautier JF, Dubois-Laforgue D, Clauin S, Beaufils S, et al. Clinical spectrum associated with hepatocyte nuclear

factor-1beta mutations. *Ann Intern Med* 2004;140(7):510–517. Epub 2004 Apr 8. PubMed PMID: 15068978

18. Malecki MT, Jhala US, Antonellis A, Fields L, Doria A, Orban T, et al. Mutations in NEUROD1 are associated with the development of type 2 diabetes mellitus. *Nat Genet* 1999;23(3):323–328. doi: 10.1038/15500. Epub 1999 Nov 5. PubMed PMID: 10545951

19. Chiang JL, Kirkman MS, Laffel LM, Peters AL. Type 1 diabetes sourcebook a. Type 1 diabetes through the life span: a position statement of the American Diabetes Association. *Diabetes Care* 2014;37(7):2034–2054. doi: 10.2337/dc14-1140. Epub 2014 Jun 18. PubMed PMID: 24935775; PubMed Central PMCID: PMCPMC5865481

20. Kordonouri O, Hartmann R, Deiss D, Wilms M, Gruters-Kieslich A. Natural course of autoimmune thyroiditis in type 1 diabetes: association with gender, age, diabetes duration, and puberty. *Arch Dis Child* 2005;90(4):411–414. doi: 10.1136/adc.2004.056424. Epub 2005 Mar 23. PubMed PMID: 15781936; PubMed Central PMCID: PMCPMC1720371

21. Kordonouri O, Klinghammer A, Lang EB, Gruters-Kieslich A, Grabert M, Holl RW. Thyroid autoimmunity in children and adolescents with type 1 diabetes: a multicenter survey. *Diabetes Care* 2002;25(8):1346–1350. doi: 10.2337/diacare.25.8.1346. Epub 2002 Jul 30. PubMed PMID: 12145233

22. Sumnik Z, Drevinek P, Snajderova M, Kolouskova S, Sedlakova P, Pechova M, et al. HLA-DQ polymorphisms modify the risk of thyroid autoimmunity in children with type 1 diabetes mellitus. *J Pediatr Endocrinol Metab* 2003;16(6):851–858. Epub 2003 Sep 2. PubMed PMID: 12948297

23. Roldan MB, Alonso M, Barrio R. Thyroid autoimmunity in children and adolescents with Type 1 diabetes mellitus. *Diabetes Nutr Metab* 1999;12(1):27–31. Epub 1999 Oct 12. PubMed PMID: 10517303

24. Kordonouri O, Deiss D, Danne T, Dorow A, Bassir C, Gruters-Kieslich A. Predictivity of thyroid autoantibodies for the development of thyroid disorders in children and adolescents with type 1 diabetes. *Diabet Med* 2002;19(6):518–521. Epub 2002 Jun 13. PubMed PMID: 12060066

25. Spaans E, Schroor E, Groenier K, Bilo H, Kleefstra N, Brand P. Thyroid disease and type 1 diabetes in Dutch children: a nationwide study (young dudes-3). *J Pediatr* 2017;187:189–193 e1. doi: 10.1016/j.jpeds.2017.05.016. Epub 2017 Jun 7. PubMed PMID: 28583704

26. Leong KS, Wallymahmed M, Wilding J, MacFarlane I. Clinical presentation of thyroid dysfunction and Addison's disease in young adults with type 1 diabetes. *Postgrad Med J* 1999;75(886):467–470. doi: 10.1136/pgmj.75.886.467. Epub 2000 Jan 26. PubMed PMID: 10646024; PubMed Central PMCID: PMCPMC1741325

27. Dost A, Rohrer TR, Frohlich-Reiterer E, Bollow E, Karges B, Bockmann A, et al. Hyperthyroidism in 276 children and adolescents with type 1 diabetes

from Germany and Austria. *Horm Res Paediatr* 2015;84(3):190–198. doi: 10.1159/000436964. Epub 2015 Jul 24. PubMed PMID: 26202175

28. Aktay AN, Lee PC, Kumar V, Parton E, Wyatt DT, Werlin SL. The prevalence and clinical characteristics of celiac disease in juvenile diabetes in Wisconsin. *J Pediatr Gastroenterol Nutr* 2001;33(4):462–465. Epub 2001 Nov 8. PubMed PMID: 11698764

29. Crone J, Rami B, Huber WD, Granditsch G, Schober E. Prevalence of celiac disease and follow-up of EMA in children and adolescents with type 1 diabetes mellitus. *J Pediatr Gastroenterol Nutr* 2003;37(1):67–71. Epub 2003 Jun 27. PubMed PMID: 12827008

30. Al-Ashwal AA, Shabib SM, Sakati NA, Attia NA. Prevalence and characteristics of celiac disease in type I diabetes mellitus in Saudi Arabia. *Saudi Med J* 2003;24(10):1113–1115. Epub 2003 Oct 28. PubMed PMID: 14578980

31. Punales M, Bastos MD, Ramos ARL, Pinto RB, Ott EA, Provenzi V, et al. Prevalence of celiac disease in a large cohort of young patients with type 1 diabetes. *Pediatr Diabetes* 2019;20(4):414–420. doi: 10.1111/pedi.12827. Epub 2019 Feb 10. PubMed PMID: 30737863

32. De Block CE, De Leeuw IH, Van Gaal LF. High prevalence of manifestations of gastric autoimmunity in parietal cell antibody-positive type 1 (insulin-dependent) diabetic patients. The Belgian Diabetes Registry. *J Clin Endocrinol Metab* 1999;84(11):4062–4067. doi: 10.1210/jcem.84.11.6095. Epub 1999 Nov 24. PubMed PMID: 10566650

33. De Block CE, De Leeuw IH, Bogers JJ, Pelckmans PA, Ieven MM, Van Marck EA, et al. Autoimmune gastropathy in type 1 diabetic patients with parietal cell antibodies: histological and clinical findings. *Diabetes Care* 2003;26(1):82–88. doi: 10.2337/diacare.26.1.82. Epub 2002 Dec 28. PubMed PMID: 12502662

34. Van den Driessche A, Eenkhoorn V, Van Gaal L, De Block C. Type 1 diabetes and autoimmune polyglandular syndrome: a clinical review. *Neth J Med* 2009;67(11):376–387. Epub 2009 Dec 17. PubMed PMID: 20009114

35. Peterson P, Salmi H, Hyoty H, Miettinen A, Ilonen J, Reijonen H, et al. Steroid 21-hydroxylase autoantibodies in insulin-dependent diabetes mellitus. Childhood Diabetes in Finland (DiMe) Study Group. *Clin Immunol Immunopathol* 1997;82(1):37–42. Epub 1997 Jan 1. PubMed PMID: 9000040

36. Insel RA, Dunne JL, Atkinson MA, Chiang JL, Dabelea D, Gottlieb PA, et al. Staging presymptomatic type 1 diabetes: a scientific statement of JDRF, the Endocrine Society, and the American Diabetes Association. *Diabetes Care* 2015;38(10):1964–1974. doi: 10.2337/dc15-1419. Epub 2015 Sep 26. PubMed PMID: 26404926; PubMed Central PMCID: PMCPMC5321245

37. Skyler JS, Bakris GL, Bonifacio E, Darsow T, Eckel RH, Groop L, et al. Differentiation of diabetes by pathophysiology, natural history, and prognosis. *Diabetes* 2017;66(2):241–255. doi: 10.2337/db16-0806. Epub 2016 Dec 17. PubMed PMID: 27980006; PubMed Central PMCID: PMCPMC5384660

38. Umpierrez GE, Smiley D, Kitabchi AE. Narrative review: ketosis-prone type 2 diabetes mellitus. *Ann Intern Med* 2006;144(5):350–357. doi: 10.7326/0003-4819-144-5-200603070-00011. Epub 2006 Mar 8. PubMed PMID: 16520476

39. Ma RC, Chan JC. Type 2 diabetes in East Asians: similarities and differences with populations in Europe and the United States. *Ann N Y Acad Sci* 2013;1281:64–91. doi: 10.1111/nyas.12098. Epub 2013 Mar 5. PubMed PMID: 23551121; PubMed Central PMCID: PMCPMC3708105

40. Gujral UP, Pradeepa R, Weber MB, Narayan KM, Mohan V. Type 2 diabetes in South Asians: similarities and differences with white Caucasian and other populations. *Ann N Y Acad Sci* 2013;1281:51–63. doi: 10.1111/j.1749-6632.2012.06838.x. Epub 2013 Jan 16. PubMed PMID: 23317344; PubMed Central PMCID: PMCPMC3715105

41. Umpierrez G, Korytkowski M. Diabetic emergencies—ketoacidosis, hyperglycaemic hyperosmolar state and hypoglycaemia. *Nat Rev Endocrinol* 2016;12(4):222–232. doi: 10.1038/nrendo.2016.15. Epub 2016 Feb 20. PubMed PMID: 26893262

42. Fadini GP, Bonora BM, Avogaro A. SGLT2 inhibitors and diabetic ketoacidosis: data from the FDA Adverse Event Reporting System. *Diabetologia* 2017;60(8):1385–1389. doi: 10.1007/s00125-017-4301-8. Epub 2017 May 14. PubMed PMID: 28500396

43. Report of the Expert Committee on the Diagnosis and Classification of Diabetes Mellitus. *Diabetes Care* 1997;20(7):1183–1197. doi: 10.2337/diacare.20.7.1183. Epub 1997 Jul 1. PubMed PMID: 9203460

44. Deputy NP, Kim SY, Conrey EJ, Bullard KM. Prevalence and changes in preexisting diabetes and gestational diabetes among women who had a live birth—United States, 2012–2016. *MMWR Morb Mortal Wkly Rep* 2018;67(43):1201–1207. doi: 10.15585/mmwr.mm6743a2. Epub 2018 Nov 2. PubMed PMID: 30383743; PubMed Central PMCID: PMCPMC6319799

45. Guariguata L, Linnenkamp U, Beagley J, Whiting DR, Cho NH. Global estimates of the prevalence of hyperglycaemia in pregnancy. *Diabetes Res Clin Pract* 2014;103(2):176–185. doi: 10.1016/j.diabres.2013.11.003. Epub 2013 Dec 5. PubMed PMID: 24300020

46. Committee on Practice B-O. ACOG practice bulletin no. 190: gestational diabetes mellitus. *Obstet Gynecol* 2018;131(2):e49–e64. doi: 10.1097/AOG.0000000000002501. Epub 2018 Jan 26. PubMed PMID: 29370047

47. Carpenter MW, Coustan DR. Criteria for screening tests for gestational diabetes. *Am J Obstet Gynecol* 1982;144(7):768–773. doi: 10.1016/0002-9378(82)90349-0. Epub 1982 Dec 1. PubMed PMID: 7148898

48. Kim C, Newton KM, Knopp RH. Gestational diabetes and the incidence of type 2 diabetes: a systematic review. *Diabetes Care* 2002;25(10):1862–1868. doi: 10.2337/diacare.25.10.1862. Epub 2002 Sep 28. PubMed PMID: 12351492

49. American Diabetes Association. 14. Management of Diabetes in Pregnancy: Standards of Medical Care in Diabetes 2020. Diabetes Care. 2020;43(Suppl 1):S183-S92. Epub 2019/12/22. doi: 10.2337/dc20-S014. PubMed PMID: 31862757

50. De Franco E, Flanagan SE, Houghton JA, Lango Allen H, Mackay DJ, Temple IK, et al. The effect of early, comprehensive genomic testing on clinical care in neonatal diabetes: an international cohort study. *Lancet* 2015;386(9997):957–963. doi: 10.1016/S0140-6736(15)60098-8. Epub 2015 Aug 2. PubMed PMID: 26231457; PubMed Central PMCID: PMCPMC4772451

51. Shepherd MH, Shields BM, Hudson M, Pearson ER, Hyde C, Ellard S, et al. A UK nationwide prospective study of treatment change in MODY: genetic subtype and clinical characteristics predict optimal glycaemic control after discontinuing insulin and metformin. *Diabetologia* 2018;61(12):2520–2527. doi: 10.1007/s00125-018-4728-6. Epub 2018 Sep 20. PubMed PMID: 30229274; PubMed Central PMCID: PMCPMC6223847

52. Lohr M, Goertchen P, Nizze H, Gould NS, Gould VE, Oberholzer M, et al. Cystic fibrosis associated islet changes may provide a basis for diabetes. An immunocytochemical and morphometrical study. *Virchows Arch A Pathol Anat Histopathol* 1989;414(2):179–185. doi: 10.1007/bf00718598. Epub 1989 Jan 1. PubMed PMID: 2492695

53. Moran A, Pillay K, Becker D, Granados A, Hameed S, Acerini CL. ISPAD clinical practice consensus guidelines 2018: management of cystic fibrosis-related diabetes in children and adolescents. *Pediatr Diabetes* 2018;19(Suppl. 27):64–74. doi: 10.1111/pedi.12732. Epub 2018 Aug 11. PubMed PMID: 30094886

54. Gilmour JA, Sykes J, Etchells E, Tullis E. Cystic fibrosis-related diabetes screening in adults: a gap analysis and evaluation of accuracy of glycated hemoglobin levels. *Can J Diabetes* 2019;43(1):13–18. doi: 10.1016/j.jcjd.2018.04.008. Epub 2018 Sep 4. PubMed PMID: 30173928

55. Gilmour JA. Response to the letter to the editor from Dr. Boudreau et al, "Validation of a stepwise approach using glycated hemoglobin levels to reduce the number of required oral glucose tolerance tests to screen for cystic fibrosis-related diabetes in adults". *Can J Diabetes* 2019;43(3):163. doi: 10.1016/j.jcjd.2019.02.002. Epub 2019 Apr 2. PubMed PMID: 30929664

56. Bismuth E, Laborde K, Taupin P, Velho G, Ribault V, Jennane F, et al. Glucose tolerance and insulin secretion, morbidity, and death in patients with cystic fibrosis. *J Pediatr* 2008;152(4):540–545. doi: 10.1016/j.jpeds.2007.09.025. Epub 2008 Mar 19. PubMed PMID: 18346512

57. Milla CE, Billings J, Moran A. Diabetes is associated with dramatically decreased survival in female but not male subjects with cystic fibrosis. *Diabetes Care* 2005;28(9):2141–2144. doi: 10.2337/diacare.28.9.2141. Epub 2005 Aug 27. PubMed PMID: 16123480

58. Onady GM, Stolfi A. Insulin and oral agents for managing cystic fibrosis-related diabetes. *Cochrane Database Syst Rev* 2016;4:CD004730. doi: 10.1002/14651858.CD004730.pub4. Epub 2016 Apr 19. PubMed PMID: 27087121

59. Abdel-Rahman O, ElHalawani H, Fouad M. Risk of endocrine complications in cancer patients treated with immune check point inhibitors: a meta-analysis. *Future Oncol* 2016;12(3):413–425. doi: 10.2217/fon.15.222. Epub 2016 Jan 19. PubMed PMID: 26775673

60. Kessing LV, Thomsen AF, Mogensen UB, Andersen PK. Treatment with antipsychotics and the risk of diabetes in clinical practice. *Br J Psychiatry* 2010;197(4):266–271. doi: 10.1192/bjp.bp.109.076935. Epub 2010 Oct 5. PubMed PMID: 20884948

61. Wilkinson A, Davidson J, Dotta F, Home PD, Keown P, Kiberd B, et al. Guidelines for the treatment and management of new-onset diabetes after transplantation. *Clin Transplant* 2005;19(3):291–298. doi: 10.1111/j.1399-0012.2005.00359.x. Epub 2005 May 10. PubMed PMID: 15877787

62. Valderhaug TG, Jenssen T, Hartmann A, Midtvedt K, Holdaas H, Reisaeter AV, et al. Fasting plasma glucose and glycosylated hemoglobin in the screening for diabetes mellitus after renal transplantation. *Transplantation* 2009;88(3):429–434. doi: 10.1097/TP.0b013e3181af1f53. Epub 2009 Aug 12. PubMed PMID: 19667949

63. Chakkera HA, Weil EJ, Castro J, Heilman RL, Reddy KS, Mazur MJ, et al. Hyperglycemia during the immediate period after kidney transplantation. *Clin J Am Soc Nephrol* 2009;4(4):853–859. doi: 10.2215/CJN.05471008. Epub 2009 Apr 3. PubMed PMID: 19339426; PubMed Central PMCID: PMCPMC2666437

64. Sharif A, Hecking M, de Vries AP, Porrini E, Hornum M, Rasoul-Rockenschaub S, et al. Proceedings from an international consensus meeting on posttransplantation diabetes mellitus: recommendations and future directions. *Am J Transplant* 2014;14(9):1992–2000. doi: 10.1111/ajt.12850. Epub 2014 Oct 14. PubMed PMID: 25307034; PubMed Central PMCID: PMCPMC4374739

65. Wallia A, Illuri V, Molitch ME. Diabetes care after transplant: definitions, risk factors, and clinical management. *Med Clin North Am* 2016;100(3):535–550. doi: 10.1016/j.mcna.2016.01.005. Epub 2016 Apr 21. PubMed PMID: 27095644

66. Kurian B, Joshi R, Helmuth A. Effectiveness and long-term safety of thiazolidinediones and metformin in renal transplant recipients. *Endocr Pract* 2008;14(8):979–984. doi: 10.4158/EP.14.8.979. Epub 2008 Dec 20. PubMed PMID: 19095596

67. Budde K, Neumayer HH, Fritsche L, Sulowicz W, Stompor T, Eckland D. The pharmacokinetics of pioglitazone in patients with impaired renal function. *Br J Clin Pharmacol* 2003;55(4):368–374. doi: 10.1046/j.1365-2125.2003.01785.x. Epub 2003 Apr 12. PubMed PMID: 12680885; PubMed Central PMCID: PMCPMC1884238

68. Luther P, Baldwin D, Jr. Pioglitazone in the management of diabetes mellitus after transplantation. *Am J Transplant* 2004;4(12):2135–2138. doi: 10.1111/j.1600-6143.2004.00613.x. Epub 2004/12/04. PubMed PMID: 15575920

69. Strom Halden TA, Asberg A, Vik K, Hartmann A, Jenssen T. Short-term efficacy and safety of sitagliptin treatment in long-term stable renal recipients with new-onset diabetes after transplantation. *Nephrol Dial Transplant* 2014;29(4):926–933. doi: 10.1093/ndt/gft536. Epub 2014 Jan 24. PubMed PMID: 24452849

70. Lane JT, Odegaard DE, Haire CE, Collier DS, Wrenshall LE, Stevens RB. Sitagliptin therapy in kidney transplant recipients with new-onset diabetes after transplantation. *Transplantation* 2011;92(10):e56–e57. doi: 10.1097/TP.0b013e3182347ea4. Epub 2011 Nov 10. PubMed PMID: 22067216

71. Centers for Disease Control and Prevention. *Promotion. National Diabetes Statistics Report, 2017* [Internet]. 2017. Available from https://dev.diabetes.org/sites/default/files/2019-06/cdc-statistics-report-2017.pdf

72. American Diabetes Association. 3. Prevention or Delay of Type 2 Diabetes: Standards of Medical Care in Diabetes 2020. Diabetes Care. 2020;43(Suppl 1):S32-S6. Epub 2019/12/22. doi: 10.2337/dc20-S003. PubMed PMID: 31862746

73. Araneta MR, Kanaya AM, Hsu WC, Chang HK, Grandinetti A, Boyko EJ, et al. Optimum BMI cut points to screen Asian Americans for type 2 diabetes. *Diabetes Care* 2015;38(5):814–820. doi: 10.2337/dc14-2071. Epub 2015 Feb 11. PubMed PMID: 25665815; PubMed Central PMCID: PMCPMC4407753

74. Hsu WC, Araneta MR, Kanaya AM, Chiang JL, Fujimoto W. BMI cut points to identify at-risk Asian Americans for type 2 diabetes screening. *Diabetes Care* 2015;38(1):150–158. doi: 10.2337/dc14-2391. Epub 2014 Dec 30. PubMed PMID: 25538311; PubMed Central PMCID: PMCPMC4392932

75. Consultation WHOE. Appropriate body-mass index for Asian populations and its implications for policy and intervention strategies. *Lancet* 2004;363(9403):157–163. doi: 10.1016/S0140-6736(03)15268-3. Epub 2004 Jan 17. PubMed PMID: 14726171

76. Chiu M, Austin PC, Manuel DG, Shah BR, Tu JV. Deriving ethnic-specific BMI cutoff points for assessing diabetes risk. *Diabetes Care* 2011;34(8):1741–1748. doi: 10.2337/dc10-2300. Epub 2011 Jun 18. PubMed PMID: 21680722; PubMed Central PMCID: PMCPMC3142051

77. Dabelea D, Mayer-Davis EJ, Saydah S, Imperatore G, Linder B, Divers J, et al. Prevalence of type 1 and type 2 diabetes among children and adolescents from 2001 to 2009. *JAMA* 2014;311(17):1778–1786. doi: 10.1001/jama.2014.3201. Epub 2014 May 6. PubMed PMID: 24794371; PubMed Central PMCID: PMCPMC4368900

78. Genuth S, Alberti KG, Bennett P, Buse J, Defronzo R, Kahn R, et al. Follow-up report on the diagnosis of diabetes mellitus. *Diabetes Care*

2003;26(11):3160–3167. doi: 10.2337/diacare.26.11.3160. Epub 2003 Oct 28. PubMed PMID: 14578255

79. Selvin E, Steffes MW, Zhu H, Matsushita K, Wagenknecht L, Pankow J, et al. Glycated hemoglobin, diabetes, and cardiovascular risk in nondiabetic adults. *N Engl J Med* 2010;362(9):800–811. doi: 10.1056/NEJMoa0908359. Epub 2010 Mar 5. PubMed PMID: 20200384; PubMed Central PMCID: PMCPMC2872990

80. Ackermann RT, Cheng YJ, Williamson DF, Gregg EW. Identifying adults at high risk for diabetes and cardiovascular disease using hemoglobin A$_{1c}$ National Health and Nutrition Examination Survey 2005–2006. *Am J Prev Med* 2011;40(1):11–17. doi: 10.1016/j.amepre.2010.09.022. Epub 2010 Dec 15. PubMed PMID: 21146762

81. Diabetes Prevention Program Research G. HbA1c as a predictor of diabetes and as an outcome in the diabetes prevention program: a randomized clinical trial. *Diabetes Care* 2015;38(1):51–58. doi: 10.2337/dc14-0886. Epub 2014 Oct 23. PubMed PMID: 25336746; PubMed Central PMCID: PMCPMC4274777

82. Zhang X, Gregg EW, Williamson DF, Barker LE, Thomas W, Bullard KM, et al. A1C level and future risk of diabetes: a systematic review. *Diabetes Care* 2010;33(7):1665–1673. doi: 10.2337/dc09-1939. Epub 2010 Jul 1. PubMed PMID: 20587727; PubMed Central PMCID: PMCPMC2890379

83. Blake DR, Meigs JB, Muller DC, Najjar SS, Andres R, Nathan DM. Impaired glucose tolerance, but not impaired fasting glucose, is associated with increased levels of coronary heart disease risk factors: results from the Baltimore Longitudinal Study on Aging. *Diabetes* 2004;53(8):2095–2100. doi: 10.2337/diabetes.53.8.2095. Epub 2004 Jul 28. PubMed PMID: 15277391

84. Lakka HM, Laaksonen DE, Lakka TA, Niskanen LK, Kumpusalo E, Tuomilehto J, et al. The metabolic syndrome and total and cardiovascular disease mortality in middle-aged men. *JAMA* 2002;288(21):2709–2716. doi: 10.1001/jama.288.21.2709. Epub 2002 Dec 4. PubMed PMID: 12460094

85. Scuteri A, Najjar SS, Morrell CH, Lakatta EG, Cardiovascular Health S. The metabolic syndrome in older individuals: prevalence and prediction of cardiovascular events: the Cardiovascular Health Study. *Diabetes Care* 2005;28(4):882–887. doi: 10.2337/diacare.28.4.882. Epub 2005 Mar 29. PubMed PMID: 15793190

86. Malik S, Wong ND, Franklin SS, Kamath TV, L'Italien GJ, Pio JR, et al. Impact of the metabolic syndrome on mortality from coronary heart disease, cardiovascular disease, and all causes in United States adults. *Circulation* 2004;110(10):1245–1250. doi: 10.1161/01.CIR.0000140677.20606.0E. Epub 2004 Aug 25. PubMed PMID: 15326067

87. Expert Panel on Detection E, Treatment of High Blood Cholesterol in A. Executive summary of the third report of the National Cholesterol Education Program (NCEP) Expert Panel on Detection, Evaluation, and Treatment of High Blood Cholesterol in Adults (Adult Treatment Panel III).

JAMA 2001;285(19):2486–2497. Epub 2001 May 23. PubMed PMID: 11368702

88. Grundy SM, Brewer HB, Jr., Cleeman JI, Smith SC, Jr., Lenfant C, American Heart A, et al. Definition of metabolic syndrome: Report of the National Heart, Lung, and Blood Institute/American Heart Association conference on scientific issues related to definition. *Circulation* 2004;109(3):433–438. doi: 10.1161/01.CIR.0000111245.75752.C6. Epub 2004 Jan 28. PubMed PMID: 14744958

89. Kahn R, Buse J, Ferrannini E, Stern M, American Diabetes Association, European Association for the Study of D. The metabolic syndrome: time for a critical appraisal: joint statement from the American Diabetes Association and the European Association for the Study of Diabetes. *Diabetes Care* 2005;28(9):2289–2304. Epub 2005 Aug 27. PubMed PMID: 16123508

90. Aguilar M, Bhuket T, Torres S, Liu B, Wong RJ. Prevalence of the metabolic syndrome in the United States, 2003–2012. *JAMA* 2015;313(19):1973–1974. doi: 10.1001/jama.2015.4260. Epub 2015 May 20. PubMed PMID: 25988468

Pathogenesis

Highlights
Pathogenesis

■ Most type 2 diabetes (~85%) develops in obese, insulin-resistant individuals who have a genetic predisposition to β-cell failure.

■ A number of genes that contribute to the risk have been identified. Likely, the genetic risk is produced by the interaction of multiple genes, each of which confers an incremental risk for the development of the disease.

■ A monogenetic cause of diabetes has been identified in a small fraction of individuals with type 2 diabetes, who usually present at a young age (<25 years old), with a strong family history of diabetes and no evidence of autoimmunity.

■ Defects in insulin action and insulin secretion are seen in most individuals with type 2 diabetes.

■ Skeletal muscle, liver, and adipose tissue are the primary sites of insulin resistance.

■ β-cell dysfunction, leading to a relative decrease in insulin levels, is a progressive process and likely results from intrinsic secretion failure and decreases in β-cell mass.

■ Abnormalities in the uptake and metabolism of fatty acids in peripheral tissues and in the β-cells may be a primary event in the development of insulin resistance and β-cell failure.

■ Inflammatory responses of tissue to excess nutrients may contribute to the insulin resistance found in type 2 diabetes.

■ Deficiency of incretin hormones (glucagon-like peptide 1, or GLP-1) and resistance to its action also contribute to development of type 2 diabetes, as do increased production of glucagon from pancreatic α-cells.

■ An increase in renal tubular absorption of glucose is seen in type 2 diabetes contributing to type 2 diabetes.

Pathogenesis

Iram Hussain, MD

Type 2 diabetes is the most common form of diabetes, accounting for >90% of cases.[1] It is a chronic condition characterized by insulin resistance in muscle, liver, and adipose tissue, and superimposed pancreatic β-cell dysfunction.[1,2] Progressive β-cell failure is essential to the development of hyperglycemia. Although abnormal carbohydrate metabolism is the defining disorder, changes in fat and protein metabolism clearly occur and contribute to the complications arising from this progressive metabolic disease. Development of diabetes is frequently due to environmental influences on a susceptible genetic background. Worldwide, the incidence of diabetes is rising rapidly in association with a variety of behavioral and environmental risk factors, mostly predisposing to obesity.[3]

The main pathophysiologic abnormalities identified in the development of type 2 diabetes are as follows (Fig. 2.1):[2]

- Resistance to the action of insulin in the peripheral tissues, particularly in the muscle and adipose tissue, as well as the liver.
- Defects in the secretion of insulin, particularly in response to glucose, and inability of pancreatic β-cells to adapt to insulin resistance.
- Increased hepatic glucose production in both fasting and fed states.
- Increased lipolysis in the adipose tissue.
- Deficiency of incretin hormones and resistance to their action.
- Increased production of glucagon from pancreatic α-cells.
- Increased renal tubular absorption of glucose in the kidney.
- Effects in the central nervous system predisposing to metabolic dysregulation and obesity.

The exact mechanisms by which genetic, environmental, and pathophysiologic factors interact to cause insulin resistance and progressive β-cell failure are not clearly understood.

GENETIC FACTORS

Multiple lines of evidence show that type 2 diabetes is a disease with genetic predisposition.[4] The incidence of type 2 diabetes is especially high among certain ethnic populations, such as Hispanics/Latinos, aboriginal peoples in the Americas and Australia, Pacific and Indian Ocean island populations, Japanese, Chinese, and

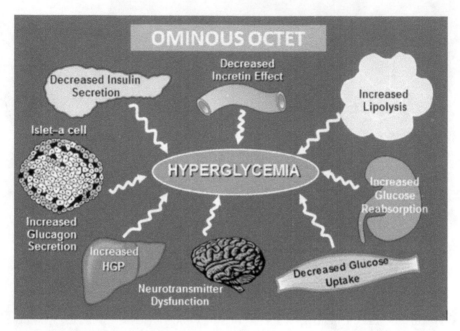

Figure 2.1 Summary of the eight principal mechanisms contributing to hyperglycemia in patients with type 2 diabetes. HGP, hepatic glucose production.

the peoples of the Indian subcontinent.[1] A family history of type 2 diabetes is an important risk factor for the development of diabetes.

Type 2 diabetes is a polygenic disease, and each individual will carry a number of alleles that increase or decrease disease risk.[5] Significant genetic pleiotropy exists, resulting in complex phenotypic manifestations of the disease. Specific genetic aberrations are present in only small subpopulations with diabetes, such as those seen in maturity-onset diabetes of the young (MODY).[1]

To date, >180 genetic loci have been identified that contribute to the risk of type 2 diabetes.[6–8] Initial genetic studies relied on the candidate gene approach or linkage studies. However, genome-wide association studies have been instrumental in identifying additional genes that show a statistically significant association with risk for type 2 diabetes.[7] Candidate gene studies have identified the E23K variant in the potassium inwardly rectifying channel, subfamily J, member 11 (KCNJ11); the P12A variant in the peroxisome proliferator–activated receptor-γ (*PPARG*) gene; common variation in the transcription factor 2, hepatic (TCF2) also called HNF1 homeobox B (HNF1B); and the Wolfram syndrome 1 (WFS1).[4] The strongest associations documented to date are for gene variants in the loci of transcription factor 7-like-2 (TCF7L2) and potassium voltage-gated channel, KQT-like subfamily, member 1 (KCNQ1).[4] TCF7L2 encodes a transcription factor that is important for β-cell development and function, while KCNQ1 codes for a pore-forming subunit of a potassium channel expressed in a variety of tissues, including pancreatic islet cells. Polymorphisms in the TCF7L2 gene are associated with decreased insulin secretion and reduced sensitivity to glucagon-like peptide 1 (GLP-1), while the E23K variant of KCNJ11 appears to affect both insulin secretion and insulin action.

Several other genes have been implicated, some of which include CDKAL1 (CDK5 regulatory subunit–associated protein 1–like 1), CDKN2 (cyclin-dependent kinase inhibitor 2A), FTO (fat mass and obesity–associated), HHEX (hematopoietically expressed homeobox), IDE (insulin-degrading enzyme), and IGF2BP2 (insulin-like growth factor 2 mRNA-binding protein 2). The most common variants are replicated across ethnic groups; however, some have a higher frequency in specific populations, such as PAX4 (paired domain gene 4) in East Asians and TBC1D4 (TBC1 domain family, member 4) in Inuit.[5] It is likely that variation in the structure or expression of other genes will be identified that modulate the risk for type 2 diabetes.

Depending on effect size, the presence of multiple at-risk polymorphisms in an individual substantially increases the risk for type 2 diabetes; however, the way in which these genetic variations interact to predispose an individual to diabetes has not been determined. Most of the genetic variants appear to inhibit insulin secretion, whereas some increase insulin resistance or the tendency to develop obesity.[9] With the identification of rare forms of type 2 diabetes and genes that confer risk, several companies are offering tests that may predict increased genetic susceptibility to type 2 diabetes. However, with the exception of the rare monogenic forms of diabetes, the clinical utility of these tests is not apparent.

ENVIRONMENTAL FACTORS

The genes that predispose an individual to diabetes have likely been selected through evolution. Until recently, humans lived in a relatively nutrient-poor environment. Possessing genes that allow for the efficient accumulation and storage of nutrients would be a distinct advantage during times of chronic or intermittent food shortage. However, these so-called "thrifty genes" are maladaptive in today's consistently food-rich environment.

There is no clear indication that ingestion of a certain type of nutrient, whether carbohydrate, fat, or protein, independent of total caloric intake, predisposes to the development of diabetes,[10] although specific dietary products, like sugar-sweetened beverages, have been implicated in obesity and diabetes risk.[11,12] The combination of a sedentary lifestyle with an increased caloric intake, leading to weight gain and the development of obesity, is the primary factor in the development of insulin resistance and ultimately type 2 diabetes.[10,13]

Genetically determined circadian rhythms also play a role in sleep-wake cycles, feeding behaviors, hormone secretion, and metabolism, and there are associations between reduction of sleep and increased obesity and other metabolic disturbances.[14] Disruption of feeding patterns attuned to circadian rhythm can result in changes in the relationship between the nutrients and their metabolizing enzymes. For example, an altered relationship between fatty acids and the lipoprotein lipase may result in lipotoxicity, causing insulin resistance and decreased secretion of leptin, increasing appetite.[15]

INSULIN RESISTANCE

Insulin resistance is defined as a decrease in the biological effect of endogenous or exogenously administered insulin to alter metabolism in target tissues. This results in decreased insulin-stimulated transport and metabolism of glucose in muscle and adipose tissue, and impaired suppression of hepatic glucose output. Insulin resistance is present years before the development of hyperglycemia and predicts the onset of diabetes.[16]

Most individuals are able to maintain normal glucose levels by increasing β-cell insulin production to compensate for the decrease in insulin action. However, in susceptible individuals, increasing insulin resistance and the failure of β-cells to maintain high levels of insulin secretion leads to progressive glucose intolerance and subsequent diabetes.[17] It is likely that genetic factors play a role both in the propensity to develop insulin resistance and in the risk for β-cell failure in response to insulin resistance.[1]

SITES OF INSULIN RESISTANCE

Insulin resistance occurs in both hepatic and peripheral tissues. Skeletal muscle is the primary site of insulin-mediated glucose uptake after a meal and is therefore the primary site of insulin resistance.[18] Impaired glucose uptake following a carbohydrate-containing meal contributes to the excessive rise in postprandial plasma glucose concentration in patients with type 2 diabetes.[17,18]

Adipose tissue also shows resistance to insulin-stimulated glucose uptake as well as resistance to inhibition of lipolysis.

In the liver, insulin resistance leads to a failure to suppress hepatic glucose production in the basal state, despite fasting hyperinsulinemia. The increase in hepatic glucose production directly correlates with the level of fasting plasma glucose. In addition, patients with type 2 diabetes do not demonstrate normal suppression of hepatic glucose production in response to the insulin secretion that follows a meal.[2]

MECHANISMS OF INSULIN RESISTANCE

The action of insulin on its target tissues is influenced by sex, age, ethnicity, physical activity, medications, and, most importantly, weight.[19,20]

Role of Obesity

Insulin resistance is known to be present to some degree in most obese individuals and is found in most individuals with type 2 diabetes.[13,19] It is important to realize that not all obese individuals develop insulin resistance, for reasons that remain unclear but are likely related to genetic factors. For example, there are some obese individuals that are metabolically healthy with no evidence of insulin resistance, dyslipidemia, or other features of the metabolic syndrome.[21] However, in general, the degree of obesity, as reflected by BMI, correlates with the degree of insulin resistance and subsequent risk for type 2 diabetes.[1] The relationship between BMI and diabetes risk is different among ethnic and racial populations.

For example, the risk for diabetes occurs at a lower BMI in Asian individuals than in most other ethnic groups.[1]

The development of obesity commonly results in the accumulation of intra-abdominal fat, which may be a stronger predictor of type 2 diabetes than overall BMI.[22] Intra-abdominal, or visceral, fat is metabolically distinct from subcutaneous fat, and its effect on glucose tolerance is independent of total adiposity. Visceral fat is more lipolytically active and less sensitive to the antilipolytic effects of insulin. This results in the increased flux of free fatty acids (FFAs) from the fat to the liver and periphery.[19] FFAs in turn inhibit insulin's antilipolytic action, resulting in a further increase in FFA levels. Excess delivery of FFAs has a number of deleterious effects, including (a) inhibition of insulin suppression of hepatic glucose production, which results acutely in increased glycogenolysis and chronically in increased gluconeogenesis, (b) decreased skeletal muscle insulin sensitivity with a subsequent decrease in uptake of glucose, and (c) blunted insulin release from β-cells.[17,19] For this reason, elevated FFAs predict progression from impaired glucose tolerance to diabetes, although in certain cases normal or minimally elevated FFA levels might not reflect true exposure to the peripheral tissues because of their efficient extraction by the liver and skeletal muscle. Levels of 11 β-hydroxysteroid dehydrogenase type I (HST11B1) in mesenteric fat may be elevated, resulting in increased conversion of cortisone to cortisol, which increases lipolysis further and alters the production of adipokines that may directly modulate glucose metabolism.[23]

Cells respond to nutrient load via a variety of pathways, integrating with hormonal signals to modulate metabolism, increasing anabolic activity in times of nutrient surplus, and switching to a catabolic state in times of perceived nutrient deficiency. Individual phenotypic response to nutrient overload is determined by interacting factors functioning within and between tissues, with genetics playing a role in these responses.

Role of Inflammation

Inflammatory response is a consistent finding in muscle and other tissues exposed to prolonged increases in nutrient load. Cellular stress activates the inflammation and cellular repair systems (innate immune system), by way of pattern recognition receptor proteins that can detect lipids and nucleic acids and initiate the increased expression of cytokines and chemokines, promoting insulin resistance in peripheral tissues. Activation also increases the production of "inflammasomes" that control the secretion of interleukins that have potent inflammatory responses and may cause disruption of β-cell function.[24] Toll-like receptors are expressed on multiple cells of the adaptive immune system and are activated by saturated fatty acids (which respond to bacterial cell wall lipids in acute infection), resulting in an inflammatory response and insulin resistance.[25] A number of studies have suggested that elaboration of inflammatory mediators may result in the infiltration of adipose tissue with macrophages, which may exacerbate adipocyte dysfunction.[26,27]

Mechanisms in Fat Cells

Adipose tissue function can be modulated by a variety of factors, including FFAs and hormones. Most excess nutrients are stored in the form of triglycerides in adipose tissue. If the storage capacity is exceeded, then nutrients enter nonstorage tissues, including myocytes, hepatocytes, vascular cells, and β-cells, resulting in both adaptive and maladaptive cellular processes leading to insulin resistance and cellular dysfunction.[28,29] An extreme example of this phenomenon is seen in individuals with lipodystrophy, who have a partial or complete absence of adipose tissue. These individuals develop extreme insulin resistance, elevated serum triglyceride and FFA levels, and an accumulation of "ectopic" triglyceride stores in muscle and liver associated with steatosis, inflammation, and cirrhosis.[30,31] The same clinical features, although not as extreme, are found in most individuals with type 2 diabetes, suggesting a similar pathophysiological mechanism resulting in insulin resistance.[32]

Mechanisms in Muscle and Liver

The cellular processes that are affected in the muscle, liver, and β-cells leading to insulin resistance are becoming clarified, but the exact mechanisms remain to be determined. Postreceptor abnormalities are primarily responsible for insulin resistance in the skeletal muscle and liver in patients with type 2 diabetes. After binding insulin, the insulin receptor initiates a complex cascade of protein phosphorylation and dephosphorylation and other processes that result in various cellular events. Increases, decreases, and the aberrant phosphorylation of specific proteins, including the insulin receptor, result in the impaired propagation of signals. This decreases the translocation of the glucose transporter proteins (GLUT4) from the cytoplasm to the cell membrane, resulting in decreased glucose transport into the myocytes, a defect in glycogen synthesis, and impaired mitochondrial oxidation of substrates.[33]

Hyperglycemia itself can also contribute to insulin resistance by way of increased flux through the hexosamine pathway. Glucosamine overproduction via this pathway disrupts the ability of insulin to cause translocation of GLUT4 to the cell surface by a mechanism that is unclear.[34]

In muscle, a small reduction in insulin binding to its cell surface receptor is observed in type 2 diabetes and is caused by downregulation of the receptor in response to hyperinsulinemia. Subsequent desensitizing of postreceptor pathways can contribute to insulin resistance. Hyperinsulinemia can also exacerbate insulin resistance as sustained hyperinsulinemia is associated with impaired glycogenesis, and suppression of insulin secretion in insulin-resistant people results in increased insulin sensitivity.[35,36] Abnormal insulin binding associated with rare mutations in the insulin gene and the insulin receptor can result in significant insulin resistance, such as in type A syndrome. The insulin resistance associated with type 2 diabetes due to insulin-signaling abnormalities is milder than that seen with these mutations.

Increased endogenous glucose production, mainly from the liver and ≤25% from the kidney, plays a significant role in the pathogenesis of type 2 diabetes.[37,38] Glucose production by the liver is regulated by the relative actions of glucagon and insulin. Glucagon increases glycogenolysis by activating protein kinase cascade pathways, and it also increases transcription of gluconeogenesis enzymes, resulting in increased glucose production. Insulin normally decreases glucagon secretion by α-cells through systemic and paracrine effects, and it also suppresses lipolysis, preventing FFAs from stimulating gluconeogenesis.[39] Portal insulin also directly suppresses glucose production by inhibiting glycogenolysis and gluconeogenesis via enzyme and transcription pathways.[40] Elevated FFAs in the liver antagonize the effects of insulin. There is a direct relationship between the fasting blood glucose and hepatic insulin resistance. In fact, hepatic glucose output in type 2 diabetes often results in an increase in fasting plasma glucose in the morning despite the overnight fasting period, a finding that confuses patients who experience a rise in glucose even without food ingestion. Failure to suppress glucagon in patients with insulin resistance also contributes to increased endogenous glucose production. Peripheral insulin resistance may also play a role in the increased glucose production by the liver. The inability of insulin to suppress the mobilization of gluconeogenic precursors from peripheral tissue results in their increased delivery to the liver.[19]

In both muscle and liver, the accumulation of intracellular stores of triglyceride strongly correlates with the degree of insulin resistance.[20] This accumulation is likely a marker of a mismatch of fatty acid uptake in the tissue (or synthesis in the liver) and the ability of these tissues to oxidize the fats. Fatty acids compete with glucose for substrate oxidation. This leads to the buildup of long-chain acyl-CoA molecules within the mitochondria, which can act as signaling molecules. The primary effect is to decrease glucose uptake into the cell, and this has been demonstrated by in vivo studies in humans.[41,42] Exercise training is also associated with increased muscle triglyceride content; however, studies suggest that acute exercise increases intramyocellular triglyceride synthesis, reducing fatty acid oxidation and preventing fatty acid–induced insulin resistance; additionally, chronic exercise increases insulin sensitivity as well as the capacity for fatty acid oxidation.[43,44] The accumulation of the acyl-CoA molecules is exacerbated by glucose and its metabolites (via glucose shunting toward glycolytic pathway), which can lead to the activation of protein kinase C isoforms or other lipid-activated proteins, resulting in insulin resistance.[45]

Studies in animals and in humans have provided evidence for both intrinsic (inherited) defects in mitochondrial metabolism and acquired mitochondrial changes that result in decreases in the oxidation of fatty acids associated with insulin resistance, obesity, and type 2 diabetes.[46] Insulin resistance is associated with a lower ratio of type I (mostly oxidative) to type II (more glycolytic) muscle fibers. Exercise can counteract some of these mechanisms by causing an increase in the number of type II fibers, increased density of mitochondria, and translocation of intracellular GLUT4 to the cell surface, enhancing glucose uptake in the skeletal muscle.[47-50]

THE FAT CELL AS AN ENDOCRINE ORGAN

Adipose tissue produces numerous proteins that act as local paracrine factors and also circulate to modulate both feeding behavior and insulin action.[19] The most well described of these is leptin, which modulates feeding behavior through interaction with specific receptors in the brain. Besides suppressing food intake, leptin plays a role in modulating glucose and lipid metabolism in the periphery and also regulates energy expenditure. These effects are primarily through the autonomic nervous system, although some actions may be direct. In addition to leptin, the fat cell expresses adiponectin, resistin, tumor necrosis factor (TNF)-α, interleukin (IL)-6, and a variety of other proteins that alter the sensitivity of tissues to insulin and may play a role in the pathogenesis of type 2 diabetes.[20]

THE KIDNEY AS AN ENDOCRINE ORGAN

There is a reciprocal relationship between renal and hepatic glucose release such that a decrease in glucose release by one organ is compensated for by an increase in glucose release by the other organ. Renal gluconeogenesis increases by approximately twofold in the postprandial state, at which point the liver and kidney are contributing equally to endogenous glucose production.[51,52] The kidneys also utilize a significant amount of glucose, ~10% after an overnight fast. In ordinary circumstances (euglycemic conditions), ~180 g of glucose is filtered by the kidneys per day, with a maximum reabsorption capacity of ~450 g of glucose per day.[53] About 90% of filtered glucose is reabsorbed by sodium–glucose co-transporter 2 (SGLT2), expressed in the S1 and S2 segment of proximal tubules, while the remainder is reabsorbed by SGLT1 in the S3 segment with a maximum capacity of ~80 g per day.[54,55] Once the glucose threshold for renal tubular reabsorption has been exceeded, glucose starts appearing in the urine.

In type 2 diabetes, renal glucose output is increased in both the fasting and the postprandial state, because of impaired suppression by insulin, possible stimulation of renal gluconeogenesis by FFAs, and the increased availability of gluconeogenesis precursors. In addition, more glucose is taken up by the kidneys; however, less is oxidized. Most importantly, there is enhanced expression of SGLT2 transporters, resulting in increased reabsorption of glucose, contributing to hyperglycemia.[56]

DEFECTS IN INSULIN SECRETION

Insulin sensitivity (the inverse of insulin resistance) is an important factor in determining the magnitude of the insulin response to β-cell stimulation by glucose, its primary secretagogue. When β-cell function is assessed, obese people who are insulin resistant manifest greater responses than lean people. This is partly mediated by an increase in β-cell mass in obesity and other insulin-resistant states, and it is associated with the increased expression of hexokinase relative to glucokinase, leading to increased insulin secretion across a wide range of glucose concentrations.[57,58] However, the pattern of insulin release in insulin resistance and early type 2 diabetes is abnormal. The first phase of insulin release is blunted or absent, whereas the second phase is enhanced and prolonged, resulting in overall hyperinsulinemia.[59] The ability of the β-cell to secrete insulin in an oscillatory manner is disrupted, and it no longer senses and responds appropriately to changes in the plasma glucose level. A defect in the normal ratio of proinsulin to insulin is observed, with decreased processing of insulin leading to relative increases in proinsulin.[20,60]

In the presence of insulin resistance, the pancreatic β-cells are required to secrete increasing amounts of insulin to maintain euglycemia. Over time, the β-cells begin to fail, resulting in decreased insulin production as well as decreased overall β-cell mass, with resultant hyperglycemia.[2] At diagnosis of type 2 diabetes,

>50%–80% of β-cell function is estimated to have already been lost.[2,20,61] With time, further deterioration occurs, and the rate of β-cell failure determines the rate of progression of the disease.[2] It appears that some stabilization of β-cell function can result from increasing insulin sensitivity by lifestyle modification, including improved diet and increased physical activity.[62,63] Additionally, pharmacotherapy with insulin-sensitizing drugs such as the thiazolidinediones and incretin therapies may also help to stabilize β-cell function,[17] at least in animal models, and compared with sulfonykureas, maintain glycemic control over a longer period of time. As a result, diabetes appears to be a progressive disorder in which secondary failure of therapeutic interventions is predictable and additional drug therapies are usually required.

There is a progressive age-related decline in β-cell function; additionally, genetic make-up, as discussed above, will make some individuals more susceptible than others to β-cell failure. No mechanistic cause of why the β-cells begin to fail after continued hypersecretion of insulin has been identified. It is hypothesized that factors that contribute to insulin resistance, such as intracellular FFAs, may also contribute to β-cell dysfunction.

In islets, FFAs are important for the normal secretion of insulin, whereas excess delivery of FFAs (lipotoxicity) results in a reduction in glucose-stimulated insulin release. Chronically elevated plasma glucose levels (glucotoxicity) also impair β-cell function by reducing the expression of a number of genes affecting these cells, including the insulin gene.[64] The accumulation of long-chain acyl-CoA molecules, leading to disrupted intracellular signaling, oxidative stress, the generation of ceramides, and hypersecretion of islet amyloid polypeptide with accumulation of amyloid protein, have all been proposed to contribute to β-cell dysfunction.[65]

Autopsy examinations have demonstrated the association of obesity with an increase in β-cell mass, whereas individuals with established type 2 diabetes have ~50% decrease in β-cell number; it has been suggested that the decrease in β-cell number is the primary factor in reduction in insulin secretion and resultant hyperglycemia.[20,66] Decreases in β-cell numbers are seen in both thin and obese individuals with type 2 diabetes. Although a longitudinal study of β-cell mass is not possible, it may be that individuals who developed diabetes have an intrinsically reduced β-cell mass that predisposed them to the disease.

FACTORS MODULATING INSULIN SECRETION

Incretin hormones (GLP-1, glucose-dependent insulinotropic peptide 1 and 2 [GIP-1, GIP-2]) are released from small intestine endocrine cells after a meal. The proteins act directly on the β-cells to increase their sensitivity to glucose but do not stimulate insulin secretion by themselves.[67] This is called the "incretin" effect and explains the significantly larger secretion of insulin from the β-cell after oral glucose as opposed to intravenous glucose administration. Patients with type 2 diabetes have a deficiency of GLP-1 and resistance to its stimulatory effect on insulin secretion.[2,67] GLP-1 also inhibits glucagon secretion so that deficiency contributes to increased hepatic glucose production. Pharmacologic doses of the native GLP-1 peptide or biologically active analogs result in a significant potentiation in insulin release in both normal individuals and individuals with type 2 diabetes. This property has been exploited by incretin mimetic medications (GLP-1 agonists), as well as inhibitors of GLP-1 degrading dipeptidyl peptidase-4 (DPP-4). In contrast, treatment with pharmacologic doses of GIP increases insulin secretion only in individuals without diabetes, as glucotoxicity causes β-cell resistance to GIP.[2]

Insulin secretion is also influenced by other gut hormones, including cholecystokinin, secretin, vasoactive intestinal polypeptide, and gastrin. What roles these hormones play in blunted insulin secretion in type 2 diabetes remains to be determined, but their effects are believed to be minor.

PHYSIOLOGICAL CONSEQUENCES OF DEFECTIVE INSULIN SECRETION

Regardless of the mechanism, the impairment in insulin secretion in type 2 diabetes after meal ingestion has physiological consequences. When the early phase of insulin secretion is reduced, portal vein insulin concentration remains low after food ingestion, and hepatic glucose production fails to be suppressed.[68] This effect may be exacerbated by a relative increase in glucagon secretion from the a-cells in the islets. Continued output of glucose by the liver plus the glucose entering the circulation from the intestinal tract after a meal lead to hyperglycemia. In addition, because of the reduced insulin secretion, glucose uptake by muscle is reduced, accentuating the hyperglycemia. Early in the progression to diabetes, the reduced first-phase insulin secretion is followed by late enhanced insulin secretion. Eventually, the plasma glucose concentration returns to normal, but only following postprandial hyperglycemia and at the expense of late hyperinsulinemia. As the defect in β-cell insulin secretion progresses, even late insulin secretion diminishes.[20] When this occurs, fasting hyperglycemia and overt diabetes develop.

CONCLUSION

Dual defects in insulin resistance and a relative decrease in insulin secretion are seen in most individuals with type 2 diabetes and are due to both genetic and environmental factors (Fig. 2.2). Increased insulin resistance is initially compensated for by an increase in insulin secretion, which may be due to increases in islet cell mass and increased production of insulin by individual β-cells.[20] With a continued oversupply of nutrients relative to energy expenditure, the progressive increase in insulin resistance cannot be adequately compensated for by increased insulin secretion, resulting first in impaired glucose tolerance and then overt diabetes. The cellular mechanisms resulting in muscle, liver, and adipose tissue resistance and β-cell failure may be similar, with alterations in intracellular metabolism as a result of the accumulation of excess energy manifested by increased intracellular triglyceride levels, abnormal mitochondrial function, and development of inflammation. The underlying genetic makeup of the individual dictates whether this prolonged energy imbalance results in hyperglycemia and the associated metabolic disorders associated with type 2 diabetes. Hyperglycemia and dyslipidemia themselves result in additional decreases in insulin action and insulin secretion, reinforcing the established defects in the tissues. Prevention and treatment of insulin resistance and diabetes are initially targeted to limit the positive energy balance and then to modulate the metabolic dysfunction once diabetes is established.

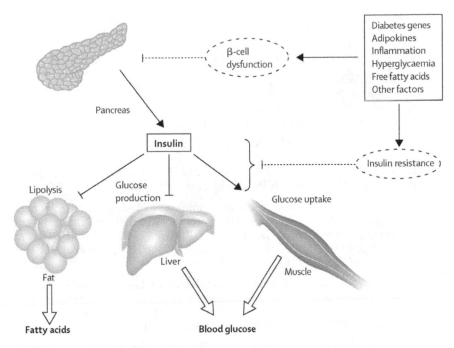

Figure 2.2 Pathogenesis of hyperglycemia in type 2 diabetes.

Source: Stumvoll.[69]

REFERENCES

1. American Diabetes Association. 2. Classification and diagnosis of diabetes: standards of medical care in diabetes 2020. *Diabetes Care* 2020;43(Suppl. 1): S14–S31. doi: 10.2337/dc20-S002. Epub 2019 Dec 22. PubMed PMID: 31862745

2. Defronzo RA. Banting lecture. From the triumvirate to the ominous octet: a new paradigm for the treatment of type 2 diabetes mellitus. *Diabetes* 2009; 58(4):773–795. doi: 10.2337/db09-9028. Epub 2009 Apr 2. PubMed PMID: 19336687; PubMed Central PMCID: PMCPMC2661582

3. Chen L, Magliano DJ, Zimmet PZ. The worldwide epidemiology of type 2 diabetes mellitus—present and future perspectives. *Nat Rev Endocrinol* 2011;8(4):228–236. doi: 10.1038/nrendo.2011.183. Epub 2011 Nov 9. PubMed PMID: 22064493

4. Frayling TM. Genome-wide association studies provide new insights into type 2 diabetes aetiology. *Nat Rev Genet* 2007;8(9):657–662. doi: 10.1038/ nrg2178. Epub 2007 Aug 19. PubMed PMID: 17703236

5. Visscher PM, Wray NR, Zhang Q, Sklar P, McCarthy MI, Brown MA, et al. 10 years of GWAS discovery: biology, function, and translation. *Am J Hum Genet* 2017;101(1):5–22. doi: 10.1016/j.ajhg.2017.06.005. Epub 2017 Jul 8. PubMed PMID: 28686856; PubMed Central PMCID: PMCPMC5501872

6. Suzuki K, Akiyama M, Ishigaki K, Kanai M, Hosoe J, Shojima N, et al. Identification of 28 new susceptibility loci for type 2 diabetes in the Japanese population. *Nat Genet* 2019;51(3):379–386. doi: 10.1038/s41588-018-0332-4. Epub 2019 Feb 6. PubMed PMID: 30718926

7. Scott RA, Scott LJ, Magi R, Marullo L, Gaulton KJ, Kaakinen M, et al. An expanded genome-wide association study of type 2 diabetes in Europeans. *Diabetes* 2017;66(11):2888–2902. doi: 10.2337/db16-1253. Epub 2017 Jun 2. PubMed PMID: 28566273; PubMed Central PMCID: PMCPMC5652602

8. Lau W, Andrew T, Maniatis N. High-resolution genetic maps identify multiple type 2 diabetes loci at regulatory hotspots in African Americans and Europeans. *Am J Hum Genet* 2017;100(5):803–816. doi: 10.1016/j.ajhg.2017.04.007. Epub 2017 May 6. PubMed PMID: 28475862; PubMed Central PMCID: PMCPMC5420350

9. Grarup N, Sandholt CH, Hansen T, Pedersen O. Genetic susceptibility to type 2 diabetes and obesity: from genome-wide association studies to rare variants and beyond. *Diabetologia* 2014;57(8):1528–1541. doi: 10.1007/s00125-014-3270-4. Epub 2014 May 27. PubMed PMID: 24859358

10. American Diabetes Association. 5. Facilitating behavior change and well-being to improve health outcomes: standards of medical care in diabetes 2020. *Diabetes Care* 2020;43(Suppl. 1):S48–S65. doi: 10.2337/dc20-S005. Epub 2019 Dec 22. PubMed PMID: 31862748

11. Malik VS, Popkin BM, Bray GA, Despres JP, Willett WC, Hu FB. Sugar-sweetened beverages and risk of metabolic syndrome and type 2 diabetes: a meta-analysis. *Diabetes Care* 2010;33(11):2477–2483. doi: 10.2337/dc10-1079. Epub 2010 Aug 10. PubMed PMID: 20693348; PubMed Central PMCID: PMCPMC2963518

12. Malik VS, Hu FB. Sweeteners and risk of obesity and type 2 diabetes: the role of sugar-sweetened beverages. *Curr Diab Rep* 2012;12:195–203. doi: 10.1007/s11892-012-0259-6. Epub 2012 Dec 1. PubMed PMID: 22289979

13. American Diabetes Association. 8. Obesity management for the treatment of type 2 diabetes: standards of medical care in diabetes 2020. *Diabetes Care* 2020;43(Suppl. 1):S89–S97. doi: 10.2337/dc20-S008. Epub 2019 Dec 22. PubMed PMID: 31862751

14. Knutson KL, Van Cauter E. Associations between sleep loss and increased risk of obesity and diabetes. *Ann N Y Acad Sci* 2008;1129:287–304. doi: 10.1196/annals.1417.033. Epub 2008 Jul 2. PubMed PMID: 18591489; PubMed Central PMCID: PMCPMC4394987

15. Maury E, Ramsey KM, Bass J. Circadian rhythms and metabolic syndrome: from experimental genetics to human disease. *Circ Res* 2010;106(3):447–462.

doi: 10.1161/CIRCRESAHA.109.208355. Epub 2010 Feb 20. PubMed PMID: 20167942; PubMed Central PMCID: PMCPMC2837358

16. Barness LA, Opitz JM, Gilbert-Barness E. Obesity: genetic, molecular, and environmental aspects. *Am J Med Genet A* 2007;143A(24):3016–3034. doi: 10.1002/ajmg.a.32035. Epub 2007 Nov 16. PubMed PMID: 18000969

17. Petersen KF, Shulman GI. Pathogenesis of skeletal muscle insulin resistance in type 2 diabetes mellitus. *Am J Cardiol* 2002;90(5A):11G–8G. Epub 2002 Sep 17. PubMed PMID: 12231074

18. DeFronzo RA, Tripathy D. Skeletal muscle insulin resistance is the primary defect in type 2 diabetes. *Diabetes Care* 2009;32(Suppl. 2):S157–S163. doi: 10.2337/dc09-S302. Epub 2009 Nov 13. PubMed PMID: 19875544; PubMed Central PMCID: PMCPMC2811436

19. Boden G. Obesity, insulin resistance and free fatty acids. *Curr Opin Endocrinol Diabetes Obes* 2011;18(2):139–143. doi: 10.1097/MED.0b013e3283444b09. Epub 2011 Feb 8. PubMed PMID: 21297467; PubMed Central PMCID: PMCPMC3169796

20. Buchanan TA. Pancreatic beta-cell loss and preservation in type 2 diabetes. *Clin Ther* 2003;25(Suppl. B):B32–B46. Epub 2003 Oct 14. PubMed PMID: 14553865

21. Karelis AD. Metabolically healthy but obese individuals. *Lancet* 2008;372(9646):1281–1283. doi: 10.1016/S0140-6736(08)61531-7. Epub 2008 Oct 22. PubMed PMID: 18929889

22. Kodama S, Horikawa C, Fujihara K, Heianza Y, Hirasawa R, Yachi Y, et al. Comparisons of the strength of associations with future type 2 diabetes risk among anthropometric obesity indicators, including waist-to-height ratio: a meta-analysis. *Am J Epidemiol* 2012;176(11):959–969. doi: 10.1093/aje/kws172. Epub 2012 Nov 13. PubMed PMID: 23144362

23. Dammann C, Stapelfeld C, Maser E. Expression and activity of the cortisol-activating enzyme 11beta-hydroxysteroid dehydrogenase type 1 is tissue and species-specific. *Chem Biol Interact* 2019;303:57–61. doi: 10.1016/j.cbi.2019.02.018. Epub 2019 Feb 24. PubMed PMID: 30796905

24. Schroder K, Tschopp J. The inflammasomes. *Cell* 2010;140(6):821–832. doi: 10.1016/j.cell.2010.01.040. Epub 2010 Mar 23. PubMed PMID: 20303873

25. Shi H, Kokoeva MV, Inouye K, Tzameli I, Yin H, Flier JS. TLR4 links innate immunity and fatty acid-induced insulin resistance. *J Clin Invest* 2006;116(11):3015–3025. doi: 10.1172/JCI28898. Epub 2006 Oct 21. PubMed PMID: 17053832; PubMed Central PMCID: PMCPMC1616196

26. Karasteigiou K, Mohamed-Ali V. The autocrine and paracrine roles of adipokines. *Mol Cell Endocrinol* 2010;318(1-2):69–78. doi: 10.1016/j.mce.2009.11.011. Epub 2009 Dec 2. PubMed PMID: 19948207

27. Iyer A, Fairlie DP, Prins JB, Hammock BD, Brown L. Inflammatory lipid mediators in adipocyte function and obesity. *Nat Rev Endocrinol* 2010;6(2):

71–82. doi: 10.1038/nrendo.2009.264. Epub 2010 Jan 26. PubMed PMID: 20098448

28. Gustafson B, Hedjazifar S, Gogg S, Hammarstedt A, Smith U. Insulin resistance and impaired adipogenesis. *Trends Endocrinol Metab* 2015;26(4):193–200. doi: 10.1016/j.tem.2015.01.006. Epub 2015 Feb 24. PubMed PMID: 25703677

29. Longo M, Zatterale F, Naderi J, Parrillo L, Formisano P, Raciti GA, et al. Adipose tissue dysfunction as determinant of obesity-associated metabolic complications. *Int J Mol Sci* 2019;20(9):E2358. doi: 10.3390/ijms20092358. Epub 2019 May 16. PubMed PMID: 31085992; PubMed Central PMCID: PMCPMC6539070

30. Brown RJ, Araujo-Vilar D, Cheung PT, Dunger D, Garg A, Jack M, et al. The diagnosis and management of lipodystrophy syndromes: a multi-society practice guideline. *J Clin Endocrinol Metab* 2016;101(12):4500–4511. doi: 10.1210/jc.2016-2466. Epub 2016 Oct 7. PubMed PMID: 27710244; PubMed Central PMCID: PMCPMC5155679

31. Hussain I, Garg A. Lipodystrophy syndromes. *Endocrinol Metab Clin North Am* 2016;45(4):783–797. doi: 10.1016/j.ecl.2016.06.012. Epub 2016 Nov 9. PubMed PMID: 27823605

32. Ficarella R, Laviola L, Giorgino F. Lipodystrophic diabetes mellitus: a lesson for other forms of diabetes? *Curr Diab Rep* 2015;15(3):12. doi: 10.1007/s11892-015-0578-5. Epub 2015 Feb 18. PubMed PMID: 25687500

33. Le Marchand-Brustel Y, Tanti JF, Cormont M, Ricort JM, Gremeaux T, Grillo S. From insulin receptor signalling to Glut 4 translocation abnormalities in obesity and insulin resistance. *J Recept Signal Transduct Res* 1999;19(1-4):217–228. doi: 10.3109/10799899909036647. Epub 1999 Mar 11. PubMed PMID: 10071760

34. Baron AD, Zhu JS, Zhu JH, Weldon H, Maianu L, Garvey WT. Glucosamine induces insulin resistance in vivo by affecting GLUT 4 translocation in skeletal muscle. Implications for glucose toxicity. *J Clin Invest* 1995; 96(6):2792–2801. doi: 10.1172/JCI118349. Epub 1995 Dec 1. PubMed PMID: 8675649; PubMed Central PMCID: PMCPMC185989

35. Del Prato S, Leonetti F, Simonson DC, Sheehan P, Matsuda M, DeFronzo RA. Effect of sustained physiologic hyperinsulinaemia and hyperglycaemia on insulin secretion and insulin sensitivity in man. *Diabetologia* 1994;37(10):1025–1035. Epub 1994 Oct 1. PubMed PMID: 7851681

36. Alemzadeh R, Langley G, Upchurch L, Smith P, Slonim AE. Beneficial effect of diazoxide in obese hyperinsulinemic adults. *J Clin Endocrinol Metab* 1998;83(6):1911–1915. doi: 10.1210/jcem.83.6.4852. Epub 1998 Jun 17. PubMed PMID: 9626118

37. Gerich JE, Meyer C, Woerle HJ, Stumvoll M. Renal gluconeogenesis: its importance in human glucose homeostasis. *Diabetes Care* 2001;24(2):382–391. Epub 2001 Feb 24. PubMed PMID: 11213896

38. Meyer C, Stumvoll M, Nadkarni V, Dostou J, Mitrakou A, Gerich J. Abnormal renal and hepatic glucose metabolism in type 2 diabetes mellitus. *J Clin Invest* 1998;102(3):619–624. doi: 10.1172/JCI2415. Epub 1998 Aug 6. PubMed PMID: 9691098; PubMed Central PMCID: PMCPMC508922

39. Chen X, Iqbal N, Boden G. The effects of free fatty acids on gluconeogenesis and glycogenolysis in normal subjects. *J Clin Invest* 1999;103(3):365–372. doi: 10.1172/JCI5479. Epub 1999 Feb 2. PubMed PMID: 9927497; PubMed Central PMCID: PMCPMC407905

40. Newgard CB, Brady MJ, O'Doherty RM, Saltiel AR. Organizing glucose disposal: emerging roles of the glycogen targeting subunits of protein phosphatase-1. *Diabetes* 2000;49(12):1967–1977. Epub 2000 Dec 16. PubMed PMID: 11117996

41. Roden M, Price TB, Perseghin G, Petersen KF, Rothman DL, Cline GW, et al. Mechanism of free fatty acid-induced insulin resistance in humans. *J Clin Invest* 1996;97(12):2859–2865. doi: 10.1172/JCI118742. Epub 1996 Jun 15. PubMed PMID: 8675698; PubMed Central PMCID: PMCPMC507380

42. Rothman DL, Magnusson I, Cline G, Gerard D, Kahn CR, Shulman RG, et al. Decreased muscle glucose transport/phosphorylation is an early defect in the pathogenesis of non-insulin-dependent diabetes mellitus. *Proc Natl Acad Sci U S A* 1995;92(4):983–987. doi: 10.1073/pnas.92.4.983. Epub 1995 Feb 14. PubMed PMID: 7862678; PubMed Central PMCID: PMCPMC42621

43. Schenk S, Horowitz JF. Acute exercise increases triglyceride synthesis in skeletal muscle and prevents fatty acid-induced insulin resistance. *J Clin Invest* 2007;117(6):1690–1698. doi: 10.1172/JCI30566. Epub 2007 May 19. PubMed PMID: 17510709; PubMed Central PMCID: PMCPMC1866251

44. Phillips SM, Green HJ, Tarnopolsky MA, Heigenhauser GF, Hill RE, Grant SM. Effects of training duration on substrate turnover and oxidation during exercise. *J Appl Physiol* (1985) 1996;81(5):2182–2191. doi: 10.1152/jappl.1996.81.5.2182. Epub 1996 Nov 1. PubMed PMID: 9053394

45. Ruderman NB, Saha AK, Vavvas D, Witters LA. Malonyl-CoA, fuel sensing, and insulin resistance. *Am J Physiol* 1999;276(1):E1–E18. doi: 10.1152/ajpendo.1999.276.1.E1. Epub 1999 Jan 14. PubMed PMID: 9886945

46. Schrauwen P, Hesselink MK. Oxidative capacity, lipotoxicity, and mitochondrial damage in type 2 diabetes. *Diabetes* 2004;53(6):1412–1417. Epub 2004 May 27. PubMed PMID: 15161742

47. Hansen PA, Nolte LA, Chen MM, Holloszy JO. Increased GLUT-4 translocation mediates enhanced insulin sensitivity of muscle glucose transport after exercise. *J Appl Physiol* (1985) 1998;85(4):1218–1222. doi: 10.1152/jappl.1998.85.4.1218. Epub 1998 Oct 7. PubMed PMID: 9760308

48. Thorell A, Hirshman MF, Nygren J, Jorfeldt L, Wojtaszewski JF, Dufresne SD, et al. Exercise and insulin cause GLUT-4 translocation in human skeletal muscle. *Am J Physiol* 1999;277(4):E733–E741. doi: 10.1152/ajpendo.1999.277.4.E733. Epub 1999 Oct 12. PubMed PMID: 10516134

49. Ebeling P, Bourey R, Koranyi L, Tuominen JA, Groop LC, Henriksson J, et al. Mechanism of enhanced insulin sensitivity in athletes. Increased blood flow, muscle glucose transport protein (GLUT-4) concentration, and glycogen synthase activity. *J Clin Invest* 1993;92(4):1623–1631. doi: 10.1172/JCI116747. Epub 1993 Oct 1. PubMed PMID: 8408617; PubMed Central PMCID: PMCPMC288320

50. Houmard JA, Egan PC, Neufer PD, Friedman JE, Wheeler WS, Israel RG, et al. Elevated skeletal muscle glucose transporter levels in exercise-trained middle-aged men. *Am J Physiol* 1991;261(4 Pt 1):E437–E443. doi: 10.1152/ajpendo.1991.261.4.E437. Epub 1991 Oct 1. PubMed PMID: 1928336

51. Mather A, Pollock C. Glucose handling by the kidney. *Kidney Int Suppl* 2011(120):S1–S6. doi: 10.1038/ki.2010.509. Epub 2011 Mar 5. PubMed PMID: 21358696

52. Meyer C, Woerle HJ, Dostou JM, Welle SL, Gerich JE. Abnormal renal, hepatic, and muscle glucose metabolism following glucose ingestion in type 2 diabetes. *Am J Physiol Endocrinol Metab* 2004;287(6):E1049–E1056. doi: 10.1152/ajpendo.00041.2004. Epub 2004 Aug 12. PubMed PMID: 15304374

53. Vallon V, Thomson SC. Targeting renal glucose reabsorption to treat hyperglycaemia: the pleiotropic effects of SGLT2 inhibition. *Diabetologia* 2017;60(2):215–225. doi: 10.1007/s00125-016-4157-3. Epub 2016 Nov 24. PubMed PMID: 27878313; PubMed Central PMCID: PMCPMC5884445

54. Rieg T, Vallon V. Development of SGLT1 and SGLT2 inhibitors. *Diabetologia* 2018;61(10):2079–2086. doi: 10.1007/s00125-018-4654-7. Epub 2018 Aug 23. PubMed PMID: 30132033; PubMed Central PMCID: PMCPMC6124499

55. Ghezzi C, Loo DDF, Wright EM. Physiology of renal glucose handling via SGLT1, SGLT2 and GLUT2. *Diabetologia* 2018;61(10):2087–2097. doi: 10.1007/s00125-018-4656-5. Epub 2018 Aug 23. PubMed PMID: 30132032; PubMed Central PMCID: PMCPMC6133168

56. Gerich JE. Role of the kidney in normal glucose homeostasis and in the hyperglycaemia of diabetes mellitus: therapeutic implications. *Diabet Med* 2010;27(2):136–142. doi: 10.1111/j.1464-5491.2009.02894.x. Epub 2010 Jun 16. PubMed PMID: 20546255; PubMed Central PMCID: PMCPMC4232006

57. Pick A, Clark J, Kubstrup C, Levisetti M, Pugh W, Bonner-Weir S, et al. Role of apoptosis in failure of beta-cell mass compensation for insulin resistance and beta-cell defects in the male Zucker diabetic fatty rat. *Diabetes* 1998;47(3):358–364. Epub 1998 Mar 31. PubMed PMID: 9519740

58. Cockburn BN, Ostrega DM, Sturis J, Kubstrup C, Polonsky KS, Bell GI. Changes in pancreatic islet glucokinase and hexokinase activities with increasing age, obesity, and the onset of diabetes. *Diabetes* 1997;46(9):1434–1439. Epub 1997 Sep 1. PubMed PMID: 9287043

59. Pratley RE, Weyer C. The role of impaired early insulin secretion in the pathogenesis of type II diabetes mellitus. *Diabetologia* 2001;44(8):929–945. doi: 10.1007/s001250100580. Epub 2001 Aug 3. PubMed PMID: 11484070

60. Kahn SE. Clinical review 135: The importance of beta-cell failure in the development and progression of type 2 diabetes. *J Clin Endocrinol Metab* 2001;86(9):4047–4058. doi: 10.1210/jcem.86.9.7713. Epub 2001 Sep 11. PubMed PMID: 11549624

61. Boden G. Pathogenesis of type 2 diabetes. Insulin resistance. *Endocrinol Metab Clin North Am* 2001;30(4):801–815. Epub 2001 Dec 1. PubMed PMID: 11727400

62. Way KL, Hackett DA, Baker MK, Johnson NA. The effect of regular exercise on insulin sensitivity in type 2 diabetes mellitus: a systematic review and meta-analysis. *Diabetes Metab J* 2016;40(4):253–271. doi: 10.4093/dmj.2016.40.4.253. Epub 2016 Aug 19. PubMed PMID: 27535644; PubMed Central PMCID: PMCPMC4995180

63. Hemmingsen B, Gimenez-Perez G, Mauricio D, Roque IFM, Metzendorf MI, Richter B. Diet, physical activity or both for prevention or delay of type 2 diabetes mellitus and its associated complications in people at increased risk of developing type 2 diabetes mellitus. *Cochrane Database Syst Rev* 2017;12:CD003054. doi: 10.1002/14651858.CD003054.pub4. Epub 2017 Dec 6. PubMed PMID: 29205264; PubMed Central PMCID: PMCPMC6486271

64. Poitout V, Robertson RP. Minireview: Secondary beta-cell failure in type 2 diabetes—a convergence of glucotoxicity and lipotoxicity. *Endocrinology* 2002;143(2):339–342. doi: 10.1210/endo.143.2.8623. Epub 2002 Jan 18. PubMed PMID: 11796484

65. Ogihara T, Mirmira RG. An islet in distress: beta cell failure in type 2 diabetes. *J Diabetes Investig* 2010;1(4):123–133. doi: 10.1111/j.2040-1124.2010.00021.x. Epub 2010 Aug 2. PubMed PMID: 24843420; PubMed Central PMCID: PMCPMC4008003

66. Butler AE, Janson J, Bonner-Weir S, Ritzel R, Rizza RA, Butler PC. Beta-cell deficit and increased beta-cell apoptosis in humans with type 2 diabetes. *Diabetes* 2003;52(1):102–110. Epub 2002 Dec 28. PubMed PMID: 12502499

67. Drucker DJ, Nauck MA. The incretin system: glucagon-like peptide-1 receptor agonists and dipeptidyl peptidase-4 inhibitors in type 2 diabetes. *Lancet* 2006;368(9548):1696–1705. doi: 10.1016/S0140-6736(06)69705-5. Epub 2006 Nov 14. PubMed PMID: 17098089

68. Del Prato S, Marchetti P, Bonadonna RC. Phasic insulin release and metabolic regulation in type 2 diabetes. *Diabetes* 2002;51(Suppl. 1):S109–S116. doi: 10.2337/diabetes.51.2007.s109. Epub 2002 Jan 30. PubMed PMID: 11815468

69. Stumvoll M, Goldstein BJ, van Haeften TW. Type 2 diabetes: principles of pathogenesis and therapy. *Lancet.* 2005;365(9467):1333–1346. doi: 10.1016/S0140-6736(05)61032-X. Epub 2005 Apr 13. PubMed PMID: 15823385.

Management

Highlights

Therapeutic Objectives and Plan

Nutrition Therapy for Adults with Type 2 Diabetes
    Effectiveness of Diabetes Nutrition Therapy
    Macronutrients
    Eating Patterns
    Energy Balance and Weight Management
    Sugar-Sweetened Beverages (SSBs) & Sugar Substitutes
    Alcohol Consumption
    Micronutrients, Herbal Supplements, and Medications
    Role of Nutrition Therapy in the Prevention and Management of
        Diabetes Complications
    Conclusion

Exercise
    The Benefits of Exercise for People with Type 2 Diabetes
    American Diabetes Association Recommendations for Exercise
    Safety Considerations
    Special Populations
    Jumping Over the Barriers to Exercise
    Conclusion

Pharmaceutical Intervention
    Overview of Pharmacologic Classes
    Biguanides
    Sulfonylureas and Meglitinides
    TZDs
    SGLT2 Inhibitors
    GLP-1 RAs
    DPP-4 Inhibitors
    Other Glucose-Lowering Classes

Highlights
Therapeutic Objectives and Plan

■ The major management goals of type 2 diabetes are as follows:
- Prevent microvascular and macrovascular complications.
- Avoid symptoms related to adverse events of medications (e.g., hypoglycemia), hyperglycemia, and its complications.

■ Specific goals of therapy are as follows:
- Eliminate symptoms.
- Optimize glycemic parameters.
- Achieve and maintain a reasonable body weight.
- Achieve and maintain blood pressure control.
- Achieve and maintain optimal lipoprotein parameters.
- Identify, prevent, and treat microvascular and macrovascular complications.
- Achieve optimal overall health and well-being.

■ Recommended treatment modalities include the following:
- Diet modification to improve glucose and lipid parameters and achieve desired body weight.

- Exercise to improve glucose control and improve cardiovascular health.
- Pharmacologic intervention.

■ Therapy should be individualized, based on patient age, co-morbidities (including cardiovascular disease risk), lifestyle, financial restrictions, self-management skills learned, and level of patient motivation.

■ Recommendations for metabolic control are found in Table 3.1.

■ Patient education that enhances self-care behaviors is essential for the successful management of type 2 diabetes.

NUTRITION THERAPY FOR ADULTS WITH TYPE 2 DIABETES

■ Nutrition therapy is an important component in the diabetes management strategy. Adults with type 2 diabetes should be referred to a registered dietitian nutritionist (RD/RDN) for individualized medical nutrition therapy (MNT) at diagnosis and as needed throughout the life span and during times of changing health status to achieve treatment goals.

- There is no "one-size-fits-all" eating plan that is ideal for all people with type 2 diabetes. Healthy eating goals should be based on individualized assessment of current eating patterns, preferences, and metabolic goals. Healthcare providers should focus on the key factors that are common among healthy eating patterns:
  - Emphasize nonstarchy vegetables;
  - Minimize added sugars and refined grains; and
  - Choose whole foods over highly processed foods to the extent possible.

- Reducing overall carbohydrate intake (particularly from added sugars and refined grains) for individuals with type 2 diabetes has demonstrated the most evidence for improving glycemia and may be applied in a variety of eating patterns that meet individual needs and preferences.

- Modest weight loss can improve A1C, CVD risk factors, and quality of life in adults with overweight/obesity and type 2 diabetes. As little as 5% weight loss shows clinical benefit; 15% weight loss or more may provide optimal outcomes if it is needed and can be feasibly and safely accomplished.

- In select individuals with type 2 diabetes, an overall healthy eating plan that results in energy deficit in conjunction with weight loss medications and/or metabolic surgery should be considered to help achieve weight loss and maintenance goals, lower A1C, and reduce CVD risk.

EXERCISE

- Unless contraindicated, appropriate physical activity is strongly recommended to maximize the effects of dietary modification.

- The potential benefits of increased physical activity include the following:
  - Improved insulin sensitivity and glucose tolerance.
  - Weight loss and maintenance of desirable body weight when combined with restricted caloric intake.
  - Improved cardiovascular risk factors.
  - Potential reduction in dosage or need for insulin or oral antidiabetic agents.
  - Enhanced work capacity.
  - Enriched quality of life and improved sense of well-being.

- In patients treated with insulin or insulin secretagogues, hypoglycemia can be precipitated by exercise and requires a specific plan of monitoring and care to minimize risk.

- In patients with labile blood glucose levels or microvascular and/or cardiovascular complications, exercise needs to be accompanied by a specific plan of monitoring and care to minimize risk.

PHARMACEUTICAL INTERVENTION

- At the time of diagnosis of type 2 diabetes, in addition to lifestyle intervention, metformin therapy should be initiated concurrently.

- When a patient is unable to achieve normal or near-normal glucose levels with dietary changes, exercise, and metformin (if not contraindicated) despite adequate education and effort, secondary pharmacologic treatment should be implemented.

- The choice among glucose-lowering agents should be individualized, taking into account patient preferences, co-morbidities/contraindications, goals, ability for self-care management, social support, and finances.

- In patients with cardiovascular disease, agents with proven cardiovascular benefit should be used as second-line treatment after metformin.

- In patients who would benefit from weight loss, glucose-lowering agents, which promote weight loss, should be used: glucagon-like peptide 1 receptor agonists (GLP-1RAs; greater effect) or sodium–glucose cotransporter 2 (SGLT2) inhibitors.

- In patients in whom hypoglycemia is a major concern, agents with low risk of hypoglycemia should be prioritized: GLP-1RAs, dipeptidyl-peptidase-4 (DPP-4) inhibitors, SGLT2 inhibitors, thiazolidinediones.

- The GLP-1 RA class should be considered before insulin in most patients with type 2 diabetes.

- Insulin should be initiated after a GLP-1 RA or in the setting of significant hyperglycemia, acute metabolic decompensation, or suspicion for type 1 diabetes.

ASSESSMENT OF TREATMENT EFFICACY

- People with diabetes and providers need to understand the rationale for different modalities to assess glycemic management.

- A1C is the primary metric for measuring effectiveness of treatment.

- Self-monitoring of blood glucose and continuous glucose monitoring are used for daily assessments and to adjust medication regimens.

- Glycemic goals should be individualized based on duration of diabetes; pregnancy status; cardiovascular disease; as well as hypoglycemia risk, age, life expectancy, patient preference and willingness, cultural factors, cognitive abilities, resources and support systems, and co-morbid conditions.

- More or less stringent glycemic goals may be appropriate for individual patients.

- Time in range (TIR) is the most important continuous glucose monitoring metric. A 70% TIR of 70–180 mg/dL (3.9–10.0 mmol/L) is recommended for most patients with type 2 diabetes.

POPULATION HEALTH AND COST EFFECTIVENESS

- Rising rates of diabetes and obesity are requiring a shift in management strategies.

- Population health is now an important framework for chronic disease management.

■ Barriers to population health delivery include lack of access to diabetes self-management, specialty referral, and fragmentation of data sharing.

■ An increasing shift to value-based payments aims to focus on preventive measures for diabetes and reduce unnecessary utilization.

■ Incorporating elements of population health in clinical practice requires restructuring of roles for the providers and clinical staff and longitudinal care of the patient.

DIABETES TECHNOLOGY

■ Real-time continuous and flash glucose monitoring can increase engagement in daily glycemic assessments, pattern recognition, and hypoglycemia awareness.

■ Smart insulin pens/caps help insulin dose tracking.

■ Patch pumps can be a simpler alternative to deliver basal bolus insulin treatment compared with regular insulin pump therapy.

■ Pump therapy can add convenience to insulin delivery for people requiring complex insulin programs and when enhanced by continuous glucose monitor integration; it can reduce hypoglycemia and improve overall glycemia.

Management

THERAPEUTIC OBJECTIVES AND PLAN

Iram Hussain, MD

A thorough medical evaluation to assess a patient's diabetes status is critical. Evaluate for the presence of complications or co-morbidities, the patient's risk of and from hypoglycemia, his or her self-management education and skill level, and his or her social support. With this information, lay out a well thought-out assessment and corresponding management plan. The elements of the medical history, physical evaluation, laboratory testing and other screening for complications or co-morbidities, and appropriate referrals are outlined in Table 3.1.

Table 3.1–Initial,* Follow-Up,^ and Annuala Medical Evaluation for the Patient with Diabetes

Medical History

- Age and characteristics of onset of diabetes (e.g., diabetic ketoacidosis, asymptomatic laboratory finding)*
- Family history of diabetes in first-degree relative and history of autoimmune disorder (especially in type 1 diabetes)*
- Eating patterns, nutritional status, and weight history; growth and development in children and adolescents*^a
- Diabetes education history*
- Review of previous treatment regimens and response to therapy (A1C records)*a
- Current treatment of diabetes, including medications, meal plans, physical activity patterns, and results of glucose monitoring and patient's use of data*^a
- Diabetic ketoacidosis frequency, severity, and cause*
- History of complications, including the following:
  - History of diabetes-related complications*a
  - Microvascular: retinopathy, nephropathy, neuropathy (sensory, including history of foot lesions; autonomic, including sexual dysfunction and gastroparesis)*a
  - Hypoglycemia awareness*^a
  - Any severe hypoglycemia: frequency and cause*^a

(continued)

Table 3.1 *(continued)*

- Macrovascular: coronary heart disease, cerebrovascular disease, peripheral arterial disease*[a]
- Other: psychosocial problems, dental disease*[a]
- Other endocrine disorders*

Physical Examination

- Height, weight, BMI*^[a]
- Blood pressure determination, including orthostatic measurements when indicated*^[a]
- Fundoscopic examination*[a]
- Thyroid palpation*[a]
- Skin examination (for acanthosis nigricans and insulin injection sites)*^[a]
- Complete foot examination*[a]
  - Inspection^ (every visit in patients with sensory loss, previous foot ulcers or amputations)
  - Palpation of dorsalis pedis and posterior tibial pulses
  - Presence/absence of patellar and Achilles reflexes
  - Determination of proprioception, vibration, and 10 g monofilament sensation

Laboratory Evaluation

- A1C, if results are not available within the past 2–3 months*^[a]

If not performed/available within past year*[a]

- Fasting lipid profile, including total, LDL, and HDL cholesterol and triglycerides (may also need to be checked after medication changes)
- Liver function tests (may also need to be checked after medication changes)
- Tests for urine albumin excretion with spot urine albumin-to-creatinine ratio
- Serum creatinine and calculated glomerular filtration rate
- Thyroid-stimulating hormone in all patients with type 1 diabetes, patients with dyslipidemia, and women >50 years (may also need to be checked after thyroid medication dose changes)
  - Vitamin B12 on metformin (when indicated)
  - Serum potassium levels in patients on ACE inhibitors, angiotensin receptor blockers, or diuretics (may need to be more frequent in patients with chronic kidney disease or medications that affect renal function and electrolytes)

Referrals*

- Annual dilated eye exam
- Family planning for women of reproductive age
- Registered dietitian for medical nutrition therapy
- Diabetes self-management education and support
- Dental examination
- Mental health professional, if needed

Performed at initial visit,* follow-up visit,^ and annual visit.[a]

The main management goals for patients with type 2 diabetes are to prevent micro- and macrovascular complications and to avoid or alleviate symptoms. Atherosclerotic cardiovascular complications, including coronary heart disease, cerebrovascular disease, and peripheral artery disease, as well as heart failure, both with preserved and reduced ejection fraction, result in increased morbidity and mortality in patients with type 2 diabetes.[1,2] Thus, management of risk factors such as blood pressure and lipids, smoking cessation, and antiplatelet therapy are essential aspects of care. Decreased atherosclerotic cardiovascular disease (ASCVD) morbidity and mortality has been shown with aggressive multimodal risk factor modification in patients with diabetes[1,3] and in high-risk patients with the use of sodium–glucose cotransporter 2 (SGLT2) inhibitors and glucagon-like protein 1 (GLP-1) receptor agonists.[4,5,6]

Meeting glycemic targets is also important, since it clearly lowers the risk of development and progression of diabetic retinopathy, nephropathy, and neuropathy.[2,7–11] A summary of recommended therapeutic targets for adults with diabetes is provided in Table 3.2.

The evidence that long-term glycemic control can prevent or ameliorate the microvascular and neuropathic complications of diabetes comes from a series of clinical trials. The Diabetes Control and Complications Trial (DCCT) demonstrated the beneficial effects of glycemic control in slowing the progression of retinopathy, nephropathy, and neuropathy in type 1 diabetes, and the Epidemiology of Diabetes Interventions and Complications (EDIC) study showed persistence of these microvascular benefits over two decades.[11,13] The UK Prospective Diabetes Study (UKPDS) demonstrated that intensive glycemic control in addition to lifestyle intervention resulted in reduction in the risk of development of combined end points, largely microvascular, with a trend toward reduction in cardiovascular events in patients with newly diagnosed type 2 diabetes.[14,15] Long-term follow-up of UKPDS cohorts showed favorable effects of early glycemic control on microvascular complications.[16] In both of these trials, the more intensively treated group exhibited an average A1C of ~7% (53 mmol/mol); thus, an A1C target of <7% (53 mmol/mol) has been adopted as the treatment target for most patients with diabetes, since the relative risks and benefits at this level of glycemic control are well established.

The absolute risk of end-stage microvascular complications (blindness, dialysis, or amputation) developing over an intermediate time frame (6–10 years) is small at an A1C of 7% (53 mmol/mol), at least in patients with no or early complications. However, there is no threshold or lower limit in A1C below which complications do not develop, thus the rationale for considering lower targets.[17] An A1C goal of less than 6.5% (48 mmol/mol) is reasonable in patients with a long life expectancy, those treated with lifestyle changes or metformin only, and those who are on medications that can achieve this without risk of hypoglycemia.[11] Patients with multiple complications or co-morbidities, with limited life expectancy, with long disease duration, with limited resources and support, and who are prone to hypoglycemia and at risk for its consequences may need to have less stringent targets such as A1C <8% (64 mmol/mol).[11]

The UKPDS and the Steno-2 Study demonstrated that more intensive blood pressure, lipid, and glycemic management resulted in substantial reduction in both micro- and macrovascular complications in younger patients with type 2 diabetes.[18,19] Findings from the Action to Control Cardiovascular Risk in Diabetes (ACCORD) trial, Veteran's Affairs Diabetes Trial (VADT), and the Action in Diabetes and Vascular Disease (ADVANCE) trial, all consistently show that trying to aggressively lower A1C levels (<6.0% [42 mmol/mol] in ACCORD, <6.5% [48 mmol/mol] in ADVANCE, and a 1.5% difference from the control group in the VADT) in patients with long-standing diabetes at high ASCVD risk, does not reduce CVD events,[20,21] and may actually be associated with higher mortality rates.[8,9] In these trials, aggressive insulin therapy was implemented in many

Table 3.2–Summary of Recommended Targets for Nonpregnant Adults with Diabetes

Glycemic control	A1C <7.0% (53 mmol/mol)*
Preprandial plasma glucose	80–130 mg/dl (4.4–7.2 mmol/l)
Postprandial plasma glucose†	<180 mg/dl (<10.0 mmol/l)
Blood pressure^	
Lower ASCVD risk	<140/90 mmHg
Higher ASCVD risk	<130/80 mmHg
Lipids	
LDL cholesterol#	Majority of patients, especially between ages 40–75 years, should be on statin therapy regardless of LDL-C levels.
Primary prevention in	
high-risk patients	Reduce LDL-C by 50% or more
Secondary prevention in	
very high-risk patients	<70 mg/dl (<1.8mmol/l)#
Triglycerides	<150 mg/dl (<1.7 mmol/l)
HDL cholesterol	≥40 mg/dl (>1.1 mmol/l) for men
	≥50 mg/dl (>1.3 mmol/l) for women

Key concepts in setting glycemic goals are as follows:

■ Goals should be individualized based on duration of diabetes, pregnancy status, age, co-morbid conditions, hypoglycemia unawareness and risk, and other individual patient considerations.[12]

■ More stringent glycemic goals (i.e., A1C <6.5% [48 mmol/mol]) may further reduce complications at the cost of increased risk of hypoglycemia (particularly in individuals with type 1 diabetes).

■ Postprandial glucose may be targeted if A1C goals are not met, despite reaching preprandial glucose goals.

*Referenced to a nondiabetic range of 4.0%–6.0% (20–42 mmol/mol) using a Diabetes Control and Complications Trial (DCCT)–based assay. More or less stringent glycemic goals may be appropriate for individual patients.

^Lower atherosclerotic cardiovascular disease (ASCVD) risk is defined as a 10-year ASCVD risk of <15%, whereas a higher ASCVD risk is defined as 10-year ASCVD risk ≥15%.

#Instead of target LDL cholesterol levels, recommendations are to treat patient with moderate-intensity or high-intensity statins based on cardiovascular risk (as calculated by the American Heart Association's ASCVD risk calculator). If patients have diabetes and ASCVD, and LDL cholesterol is ≥70 mg/dL on maximally tolerated statin dose, then additional LDL-lowering therapy (ezetimibe or PCSK9 inhibitor) may be considered.

†Postprandial glucose measurements should be made 1–2 h after the beginning of the meal, generally peak levels in patients with diabetes.

Source: Davies,[1] American Diabetes Association,[2] and American Diabetes Association.[11]

patients in order to try and achieve these tight glycemic targets.[7,20] Taken in total, the most effective approach for prevention of macrovascular complications appears to be multifactorial risk factor management, with glycemic goals that are personalized based upon patient characteristics and risk factors. Additionally, over the past several years a number of cardiovascular outcome trials have demonstrated the benefit in CVD event reduction with the use of long-acting GLP-1 receptor agonists and SGLT-2 inhibitors, prompting a revision in the recommendations for glycemic management in high-risk patients.[1] More recent trials are also focusing on the renovascular benefits of SGLT-2 inhibitors in patients with diabetic nephropathy.[22–24] A more specific discussion of cardiovascular risk reduction strategies is given in Chapter 5: Detection and Treatment of Chronic Complications.

A rational approach to the treatment of elevated blood glucose in patients with type 2 diabetes should include measures that will specifically reverse the underlying pathogenic metabolic disturbances that result in hyperglycemia (i.e., insulin resistance and impaired β-cell function). It is critical to educate patients and their families on self-care practices necessary to manage diabetes.[1,25] National standards exist for diabetes education programs, and these should be followed.[1,25] The initial evaluation should include: development of a meal plan and exercise program, identification of complications and potential co-morbid conditions, initiation of appropriate pharmacologic therapy, and a monitoring program both at home and in the healthcare setting to assess disease control.[12] Within this scheme, careful attention to psychosocial influences and/or behavior modification techniques is valuable, as outlined in Diabetes Self-Management Education and Behavior Change (page 303).

REFERENCES

1. Davies MJ, D'Alessio DA, Fradkin J, Kernan WN, Mathieu C, Mingrone G, et al. Management of hyperglycemia in type 2 diabetes, 2018. A consensus report by the American Diabetes Association (ADA) and the European Association for the Study of Diabetes (EASD). *Diabetes Care* 2018;41(12):2669–2701. doi: 10.2337/dci18-0033. Epub 2018 Oct 7. PubMed PMID: 30291106; PubMed Central PMCID: PMCPMC6245208

2. American Diabetes Association. 10. Cardiovascular disease and risk management: standards of medical care in diabetes 2020. *Diabetes Care* 2020;43(Suppl. 1):S111–S134. doi: 10.2337/dc20-S010. Epub 2019 Dec 22. PubMed PMID: 31862753

3. Gaede P, Lund-Andersen H, Parving HH, Pedersen O. Effect of a multifactorial intervention on mortality in type 2 diabetes. *N Engl J Med* 2008;358(6):580–591. doi: 10.1056/NEJMoa0706245. Epub 2008 Feb 8. PubMed PMID: 18256393

4. Udell JA, Yuan Z, Rush T, Sicignano NM, Galitz M, Rosenthal N. Cardiovascular outcomes and risks after initiation of a sodium glucose cotransporter 2 inhibitor: results from the EASEL population-based cohort study (evidence for cardiovascular outcomes with sodium glucose cotransporter 2 inhibitors in the real world). *Circulation* 2018;137(14):1450–1459. doi:

10.1161/CIRCULATIONAHA.117.031227. Epub 2017 Nov 15. PubMed PMID: 29133607; PubMed Central PMCID: PMCPMC5895161

5. Birkeland KI, Jorgensen ME, Carstensen B, Persson F, Gulseth HL, Thuresson M, et al. Cardiovascular mortality and morbidity in patients with type 2 diabetes following initiation of sodium-glucose co-transporter-2 inhibitors versus other glucose-lowering drugs (CVD-REAL Nordic): a multinational observational analysis. *Lancet Diabetes Endocrinol* 2017;5(9):709–717. doi: 10.1016/S2213-8587(17)30258-9. Epub 2017 Aug 7. PubMed PMID: 28781064

6. Bethel MA, Patel RA, Merrill P, Lokhnygina Y, Buse JB, Mentz RJ, et al. Cardiovascular outcomes with glucagon-like peptide-1 receptor agonists in patients with type 2 diabetes: a meta-analysis. *Lancet Diabetes Endocrinol* 2018;6(2):105–113. doi: 10.1016/S2213-8587(17)30412-6. Epub 2017 Dec 10. PubMed PMID: 29221659

7. The ADVANCE Collaborative Group, Patel A, MacMahon S, Chalmers J, Neal B, Billot L, et al. Intensive blood glucose control and vascular outcomes in patients with type 2 diabetes. *N Engl J Med* 2008;358(24):2560–2572. doi: 10.1056/NEJMoa0802987. Epub 2008 Jun 10. PubMed PMID: 18539916

8. Ismail-Beigi F, Craven T, Banerji MA, Basile J, Calles J, Cohen RM, et al. Effect of intensive treatment of hyperglycaemia on microvascular outcomes in type 2 diabetes: an analysis of the ACCORD randomised trial. *Lancet* 2010;376(9739):419–430. doi: 10.1016/S0140-6736(10)60576-4. Epub 2010 Jul 03. PubMed PMID: 20594588; PubMed Central PMCID: PMCPMC4123233

9. Action to Control Cardiovascular Risk in Diabetes Study Group, Gerstein HC, Miller ME, Byington RP, Goff DC, Jr., Bigger JT, et al. Effects of intensive glucose lowering in type 2 diabetes. *N Engl J Med* 2008;358(24):2545–2559. doi: 10.1056/NEJMoa0802743. Epub 2008 Jun 10. PubMed PMID: 18539917; PubMed Central PMCID: PMCPMC4551392

10. Stratton IM, Adler AI, Neil HA, Matthews DR, Manley SE, Cull CA, et al. Association of glycaemia with macrovascular and microvascular complications of type 2 diabetes (UKPDS 35): prospective observational study. *BMJ* 2000;321(7258):405–412. Epub 2000 Aug 11. PubMed PMID: 10938048; PubMed Central PMCID: PMCPMC27454

11. American Diabetes Association. 6. Glycemic targets: Standards of medical care in diabetes 2020. *Diabetes Care* 2020;43(Suppl. 1):S66–S76. doi: 10.2337/dc20-S006. Epub 2019 Dec 22. PubMed PMID: 31862749

12. American Diabetes Association. 4. Comprehensive medical evaluation and assessment of co-morbidities: standards of medical care in diabetes 2020. *Diabetes Care* 2020;43(Suppl. 1):S37–S47. doi: 10.2337/dc20-S004. Epub 2019 Dec 22. PubMed PMID: 31862747

13. Diabetes Control Complications Trial (DCCT)/Epidemiology of Diabetes Interventions and Complications (EDIC) Research Group, Lachin JM, White NH, Hainsworth DP, et al. Effect of intensive diabetes therapy on the

progression of diabetic retinopathy in patients with type 1 diabetes: 18 years of follow-up in the DCCT/EDIC. *Diabetes* 2015;64(2):631–642. doi: 10.2337/db14-0930. Epub 2014 Sep 11. PubMed PMID: 25204977; PubMed Central PMCID: PMCPMC4303965

14. UK Prospective Diabetes Study (UKPDS) Group. Effect of intensive blood-glucose control with metformin on complications in overweight patients with type 2 diabetes (UKPDS 34). *Lancet* 1998;352(9131):854–865. Epub 1998 Sep 22. PubMed PMID: 9742977

15. UK Prospective Diabetes Study (UKPDS) Group. Intensive blood-glucose control with sulphonylureas or insulin compared with conventional treatment and risk of complications in patients with type 2 diabetes (UKPDS 33). *Lancet* 1998;352(9131):837–853. Epub 1998 Sep 22. PubMed PMID: 9742976

16. Holman RR, Paul SK, Bethel MA, Matthews DR, Neil HA. 10-year follow-up of intensive glucose control in type 2 diabetes. *N Engl J Med* 2008;359(15):1577–1589. doi: 10.1056/NEJMoa0806470. Epub 2008 Sep 12. PubMed PMID: 18784090

17. American Diabetes Association. 3. Prevention or delay of type 2 diabetes: standards of medical care in diabetes 2020. *Diabetes Care* 2020;43(Suppl. 1):S32–S36. doi: 10.2337/dc20-S003. Epub 2019 Dec 22. PubMed PMID: 31862746

18. Gaede P, Vedel P, Larsen N, Jensen GV, Parving HH, Pedersen O. Multifactorial intervention and cardiovascular disease in patients with type 2 diabetes. *N Engl J Med* 2003;348(5):383–393. doi: 10.1056/NEJMoa021778. Epub 2003 Jan 31. PubMed PMID: 12556541

19. UK Prospective Diabetes (UKPDS) Study Group. Tight blood pressure control and risk of macrovascular and microvascular complications in type 2 diabetes: UKPDS 38. *BMJ* 1998;317(7160):703–713. Epub 1998 Sep 11. PubMed PMID: 9732337; PubMed Central PMCID: PMCPMC28659

20. Duckworth W, Abraira C, Moritz T, Reda D, Emanuele N, Reaven PD, et al. Glucose control and vascular complications in veterans with type 2 diabetes. *N Engl J Med* 2009;360(2):129–139. doi: 10.1056/NEJMoa0808431. Epub 2008 Dec 19. PubMed PMID: 19092145

21. Skyler JS, Bergenstal R, Bonow RO, Buse J, Deedwania P, Gale EA, et al. Intensive glycemic control and the prevention of cardiovascular events: implications of the ACCORD, ADVANCE, and VA diabetes trials: a position statement of the American Diabetes Association and a scientific statement of the American College of Cardiology Foundation and the American Heart Association. *Diabetes Care* 2009;32(1):187–192. doi: 10.2337/dc08-9026. Epub 2008 Dec 19. PubMed PMID: 19092168; PubMed Central PMCID: PMCPMC2606812

22. Neal B, Perkovic V, Matthews DR. Canagliflozin and cardiovascular and renal events in type 2 diabetes. *N Engl J Med* 2017;377(21):2099. doi: 10.1056/NEJMc1712572. Epub 2017 Nov 23. PubMed PMID: 29166232

23. Perkovic V, Jardine MJ, Neal B, Bompoint S, Heerspink HJL, Charytan DM, et al. Canagliflozin and renal outcomes in type 2 diabetes and nephropathy. *N Engl J of Med* 2019;380(24):2295–2306. doi: 10.1056/NEJMoa1811744. Epub 2019 Apr 17. PubMed PMID: 30990260

24. Zelniker TA, Wiviott SD, Raz I, Im K, Goodrich EL, Bonaca MP, et al. SGLT2 inhibitors for primary and secondary prevention of cardiovascular and renal outcomes in type 2 diabetes: a systematic review and meta-analysis of cardiovascular outcome trials. *Lancet* 2019;393(10166):31–39. doi: 10.1016/S0140-6736(18)32590-X. Epub 2018 Nov 15. PubMed PMID: 30424892

25. American Diabetes Association. 5. Facilitating behavior change and well-being to improve health outcomes: standards of medical care in diabetes 2020. *Diabetes Care* 2020;43(Suppl. 1):S48–S65. doi: 10.2337/dc20-S005. Epub 2019 Dec 22. PubMed PMID: 31862748

NUTRITION THERAPY FOR ADULTS WITH TYPE 2 DIABETES[1]

Janice MacLeod, MA, RDN, LD, CDE, FAADE
Fredrick Dunn, MD

Nutrition therapy is the cornerstone of care for people with type 2 diabetes and related metabolic diseases; therefore, it is important that all members of the healthcare team know and champion the benefits of nutrition therapy and key nutrition messages. Nutrition counseling that works toward achieving and maintaining individualized treatment goals, such as glycemic targets, cardiovascular risk factors (e.g., lipids, blood pressure), and/or weight management is recommended for all adults with type 2 diabetes. Despite the recent introduction of powerful medications to control hyperglycemia and prevent micro- and macro-vascular complications, medical nutrition therapy (MNT) remains fundamental in the overall diabetes management plan.

Furthermore, a "one-size-fits-all" eating plan is no longer optimal for management of type 2 diabetes. It is unrealistic to expect a single meal plan to be acceptable to all people with diabetes, given the broad spectrum affected by type 2 diabetes (i.e., cultural background, personal preferences, co-morbidities, and socioeconomic settings in which they live). It is therefore important for clinicians to understand the rationale for variations in dietary therapy. The American Diabetes Association (ADA) emphasizes that medical nutrition therapy (MNT) is fundamental in the overall diabetes management plan, and the need for MNT should be reassessed frequently by healthcare providers in collaboration with people with diabetes across the life span, with special attention during times of changing health status and life stages.[1-3]

EFFECTIVENESS OF DIABETES NUTRITION THERAPY

Highlights

- Refer adults living with type 2 diabetes to individualized, diabetes-focused MNT at diagnosis and as needed throughout the life span and during times of changing health status to achieve treatment goals. Coordinate and align the MNT plan with the overall management strategy, including use of medications, physical activity, etc., on an ongoing basis.
- Refer adults with type 2 diabetes to comprehensive diabetes self-management education and support (DSMES) services according to national standards.
- Diabetes-focused MNT is provided by a registered dietitian nutritionist/registered dietitian (RDN), preferably one who has comprehensive knowledge and experience in diabetes care.
- Diabetes MNT is a covered Medicare benefit and should be adequately reimbursed by insurance and other payers or bundled in evolving value-based care and payment models.

---

[1]The content of this section has been adapted from Evert AB, Dennison M, Gardner CD, et al. Nutrition therapy for adults with diabetes or prediabetes: a consensus report. *Diabetes Care* 2019;42(5):731–754. For a full literature review and additional reference, refer to the report.

Diabetes Nutrition Therapy Definition and Delivery

MNT is an evidence-based application of the nutrition care process provided by an RDN and is the legal definition of nutrition counseling by an RDN in the U.S.[4, 5] Essential components of MNT are assessment; nutrition diagnosis; interventions (e.g., education and counseling); and monitoring with ongoing follow-up to support long-term lifestyle changes, evaluate outcomes, and modify interventions as needed.[4] The goals of nutrition therapy are described in Table 3.3. See Table 3.4 for the recommended structure for the implementation of MNT for adults with diabetes.

Table 3.3–Goals of Nutrition Therapy

- To promote and support healthful eating patterns, emphasizing a variety of nutrient-dense foods in appropriate portion sizes, in order to improve overall health and specifically to:
  - o Improve A1C, blood pressure, and cholesterol levels (goals differ for individuals based on age, duration of diabetes, health history, and other present health conditions). Further recommendations for individualization of goals can be found in the American Diabetes Association Standards of Medical Care in Diabetes.
  - o Achieve and maintain body weight goals
  - o Delay or prevent complications of diabetes

- To address individual nutrition needs based on personal and cultural preferences, health literacy and numeracy, access to healthful food choices, willingness and ability to make behavioral changes, as well as barriers to change

- To maintain the pleasure of eating by providing positive messages about food choices, while limiting food choices only when indicated by scientific evidence

- To provide the individual with diabetes with practical tools for day-to-day meal planning

Source: Evert AB, Dennison M, Gardner CD, et al. Nutrition therapy for adults with diabetes or prediabetes: a consensus report. *Diabetes Care* 2019;42(5):731–754

Table 3.4–Academy of Nutrition and Dietetics Evidence-Based Nutrition Practice Guidelines–Recommended Structure for the Implementation of MNT for Adults with Diabetes

Initial series of MNT encounters: The RDN should implement three to six MNT encounters during the first 6 months following diagnosis and determine if additional MNT encounters are needed based on an individualized assessment.

MNT follow-up encounters: The RDN should implement a minimum of one annual MNT follow-up encounter.

Source: Franz.[4]

The unique academic preparation, training, skills, and expertise make the RDN the preferred member of the healthcare team to provide diabetes MNT and leadership in interprofessional team–based nutrition and diabetes care.[1,4,6] To complement diabetes nutrition therapy, members of the healthcare team can and should provide evidence-based guidance that allows people with diabetes to make healthy food choices that meet their individual needs and optimize their overall health.

In addition to diabetes MNT, DSMES is important for people with type 2 diabetes to improve cardiometabolic and microvascular outcomes in a disease that is largely self-managed.[1,7] DSMES includes the ongoing process that facilitates the knowledge, skills, and abilities necessary for diabetes self-care throughout the life span, with nutrition as one of the core curriculum topics taught in comprehensive programs.[7]

Healthcare professionals can use the education algorithm suggested by the American Diabetes Association, the American Association of Diabetes Educators, and the Academy of Nutrition and Dietetics[1] that defines and describes the four critical times to assess, provide, and adjust care. New remote, continuous (versus episodic), data-driven care models are evolving, made possible by a growing suite of connected devices including glucose monitoring devices and smart insulin delivery devices.

MNT Effectiveness in Improving Outcomes

Reported A1C reductions from MNT can be similar to or greater than what would be expected with treatment using currently available medication for type 2 diabetes.[4] Strong evidence supports the effectiveness of MNT interventions provided by RDNs for improving A1C, with absolute decreases up to 2.0% in type 2 diabetes at 3–6 months. Ongoing MNT support is helpful in maintaining glycemic improvements.[4]

Cost-effectiveness of lifestyle interventions and MNT for the management of type 2 diabetes has been documented in multiple studies.[5,6,8] The National Academy of Medicine recommends individualized MNT, provided by an RDN upon physician referral, as part of the multidisciplinary approach to diabetes care.[9] Diabetes MNT is a covered Medicare benefit and should also be adequately reimbursed by insurance and other payers, or bundled in evolving value-based care and payment models, because it can result in improved outcomes such as reduced A1C and cost savings.[5,6,8]

MACRONUTRIENTS

Highlights

- Evidence suggests that there is not an ideal percentage of calories from carbohydrate, protein, and fat for all people with type 2 diabetes; therefore, macronutrient distribution should be based on individualized assessment of current eating patterns, preferences, and metabolic goals.
- A key strategy to achieve glycemic targets through dietary changes should include an assessment of current dietary intake followed by individualized

guidance on self-monitoring carbohydrate intake to optimize meal timing and food choices and to guide medication and physical activity recommendations.

- People with type 2 diabetes are encouraged to consume at least the amount of dietary fiber recommended for the general public. Increasing fiber intake, especially through food (vegetables, pulses [beans, peas, and lentils], fruits, and whole intact grains), may help in modestly lowering A1C, along with providing other potential health benefits.

Macronutrient Needs for People with Type 2 Diabetes Compared with the General Population

Although numerous studies have attempted to identify the optimal mix of macronutrients for the eating plans of people with type 2 diabetes, a systematic review[10] found that there is no ideal mix that applies broadly to all people with type 2 diabetes and that macronutrient proportions should be individualized. It has been observed that people with diabetes, on average, eat about the same proportions of macronutrients as the general public: ~45% of their calories from carbohydrate, ~36%–40% of calories from fat, and the remainder (~16%–18%) from protein.[11] Regardless of the macronutrient mix, total energy intake should be appropriate to attain weight management goals. Further, individualization of the macronutrient composition will depend on the status of the individual, including metabolic goals (glycemia, lipid profile, etc.), physical activity, and food preferences and availability. The source of the macronutrients may be more relevant to health than their distribution; patients with diabetes should be encouraged to choose whole foods over processed foods as often as possible.

Carbohydrate Needs for People with Type 2 Diabetes Compared with the General Population

Carbohydrate is a readily used source of energy and the primary dietary influence on postprandial blood glucose.[12, 13] Foods containing carbohydrate—with various proportions of sugars, starches, and fiber—have a wide range of effects on the glycemic response. Some result in an extended rise and slow fall of blood glucose concentrations, while others result in a rapid rise followed by a rapid fall.[14] The quality of carbohydrate foods selected—ideally those rich in dietary fiber, vitamins, and minerals and low in added sugars, fats, and sodium—should be addressed as part of an individualized eating plan that includes all components necessary for optimal nutrition.[4] Carbohydrate from whole food sources such as whole grains, beans and legumes, starchy vegetables, fruit, and dairy should be emphasized over processed foods containing added sugars and refined grains.

The amount of carbohydrate intake required for optimal health in humans is unknown. Although the recommended dietary allowance for carbohydrate for adults without diabetes (19 years and older) is 130 g/day and is determined in part by the brain's requirement for glucose, this energy requirement can be fulfilled by the body's metabolic processes, which include glycogenolysis, gluconeogenesis (via metabolism of the glycerol component of fat or gluconeogenic amino acids in protein), and/or ketogenesis in the setting of very low dietary carbohydrate intake.[13]

Dietary Fiber Needs of People with Diabetes

The regular intake of sufficient dietary fiber is associated with lower all-cause mortality in people with diabetes. Therefore, people with type 2 diabetes should consume at least the amount of fiber recommended by the *2015–2020 Dietary Guidelines for Americans* (a minimum of 14 g of fiber per 1,000 kcal) with at least half of grain consumption being whole intact grains.[12] Other sources of dietary fiber include nonstarchy vegetables, avocados, fruits and berries, as well as pulses such as beans, peas, and lentils. Meeting the recommended fiber intake through foods that are naturally high in dietary fiber, as compared with supplementation, is encouraged for the additional benefits of coexisting micronutrients and phytochemicals.[15]

Glycemic Index and Glycemic Load Impact on Glycemia

The use of the glycemic index (GI) and glycemic load (GL) to rank carbohydrate foods according to their effects on glycemia continues to be of interest for people with diabetes, especially those needing insulin for prandial coverage. As defined by Brand-Miller et al.,[16] "the GI provides a good summary of postprandial glycemia. It predicts the peak (or near peak) response, the maximum glucose fluctuation, and other attributes of the response curve." Two systematic reviews of the literature regarding GI and GL in individuals with diabetes and at risk for diabetes reported no significant impact on A1C and mixed results on fasting glucose.[4, 14] Further, studies have used varying definitions of low- and high-GI foods, leading to uncertainty in the utility of GI and GL in clinical care.[10]

Protein Needs of People with Diabetes

There is limited research in people with type 2 diabetes without kidney disease on the impact of various amounts of protein consumed. Research indicates potential improvements in weight with increased protein consumption but inconsistent or statistically insignificant changes in other diabetes-related outcomes with varying protein intake.[17]

Dietary Fat and Cholesterol Goals for People with Diabetes

The National Academy of Medicine has defined an acceptable macronutrient distribution for total fat for all adults to be 20%–35% of total calorie intake.[13] Eating patterns that replace certain carbohydrate foods with those higher in total fat, however, have demonstrated greater improvements in glycemia and certain CVD risk factors (serum HDL cholesterol [HDL-C] and triglycerides) compared with lower-fat diets. The types or quality of fats in the eating plans may influence CVD outcomes beyond the total amount of fat.[18] Foods containing synthetic sources of trans fats should be minimized to the greatest extent possible.[12]

The body makes enough cholesterol for physiological and structural functions such that people do not need to obtain cholesterol through foods. Although the *2015–2020 Dietary Guidelines for Americans* concluded that available evidence does not support the recommendation to limit dietary cholesterol for the general population, exact recommendations for dietary cholesterol for other populations, such as people with diabetes, are not as clear.[12] Whereas cholesterol intake has cor-related with serum cholesterol levels, it has not correlated well with CVD events.[19] More research is needed regarding the relationship among dietary cholesterol, blood cholesterol, and CVD events in people with type 2 diabetes.

EATING PATTERNS

Highlights

- A variety of eating patterns (combinations of different foods or food groups) are acceptable for the management of type 2 diabetes.
- Until the evidence surrounding comparative benefits of different eating patterns in specific individuals strengthens, healthcare providers should focus on the key factors that are common among the patterns:
  - Emphasize nonstarchy vegetables;
  - Minimize added sugars and refined grains; and
  - Choose whole foods over highly processed foods to the extent possible.
- Reducing overall carbohydrate intake (particularly from added sugars and refined grains) for individuals with type 2 diabetes has demonstrated the most evidence for improving glycemia and may be applied in a variety of eating patterns that meet individual needs and preferences.
- For select adults with type 2 diabetes not meeting glycemic targets or where reducing antiglycemic medications is a priority, reducing overall carbohydrate intake with low- or very low–carbohydrate eating plans is a viable approach. However, patients should be counseled on replacing carbohydrate with healthy sources of fat and protein.

Evidence for Specific Eating Patterns to Manage Type 2 Diabetes

An eating pattern represents the totality of all foods and beverages consumed.[12] An eating plan is a guide to help individuals plan when, what, and how much to eat on a daily basis and applies to the foods emphasized in the individual's selected eating pattern.

A number of eating patterns have been studied for their benefits in managing or preventing type 2 diabetes. Table 3.5 provides a summary of some of the most common eating patterns studied and their potential benefits. Emphasis is given to evidence from randomized trials in people with type 2 diabetes with at least 10 people in each dietary group and a retention rate of >50%. Overall, few long-term (2 years or longer) randomized trials have been conducted of any of the dietary patterns in any of the conditions examined.

Low-Carbohydrate or Very Low–Carbohydrate Eating Patterns

Low-carbohydrate eating patterns, especially very low–carbohydrate (VLC) eating patterns, have been shown to reduce A1C and the need for antihyperglyce-mic medications. These eating patterns are among the most studied eating patterns for type 2 diabetes; however, the definitions of "low carbohydrate" and "very low

Table 3.5–Eating Patterns and Their Potential Benefits in Type 2 Diabetes

Type of eating pattern	Description	Potential benefits reported*
USDA Dietary Guidelines For Americans[12]	Emphasizes a variety of vegetables from all of the subgroups; fruits, especially whole fruits; grains, at least half of which are whole intact grains; lower-fat dairy; a variety of protein foods; and oils. This eating pattern limits saturated fats and *trans* fats, added sugars, and sodium.	DGA added to the table for reference; not reviewed as part of the American Diabetes Association's Nutrition Consensus Report
Mediterranean-style	Emphasizes plant-based food (vegetables, beans, nuts and seeds, fruits, and whole intact grains); fish and other seafood; olive oil as the principal source of dietary fat; dairy products (mainly yogurt and cheese) in low to moderate amounts; typically fewer than four eggs/week; red meat in low frequency and amounts; wine in low to moderate amounts; and concentrated sugars or honey rarely.	■ Reduced risk of diabetes ■ A1C reduction ■ Lowered triglycerides ■ Reduced risk of major cardiovascular events
Vegetarian or vegan	The two most common approaches found in the literature emphasize plant-based vegetarian eating devoid of all flesh foods but including egg (ovo) and/or dairy (lacto) products, or vegan eating devoid of all flesh foods and animal-derived products.	■ Reduced risk of diabetes ■ A1C reduction ■ Weight loss ■ Lowered LDL cholesterol (LDL-C) and non–HDL-C
Low-fat[10, 20, 21]	Emphasizes vegetables, fruits, starches (e.g., breads/crackers, pasta, whole intact grains, starchy vegetables), lean protein sources (including beans), and low-fat dairy products. In this review, a low-fat eating pattern is defined as total fat intake ≤30% of total calories and saturated fat intake ≤10%.	■ Reduced risk of diabetes ■ Weight loss
Very low–fat	Emphasizes fiber-rich vegetables, beans, fruits, whole intact grains, nonfat dairy, fish, and egg whites and comprises 70%–77% carbohydrate (including 30–60 g fiber), 10% fat, 13%–20% protein.	■ Weight loss ■ Lowered blood pressure

(continued)

Table 3.5 *(continued)*

Type of eating pattern	Description	Potential benefits reported*
Low-carbohydrates[22–24]	Emphasizes vegetables low in carbohydrate (such as salad greens, broccoli, cauliflower, cucumber, cabbage, and others); fat from animal foods, oils, butter, and avocado; and protein in the form of meat, poultry, fish, shellfish, eggs, cheese, nuts, and seeds. Some plans include fruit (e.g., berries) and a greater array of nonstarchy vegetables. Avoids starchy and sugary foods such as pasta, rice, potatoes, bread, and sweets. There is no consistent definition of "low" carbohydrate. In this review, a low-carbohydrate eating pattern is defined as reducing carbohydrate to 26%–45% of total calories.	■ A1C reduction ■ Weight loss ■ Lowered blood pressure ■ Increased HDL-C and lowered triglycerides
Very low–carbohydrate (VLC)[22–24]	Similar to the low-carbohydrate pattern but further limits carbohydrate-containing foods, and meals typically derive more than half of calories from fat. Often has a goal of 20–50 g of nonfiber carbohydrate per day to induce nutritional ketosis. In this review, a VLC eating pattern is defined as reducing carbohydrate to <26% of total calories.	■ A1C reduction ■ Weight loss ■ Lowered blood pressure ■ Increased HDL-C and lowered triglycerides
Dietary Approaches to Stop Hypertension (DASH)	Emphasizes vegetables, fruits, and low-fat dairy products; includes whole intact grains, poultry, fish, and nuts; reduced in saturated fat, red meat, sweets, and sugar-containing beverages. May also be reduced in sodium.	■ Reduced risk of diabetes ■ Weight loss ■ Lowered blood pressure
Paleo	Emphasizes foods theoretically eaten regularly during early human evolution, such as lean meat, fish, shellfish, vegetables, eggs, nuts, and berries. Avoids grains, dairy, salt, refined fats, and sugar.	■ Mixed results ■ Inconclusive evidence

Source: Randomized controlled trials, meta-analyses, observational studies, nonrandomized single-arm studies, cohort studies. USDA, U.S. Department of Agriculture. For full literature review and references, refer to Evert AB, Dennison M, Gardner CD, et al. Nutrition therapy for adults with diabetes or prediabetes: a consensus report. Diabetes Care 2019;42(5):731–754

carbohydrate" are not consistent in all studies. They are typically defined by the percent of calories from carbohydrate. See Table 3.6 for a conversion of percent calories from carbohydrate to grams of carbohydrate per day.

One meta-analysis of randomized controlled trials (RCTs) that compared low-carbohydrate eating patterns (defined as ≤45% of calories from carbohydrate) to high-carbohydrate eating patterns (defined as >45% of calories from carbohydrate) found that A1C benefits were more pronounced in the VLC interventions (where <26% of calories came from carbohydrate) at 3 and 6 months but not at 12 and 24 months.[22]

Another meta-analysis of RCTs compared a low-carbohydrate eating pattern (defined as <40% of calories from carbohydrate) to a low-fat eating pattern (defined as <30% of calories from fat). In trials up to 6 months long, the low-carbohydrate eating pattern improved A1C more, and in trials of varying lengths, lowered triglycerides, raised HDL-C, lowered blood pressure, and resulted in greater reductions in diabetes medication.[23] Finally, in another meta-analysis comparing low-carbohydrate to high-carbohydrate eating patterns, the larger the carbohydrate restriction, the greater the reduction in A1C, though A1C was similar at durations of 1 year and longer for both eating patterns.[24]

Because of theoretical concerns regarding use of VLC eating plans in people with chronic kidney disease, disordered eating patterns, and in women who are pregnant, further research is needed before recommendations can be made for these subgroups. Adopting a VLC eating plan can cause diuresis and swiftly reduce blood glucose; therefore, consultation with a knowledgeable practitioner at the onset is necessary to prevent dehydration and reduce insulin and hypoglycemic medications to prevent hypoglycemia.

No randomized trials were found in people with type 2 diabetes that varied the saturated fat content of the low-carbohydrate or VLC eating patterns to examine effects on glycemia, CVD risk factors, or clinical events. Most of the trials using a carbohydrate-restricted eating pattern did not restrict saturated fat; from the current evidence, this eating pattern does not appear to increase overall cardiovascular risk, but long-term studies with clinical event outcomes are needed.[25-29]

Intermittent Fasting

While intermittent fasting is not an eating pattern by definition, it has been included because of increased interest from the diabetes community. Fasting means to go without food, drink, or both for a period of time. People fast for reasons rang-

Table 3.6–Quick Reference Conversion of Percent Calories from Carbohydrate Shown in Grams Per Day

Calories	10%	20%	30%	40%	50%	60%	70%
1,200	30 g	60 g	90 g	120 g	150 g	180 g	210 g
1,500	38 g	75 g	113 g	150 g	188 g	225 g	263 g
2,000	50 g	100 g	150 g	200 g	250 g	300 g	350 g
2,500	63 g	125 g	188 g	250 g	313 g	375 g	438 g

Source: Evert AB, Dennison M, Gardner CD, et al. Nutrition therapy for adults with diabetes or prediabetes: a consensus report. *Diabetes Care* 2019;42(5):731–754

ing from weight management to upcoming medical visits to religious and spiritual practice. Intermittent fasting is a way of eating that focuses more on when you eat (i.e., consuming all daily calories within set hours during the day) than what you eat. While it usually involves set times for eating and set times for fasting, people can approach intermittent fasting in many different ways.

Published intermittent fasting studies involving diabetes and diabetes prevention demonstrate a variety of approaches, including restricting food intake for 18–20 h per day, alternate-day fasting, and severe calorie restriction for up to 8 consecutive days or longer.[30] Four fasting studies of participants with type 2 diabetes were small (≤63 participants) and of short duration (≤20 weeks). Three of the studies[31-33] demonstrated that intermittent fasting, either in consecutive days of restriction or by fasting 16 h per day or more, may result in weight loss; however, there was no improvement in A1C compared with a nonfasting eating plan. One of the studies[34] showed similar reductions in A1C, weight, and medication doses when 2 days of severe energy restriction were compared with chronic energy restriction. The safety of intermittent fasting in people with special health situations, including pregnancy and disordered eating, has not been studied.

Eating Pattern Recommendations for Type 2 Diabetes

Until the evidence surrounding comparative benefits of different eating patterns in specific individuals strengthens, healthcare providers should focus on the key factors that are common among the patterns: 1) emphasize nonstarchy vegetables, 2) minimize added sugars and refined grains, and 3) choose whole foods over highly processed foods to the extent possible.[35]

Multiple trials and meta-analyses have been published addressing the comparative effects of specific eating patterns for diabetes. Whereas no single eating pattern has emerged as being clearly superior to all others for all diabetes-related outcomes, evidence suggests certain eating patterns are better for specific outcomes.

All eating patterns include a range of more-healthy versus less-healthy options. For example, lentils and sugar-sweetened beverages are both considered part of a vegan eating pattern; fish and processed red meats are both considered part of a low-carbohydrate eating pattern; and removing the bun from a fast food burger might make it part of a paleo eating pattern but does not necessarily make it healthier. Further, studies comparing the same two or more eating patterns could easily differ in the investigators' definition of the patterns, the effectiveness of the research team in fostering pattern adherence among study participants, the accuracy of assessing pattern adherence, study duration, and participant population characteristics.

ENERGY BALANCE AND WEIGHT MANAGEMENT

Highlights

- To support weight loss and improve A1C, CVD risk factors, and quality of life in adults with overweight/obesity and type 2 diabetes, MNT and DSMES services should include an individualized eating plan in a format that results in an energy deficit in combination with enhanced physical activity.

- For adults with type 2 diabetes who are not taking insulin and who have limited health literacy or numeracy, or who are older and prone to hypoglycemia, a simple and effective approach to glycemia and weight management emphasizing appropriate portion sizes and healthy eating may be considered.

- In overweight or obese type 2 diabetes patients, 5% weight loss is recommended to achieve clinical benefit, and the benefits are progressive. The goal for optimal outcomes is 15% weight loss or more when needed and can be feasibly and safely accomplished. In prediabetes, the goal is 7%–10% for preventing progression to type 2 diabetes.

- In select individuals with type 2 diabetes, an overall healthy eating plan that results in energy deficit in conjunction with weight loss medications and/or metabolic surgery should be considered to help achieve weight loss and maintenance goals, lower A1C, and reduce CVD risk.

- In conjunction with lifestyle therapy, medication-assisted weight loss can be considered for people at risk for type 2 diabetes when needed to achieve and sustain 7%–10% weight loss.

- People with type 2 diabetes should be screened and evaluated during DSMES and MNT encounters for disordered eating, and nutrition therapy should accommodate these disorders.

What Is the Role of Weight Loss Therapy in People with Type 2 Diabetes with Overweight or Obesity?

There is substantial evidence indicating that weight loss is highly effective in managing cardiometabolic health in people with type 2 diabetes.

Eating plans that create an energy deficit and are customized to fit the person's preferences and resources can help with long-term sustainment and are the cornerstone of weight loss therapy. Regular physical activity, which can contribute to both weight loss and prevention of weight regain, and behavioral strategies are also important components of lifestyle therapy for weight management.[36,37] Structured weight loss programs with regular visits and use of meal replacements have been shown to enhance weight loss in people with diabetes.[38]

The combined data do not point to a threshold of weight loss for maximal clinical benefits in people with diabetes; rather, the greater the weight loss, the greater the benefits. Previous recommendations of weight loss of 5% or ≥7% for people with overweight or obesity are based on the threshold needed for therapeutic advantages; however, weight loss targeted at ≥15%, when such can feasibly and safely be accomplished, is associated with even better outcomes in type 2 diabetes.[38,39]

A meta-analysis conducted by Franz et al.[37] found that lifestyle interventions producing <5% weight loss had less effect on A1C, lipids, or blood pressure compared with studies achieving weight loss of ≥5%. Other meta-analyses focusing on nonmedicine or medicine-assisted weight loss interventions in type 2 diabetes support this finding. More recently, the Look AHEAD trial[39] compared standard DSMES to a more intensive lifestyle intervention and reduced-calorie eating plan. The intensive lifestyle intervention resulted in 8.6% weight loss at 1 year, and the downstream therapeutic benefits were far-ranging even though benefits were not seen for the primary cardiovascular outcomes.[20]

A systematic review of the effectiveness of MNT revealed mixed weight loss outcomes in participants with type 2 diabetes.[4] Similarly, while DSMES is a fundamental component of diabetes care,[1] it does not consistently produce sufficient weight loss to achieve optimal therapeutic benefits in people with diabetes.[36, 40] For these reasons, diabetes MNT and DSMES should emphasize a targeted and concerted plan for weight management.

The addition of metabolic surgery, weight loss medications, and glucose-lowering agents that promote weight loss can also be used as an adjunct to lifestyle interventions, resulting in greater weight loss that is maintained for a longer period of time. See Table 3.7 for an overview of the treatment options for overweight and obesity in people with type 2 diabetes.

What Is the Best Weight Loss Plan for Individuals with Diabetes?

For purposes of weight loss, the ability to sustain and maintain an eating plan that results in an energy deficit, irrespective of macronutrient composition or eating pattern, is critical for success. Studies investigating specific weight loss eating plans using a broad range of macronutrient composition in people with diabetes have shown mixed results regarding effects on weight, A1C, serum lipids, and blood pressure.[21] As a result, the evidence does not identify one eating plan that is clearly superior to others and that can be generally recommended for weight loss for people with diabetes. Individualized eating plans should support calorie reduction (e.g., employing use of appropriate portion sizes, meal replacements, and/or behavioral interventions) in the context of a lifestyle program, with appropriate modifications in the medication plan to minimize associated adverse effects such as weight gain, hypoglycemia, and hypotension.

Weight loss interventions can be implemented in usual care settings and alternately in telehealth programs. In general, the intervention intensity and degree of individual participation in the program are important factors for successful weight loss.

Table 3.7–Treatment Options for Overweight and Obesity in Type 2 Diabetes

Treatment	BMI category (kg/m²)		
	25.0–26.9 (or 23.0–24.9*)	27.0–29.9 (or 25.0–27.4*)	≥30.0 (or ≥27.5*)
Diet, physical activity, and behavioral therapy	†	†	†
Pharmacotherapy		†	†
Metabolic surgery			†

*Recommended cut points for Asian American individuals (expert opinion). †Treatment may be indicated for select motivated patients. *Source*: American Diabetes Association.[41]

Role of Weight Loss on Potential for Type 2 Diabetes Remission

The Look AHEAD trial[42] and the Diabetes Remission Clinical Trial (DiRECT)[38] highlight the potential for type 2 diabetes remission—defined as the maintenance of euglycemia (complete remission) or prediabetes level of glycemia (partial remission) with no diabetes medication for at least 1 year[42, 43]—in people undergoing weight loss treatment. In the Look AHEAD trial, when compared with the control group, the intensive lifestyle arm resulted in at least partial diabetes remission in 11.5% of participants as compared with 2% in the control group.[42] The DiRECT trial showed that at 1 year, weight loss associated with the lifestyle intervention resulted in diabetes remission in 46% of participants.[38] Remission rates were related to magnitude of weight loss, rising progressively from 7% to 86% as weight loss at 1 year increased from <5% to ≥15%.[38] Diet composition may also play a role; in an RCT by Esposito et al.,[44] despite only a 2-kg difference in weight loss, the group following a low-carbohydrate Mediterranean-style eating pattern experienced greater rates of at least partial diabetes remission, with rates of 14.7% at year 1 and 5% at year 6 compared with 4.7% and 0%, respectively, in the group following a low-fat eating plan.

SUGAR-SWEETENED BEVERAGES (SSBs) & SUGAR SUBSTITUTES

SSB Consumption and Risk of Diabetes

SSB consumption in the general population contributes to a significantly increased risk of type 2 diabetes, weight gain, heart disease, kidney disease, nonalcoholic liver disease, and tooth decay.[45] For example, a meta-analysis reported that consumption of at least one serving of SSBs per day increased the risk of type 2 diabetes in adults with prediabetes by 26%.[46] Since SSBs can be a substantial source of calories and sugar in a person's diet, healthcare professionals should assess patients' beverage intake and recommend replacing SSBs with water as often as possible.

Impact of Sugar Substitutes

The term "sugar substitutes" refers to high-intensity sweeteners, artificial sweeteners, nonnutritive sweeteners, and low-calorie sweeteners. These include saccharin, neotame, acesulfame-K, aspartame, sucralose, advantame, stevia, and luo han guo (or monk fruit). The U.S. Food and Drug Administration (FDA) has reviewed several types of sugar substitutes for safety and approved them for consumption by the general public, including people with type 2 diabetes.[47]

Replacing added sugars with sugar substitutes could decrease daily intake of carbohydrate and calories, which could beneficially affect glycemic, weight, and cardiometabolic control. Importantly, when sugar substitutes are used to reduce overall calorie and carbohydrate intake, people should be counseled to avoid compensating with intake of additional calories from other food sources.

Although nonnutritive sweeteners do not appear to affect glycemia, they have been shown to induce changes in the gut microbiome that can potentially translate into metabolic disturbances.[48] A growing body of research is exploring the effect of nonnutritive sweeteners on the gut and the potential metabolic consequences.

An American Heart Association science advisory on the consumption of beverages containing sugar substitutes that was supported by the American Diabetes Association concluded there is not enough evidence to determine whether sugar substitute use definitively leads to long-term reduction in body weight or cardiometabolic risk factors, including glycemia.[49]

Sugar alcohols represent a separate category of sweeteners. Like sugar substitutes, sugar alcohols have been approved by the FDA for consumption by the general public and people with diabetes. Whereas sugar alcohols have fewer calories per gram than sugars, they are not as sweet. Therefore, a higher amount is required to match the degree of sweetness of sugars, generally bringing the calorie content to a level similar to that of sugars.[50] Use of sugar alcohols needs to be balanced with their potential to cause gastrointestinal effects in sensitive individuals. Currently, there is little research on the potential benefits of sugar alcohols for people with diabetes.

ALCOHOL CONSUMPTION

Effects of Alcohol Consumption on Diabetes-Related Outcomes

It is important that healthcare providers counsel people with diabetes about alcohol consumption and encourage no more than moderate use for people choosing to consume alcohol. Moderate alcohol consumption (one drink or less per day for adult women and two drinks or less per day for adult men) has minimal acute and/or long-term detrimental effects on glycemia in people with type 2 diabetes.[51,52] One alcohol-containing beverage is defined as 12 oz of beer, 5 oz of wine, or 1.5 oz of distilled spirits, each containing approximately 15 g of alcohol.[12] Some epidemiologic data shows improved glycemia and improved insulin sensitivity with moderate intake; however, people who choose not to drink should not be encouraged to start. It is important to note that even light drinking has been associated with an increased risk for certain cancers (breast, oropharyngeal and esophageal).[53]

Effects of Alcohol Consumption on Hypoglycemia Risk in People with Type 2 Diabetes

People with diabetes, particularly those using insulin or insulin secretagogues, may be at increased risk for delayed hypoglycemia after consuming alcohol. It is essential that people with diabetes receive education regarding the recognition and management of delayed hypoglycemia and the potential need for more frequent glucose monitoring after consuming alcohol.[54]

MICRONUTRIENTS, HERBAL SUPPLEMEMENTS, AND MEDICATIONS

Effectiveness of Micronutrient and Herbal Supplements in the Management of Diabetes

Healthcare providers should ask about the use of supplements and herbal products, and providers and people with type 2 diabetes should discuss the potential benefit of these products weighed against the cost and possible adverse effects and drug interactions. It is important to consider that nutritional supplements and herbal products are not standardized or regulated.[55] The variability of herbal and micronutrient supplements makes research in this area challenging and makes it difficult to conclude effectiveness.

Overall scientific evidence does not support the use of dietary supplements in the form of vitamins or minerals to meet glycemic targets or improve CVD risk factors in people with type 2 diabetes in the absence of an underlying deficiency.[56] Similarly, the use of herbal supplements such as cinnamon, curcumin, or aloe vera is not supported by evidence, and therefore routine use is not recommended.

However, for special populations, including women planning pregnancy, people with celiac disease, older adults, vegetarians, and people following an eating plan that restricts overall calories or one or more macronutrients, a multivitamin supplement may be justified.

Metformin Affects Vitamin B12 Status

Metformin is associated with vitamin B12 deficiency, with a recent systematic review recommending that annual blood testing of vitamin B12 levels be considered in metformin-treated people, especially in those with anemia or peripheral neuropathy.[57] This study found that even in the absence of anemia, B12 deficiency was prevalent. The exact cause of B12 deficiency in people taking metformin is not known, but some research points to malabsorption caused by metformin, with other studies suggesting improvements in B12 status with calcium supplementation. The standard of treatment has been B12 injections, but new research suggests that high-dose oral supplementation may be as effective. More research is needed in this area.

MNT and Antihyperglycemic Medications (Including Insulin)

RDNs providing MNT in diabetes care should assess and monitor medication changes in relation to the nutrition care plan. Along with other diabetes care providers, RDNs who possess advanced practice training and clinical expertise should take an active role in facilitating and maintaining organization-approved diabetes medication protocols. Use of organization-approved protocols for insulin and other glucose-lowering medications can help reduce therapeutic inertia and/or reduce the risk of hypoglycemia and hyperglycemia.[5,58]

ROLE OF NUTRITION THERAPY IN THE PREVENTION AND MANAGEMENT OF DIABETES COMPLICATIONS

Cardiovascular Disease

Highlights

- In general, replacing saturated fat with unsaturated fats reduces both total cholesterol and LDL-C and also benefits CVD risk.
- In type 2 diabetes, replacing foods high in carbohydrate with foods lower in carbohydrate and higher in fat may improve glycemia, triglycerides, and HDL-C; emphasizing foods higher in unsaturated fat instead of saturated fat may additionally improve LDL-C.

- People with type 2 diabetes are encouraged to consume <2,300 mg/day of sodium, the same amount that is recommended for the general population.
- The recommendation for the general public to eat a serving of fish (particularly fatty fish) at least two times per week is also appropriate for people with type 2 diabetes.

Nutrition therapy that includes the development of an eating plan designed to optimize blood glucose trends, blood pressure, and lipid profiles is important in the management of diabetes and can lower the risk of CVD, coronary heart disease, and stroke.[4] Findings from clinical trials support the role of nutrition therapy for achieving glycemic targets and decreasing various markers of cardiovascular and hypertension risk.[4]

Dietary Fats

Increasing evidence shows that the types of fat consumed are more important for CVD risk than total fat. Saturated fat is often considered "bad fat" due to its effect in raising LDL-C, a contributing factor in atherosclerosis. Saturated fat is found primarily in animal-based foods, like meat and dairy, and tropical oils such as coconut and palm oil. The *2015–2020 Dietary Guidelines for Americans* recommends consuming <10% of calories from saturated fat by replacing it with monounsaturated and polyunsaturated fatty acids.[12]

In contrast to saturated fat, mono- and polyunsaturated fats are thought to be protective against CVD. Unsaturated fats are found primarily in plant-based foods such as liquid oils (canola, corn, soybean, olive, etc.), nuts, seeds, and avocados, as well as fatty fish.

In a Presidential Advisory on dietary fat and CVD, the American Heart Association concluded that lowering the intake of saturated fat and replacing it with unsaturated fats, especially polyunsaturated fats, will lower the incidence of CVD.[59] Replacing saturated fat with unsaturated fats, especially polyunsaturated fat, significantly reduces both total cholesterol and LDL-C, and replacement with monounsaturated fat from plant sources, such as olive oil and nuts, reduces CVD risk. Replacing saturated fat with whole food sources of carbohydrate also reduces total cholesterol and LDL-C, but significantly increases triglycerides and reduces HDL-C.[60, 61]

As is recommended for the general public, an increase in foods containing the long-chain omega-3 fatty acids eicosapentaenoic acid (EPA) and docosahexaenoic acid (DHA), such as are found in fatty fish, is recommended for individuals with diabetes because of their beneficial effects on lipoproteins, prevention of heart disease, and associations with positive health outcomes in observational studies. For people following a vegetarian or vegan eating pattern, plant food sources of omega-3 α-linoleic acid (ALA), such as flax, walnuts, and soy, are reasonable replacements for foods high in saturated fat and may provide some CVD benefits, though the evidence is inconclusive.

Lowering the Effect of Sodium Intake on Blood Pressure and Other Cardiovascular Risk Factors

Many health groups acknowledge that the current average intake of sodium, which is >3,500 mg daily, should be reduced to prevent and manage hypertension.

While reducing sodium to the general recommendation of <2,300 mg/day demonstrates beneficial effects on blood pressure, research is less clear on the benefits of significantly lower sodium intake goals for people with combined type 2 diabetes and hypertension. Therefore, sodium intake goals that are significantly lower than 2,300 mg/day should be considered only on an individual basis.[12, 62, 63]

Other Complications

MNT can be helpful in the prevention and management of many diabetes complications such as diabetic kidney disease and gastroparesis. Patients exhibiting these complications should be referred to a dietitian for MNT.

CONCLUSIONS

Ideally, an eating plan should be developed in collaboration with the person with type 2 diabetes and an RDN through participation in DSMES when the diagnosis of type 2 diabetes is made. Nutrition therapy recommendations need to be adjusted regularly based on changes in an individual's life circumstances, preferences, and disease course.[1] Regular follow-up with a diabetes healthcare provider is also critical to adjust other aspects of the treatment plan as indicated.

Unfortunately, national data indicate that most people with diabetes do not receive any nutrition therapy or formal diabetes education.[4] Strategies to improve access, clinical outcomes, and cost effectiveness of nutrition therapy include the following:

- Reducing barriers to referrals and allowing self-referrals to MNT and DSMES;
- Providing in-person or technology-enabled diabetes nutrition therapy and education integrated with medical management;
- Engineering solutions that include two-way communication between the individual and his or her healthcare team to provide individualized feedback and tailored education based on the analyzed patient-generated health data;
- Increasing the use of community health workers and peer coaches to provide culturally appropriate, ongoing support and clinically linked care coordination and improve the reach of MNT and DSMES.

REFERENCES

1. Powers MA, Bardsley J, Cypress M, et al. Diabetes self-management education and support in type 2 diabetes: a joint position statement of the American Diabetes Association, the American Association of Diabetes Educators, and the Academy of Nutrition and Dietetics. *Diabetes Care* 2015;38: 1372–1382. PMID:26048904

2. Inzucchi SE, Bergenstal RM, Buse JB, et al. Management of hyperglycemia in type 2 diabetes, 2015: a patient-centered approach: update to a position

statement of the American Diabetes Association and the European Association for the Study of Diabetes. *Diabetes Care* 2015;38:140–149. PMID:25538310

3. American Diabetes Association. 5. Lifestyle management: standards of medical care in diabetes—2019. *Diabetes Care* 2019;42(Suppl. 1):S46–S60. PMID:30559231

4. Franz MJ, MacLeod J, Evert A, et al. Academy of Nutrition and Dietetics nutrition practice guideline for type 1 and type 2 diabetes in adults: systematic review of evidence for medical nutrition therapy effectiveness and recommendations for integration into the nutrition care process. *J Acad Nutr Diet* 2017;117:1659–1679. PMID:28533169

5. Davidson P, Ross T, Castor C. Academy of Nutrition and Dietetics: revised 2017 standards of practice and standards of professional performance for registered dietitian nutritionists (competent, proficient, and expert) in Diabetes Care. *J Acad Nutr Diet* 2018;118:932–946.e48. PMID:29703344

6. Briggs Early K, Stanley K. Position of the Academy of Nutrition and Dietetics: the role of medical nutrition therapy and registered dietitian nutritionists in the prevention and treatment of prediabetes and type 2 diabetes. *J Acad Nutr Diet* 2018;118:343–353. PMID:29389511

7. Beck J, Greenwood DA, Blanton L, et al.; 2017 Standards Revision Task Force. 2017 national standards for diabetes self-management education and support. *Diabetes Care* 2017;40:1409–1419. PMID:28754780

8. Academy of Nutrition and Dietetics Evidence Analysis Library. MNT: cost effectiveness, cost-benefit, or economic savings of MNT (2009) [Internet]. Available from https://www.andeal.org/topic.cfm?cat=4085&conclusion_statement_id=251001. Accessed 2 October 2018

9. Institute of Medicine. The role of nutrition in maintaining health in the nation's elderly: evaluating coverage of nutrition services for the medicare population [Internet], 1999. Available from https://www.nap.edu/catalog/9741/the-role-of-nutrition-in-maintaining-health-in-the-nations-elderly. Accessed 2 October 2018

10. Wheeler ML, Dunbar SA, Jaacks LM, et al. Macronutrients, food groups, and eating patterns in the management of diabetes: a systematic review of the literature, 2010. *Diabetes Care* 2012;35:434–445. PMID:22275443

11. Vitolins MZ, Anderson AM, Delahanty L, et al.; Look AHEAD Research Group. Action for Health in Diabetes (Look AHEAD) trial: baseline evaluation of selected nutrients and food group intake. *J Am Diet Assoc* 2009;109:1367–1375. PMID:19631042

12. U.S. Department of Health and Human Service; U.S. Department of Agriculture. 2015–2020 Dietary Guidelines for Americans, 8th edition [Internet], 2015. Available from https://health.gov/dietaryguidelines/2015/guidelines/. Accessed 18 January 2019

13. Institute of Medicine. Dietary reference intakes for energy, carbohydrate, fiber, fat, fatty acids, cholesterol, protein, and amino acids [Internet]. Washington, DC, National Academies Press, 2005 [cited 2014 Oct 1]. Available from https://www.nap.edu/catalog/10490/dietary-reference-intakes-for-energy-carbohydrate-fiber-fat-fatty-acids-cholesterol-protein-and-amino-acids. Accessed 1 October 2014

14. Vega-López S, Venn BJ, Slavin JL. Relevance of the glycemic index and glycemic load for body weight, diabetes, and cardiovascular disease. *Nutrients* 2018;10:E1361. PMID:30249012

15. Dahl WJ, Stewart ML. Position of the Academy of Nutrition and Dietetics: health implications of dietary fiber. *J Acad Nutr Diet* 2015;115:1861–1870. PMID:26514720

16. Brand-Miller JC, Stockmann K, Atkinson F, Petocz P, Denyer G. Glycemic index, postprandial glycemia, and the shape of the curve in healthy subjects: analysis of a database of more than 1,000 foods. *Am J Clin Nutr* 2009;89:97–105. PMID:19056599

17. Dong J-Y, Zhang Z-L, Wang P-Y, Qin L-Q. Effects of high-protein diets on body weight, glycaemic control, blood lipids and blood pressure in type 2 diabetes: meta-analysis of randomised controlled trials. *Br J Nutr* 2013;110:781–789. PMID:23829939

18. Qian F, Korat AA, Malik V, Hu FB. Metabolic effects of monounsaturated fatty acid–enriched diets compared with carbohydrate or polyunsaturated fatty acid–enriched diets in patients with type 2 diabetes: a systematic review and meta-analysis of randomized controlled trials. *Diabetes Care* 2016;39:1448–1457. PMID:27457635

19. Berger S, Raman G, Vishwanathan R, Jacques PF, Johnson EJ. Dietary cholesterol and cardiovascular disease: a systematic review and meta-analysis. *Am J Clin Nutr* 2015;102:276–294. PMID:26109578

20. Wing RR, Bolin P, Brancati FL, et al.; Look AHEAD Research Group. Cardiovascular effects of intensive lifestyle intervention in type 2 diabetes. *N Engl J Med* 2013;369:145–154. PMID:23796131

21. Kodama S, Saito K, Tanaka S, et al. Influence of fat and carbohydrate proportions on the metabolic profile in patients with type 2 diabetes: a meta-analysis. *Diabetes Care* 2009;32:959–965. PMID:19407076

22. Sainsbury E, Kizirian NV, Partridge SR, Gill T, Colagiuri S, Gibson AA. Effect of dietary carbohydrate restriction on glycemic control in adults with diabetes: a systematic review and meta-analysis. *Diabetes Res Clin Pract* 2018;139:239–252. PMID:29522789

23. van Zuuren EJ, Fedorowicz Z, Kuijpers T, Pijl H. Effects of low-carbohydrate- compared with low-fat-diet interventions on metabolic control in people with type 2 diabetes: a systematic review including GRADE assessments. *Am J Clin Nutr* 2018;108:300–331. PMID:30007275

24. Snorgaard O, Poulsen GM, Andersen HK, Astrup A. Systematic review and meta-analysis of dietary carbohydrate restriction in patients with type 2 diabetes. *BMJ Open Diabetes Res Care* 2017;5:e000354

25. Bhanpuri NH, Hallberg SJ, Williams PT, et al. Cardiovascular disease risk factor responses to a type 2 diabetes care model including nutritional ketosis induced by sustained carbohydrate restriction at 1 year: an open label, non-randomized, controlled study. *Cardiovasc Diabetol* 2018;17:56. PMID:29712560

26. Forsythe CE, Phinney SD, Fernandez ML, et al. Comparison of low fat and low carbohydrate diets on circulating fatty acid composition and markers of inflammation. *Lipids* 2008;43:65–77. PMID:18046594

27. Tay J, Luscombe-Marsh ND, Thompson CH, et al. Comparison of low- and high-carbohydrate diets for type 2 diabetes management: a randomized trial. *Am J Clin Nutr* 2015;102:780–790. PMID:26224300

28. Wycherley TP, Thompson CH, Buckley JD, et al. Long-term effects of weight loss with a very-low carbohydrate, low saturated fat diet on flow mediated dilatation in patients with type 2 diabetes: a randomised controlled trial. *Atherosclerosis* 2016;252:28–31. PMID:27494448

29. Tay J, Thompson CH, Luscombe-Marsh ND, et al. Effects of an energy-restricted low-carbohydrate, high unsaturated fat/low saturated fat diet versus a high-carbohydrate, low-fat diet in type 2 diabetes: a 2-year randomized clinical trial. *Diabetes Obes Metab* 2018;20:858–871. PMID:29178536

30. McCue, MD (Ed.). *Comparative Physiology of Fasting, Starvation, and Food Limitation* [Internet]. Berlin, Springer-Verlag, 2012. Available from https://www.nhbs.com/comparative-physiology-of-fasting-starvation-and-food-limitation-book. Accessed 19 November 2018

31. Corley BT, Carroll RW, Hall RM, Weatherall M, Parry-Strong A, Krebs JD. Intermittent fasting in type 2 diabetes mellitus and the risk of hypoglycaemia: a randomized controlled trial. *Diabet Med* 2018;35:588–594. PMID:29405359

32. Li C, Sadraie B, Steckhan N, et al. Effects of a one-week fasting therapy in patients with type-2 diabetes mellitus and metabolic syndrome—a randomized controlled explorative study. *Exp Clin Endocrinol Diabetes* 2017;125:618–624. PMID:28407662

33. Williams KV, Mullen ML, Kelley DE, Wing RR. The effect of short periods of caloric restriction on weight loss and glycemic control in type 2 diabetes. *Diabetes Care* 1998;21:2–8. PMID:9538962

34. Carter S, Clifton PM, Keogh JB. The effects of intermittent compared to continuous energy restriction on glycaemic control in type 2 diabetes; a pragmatic pilot trial. *Diabetes Res Clin Pract* 2016;122:106–112. PMID:27833048

35. Gardner CD, Trepanowski JF, Del Gobbo LC, et al. Effect of low-fat vs low-carbohydrate diet on 12-month weight loss in overweight adults and the association with genotype pattern or insulin secretion: the DIETFITS randomized clinical trial [published corrections appear in *JAMA* 2018;319:1386 and 1728]. *JAMA* 2018;319:667–679

36. Wadden TA, Neiberg RH, Wing RR, et al.; Look AHEAD Research Group. Four-year weight losses in the Look AHEAD study: factors associated with long-term success. *Obesity* (Silver Spring) 2011;19:1987–1998. PMID:21779086

37. Franz MJ, Boucher JL, Rutten-Ramos S, VanWormer JJ. Lifestyle weight-loss intervention outcomes in overweight and obese adults with type 2 diabetes: a systematic review and meta-analysis of randomized clinical trials. *J Acad Nutr Diet* 2015;115:1447–1463. PMID:25935570

38. Lean ME, Leslie WS, Barnes AC, et al. Primary care-led weight management for remission of type 2 diabetes (DiRECT): an open-label, cluster-randomised trial. *Lancet* 2018;391:541–551. PMID:29221645

39. Wing RR, Lang W, Wadden TA, et al.; Look AHEAD Research Group. Benefits of modest weight loss in improving cardiovascular risk factors in overweight and obese individuals with type 2 diabetes. *Diabetes Care* 2011;34:1481–1486. PMID:21593294

40. American Diabetes Association. 4. Lifestyle management: standards of medical care in diabetes—2018. *Diabetes Care* 2018;41(Suppl. 1):S38–S50. PMID:29222375

41. American Diabetes Association. 8. Obesity management for the treatment of type 2 diabetes: standards of medical care in diabetes—2020. *Diabetes Care* 2020;43(Suppl. 1):S89–S97

42. Gregg EW, Chen H, Wagenknecht LE, et al.; Look AHEAD Research Group. Association of an intensive lifestyle intervention with remission of type 2 diabetes. *JAMA* 2012;308:2489–2496. PMID:23288372

43. Buse JB, Caprio S, Cefalu WT, et al. How do we define cure of diabetes? *Diabetes Care* 2009;32:2133–2135. PMID:19875608

44. Esposito K, Maiorino MI, Petrizzo M, Bellastella G, Giugliano D. The effects of a Mediterranean diet on the need for diabetes drugs and remission of newly diagnosed type 2 diabetes: follow-up of a randomized trial. *Diabetes Care* 2014;37:1824–1830. PMID:24722497

45. Malik VS. Sugar sweetened beverages and cardiometabolic health. *Curr Opin Cardiol* 2017;32:572–579. PMID:28639973

46. Malik VS, Hu FB. Fructose and cardiometabolic health: what the evidence from sugar-sweetened beverages tells us. *J Am Coll Cardiol* 2015;66:1615–1624. PMID:26429086

47. Food & Nutrition Information Center, National Agricultural Library, U.S. Department of Agriculture. Nutritive and nonnutritive sweetener resources [Internet]. Available from https://www.nal.usda.gov/fnic/nutritive-and-non-nutritive-sweetener-resources. Accessed 20 November 2018

48. Suez J, Korem T, Zilberman-Schapira G, Segal E, Elinav E. Non-caloric artificial sweeteners and the microbiome: findings and challenges. *Gut Microbes* 2015;6(2):149-155

49. Johnson RK, Lichtenstein AH, Anderson CAM, et al.; American Heart Association Nutrition Committee of the Council on Lifestyle and Cardiometabolic Health; Council on Cardiovascular and Stroke Nursing; Council on Clinical Cardiology; Council on Quality of Care and Outcomes Research; Stroke Council. Low-calorie sweetened beverages and cardiometabolic health: a science advisory from the American Heart Association. *Circulation* 2018;138:e126–e140.

50. Fitch C, Keim KS; Academy of Nutrition and Dietetics. Position of the Academy of Nutrition and Dietetics: use of nutritive and nonnutritive sweeteners. *J Acad Nutr Diet* 2012;112:739–758. PMID:22709780

51. Shai I, Wainstein J, Harman-Boehm I, et al. Glycemic effects of moderate alcohol intake among patients with type 2 diabetes: a multicenter, randomized, clinical intervention trial. *Diabetes Care* 2007;30:3011–3016. PMID:17848609

52. Ahmed AT, Karter AJ, Warton EM, Doan JU, Weisner CM. The relationship between alcohol consumption and glycemic control among patients with diabetes: the Kaiser Permanente Northern California Diabetes Registry. *J Gen Intern Med* 2008;23:275–282. PMID:18183468

53. Bagnardi V, Rota M, Botteri E, Tramacere I, Islami F, Fedirko V, et al. Light alcohol drinking and cancer: a meta-analysis. *Ann Oncol* 2013;24(2):301-308

54. Franz MJ, Evert AB (Eds.). American Diabetes Association Guide to Nutrition Therapy for Diabetes. 3rd edition. Alexandria, VA, American Diabetes Association, 2017

55. U.S. Food and Drug Administration. Dietary supplements [Internet], 2018. Available from https://www.fda.gov/food/dietarysupplements/. Accessed 20 November 2018

56. Bantle JP, Wylie-Rosett J, Albright AL, et al.; American Diabetes Association. Nutrition recommendations and interventions for diabetes: a position statement of the American Diabetes Association. *Diabetes Care* 2008;31(Suppl. 1):S61–S78. PMID:18165339

57. Aroda VR, Edelstein SL, Goldberg RB, et al.; Diabetes Prevention Program Research Group. Long-term metformin use and vitamin B12 deficiency in the Diabetes Prevention Program Outcomes Study. *J Clin Endocrinol Metab* 2016;101:1754–1761. PMID:26900641

58. Garber AJ, Abrahamson MJ, Barzilay JI, et al. Consensus statement by the American Association of Clinical Endocrinologists and American College of Endocrinology on the comprehensive type 2 diabetes management algorithm—2017 executive summary. *Endocr Pract* 2017;23:207–238. PMID:28095040

59. Sacks FM, Lichtenstein AH, Wu JHY, et al.; American Heart Association. Dietary fats and cardiovascular disease: a presidential advisory from the American Heart Association. *Circulation* 2017;136:e1–e23. PMID:28620111

60. Guasch-Ferré M, Babio N, Martínez-González MA, et al.; PREDIMED Study Investigators. Dietary fat intake and risk of cardiovascular disease and all-cause mortality in a population at high risk of cardiovascular disease. *Am J Clin Nutr* 2015;102:1563–1573. PMID:26561617

61. Dietary Guidelines Advisory Committee. Scientific Report of the 2015 Dietary Guidelines Advisory Committee: Advisory Report to the Secretary of Health and Human Services and the Secretary of Agriculture [Internet], 2015. Washington, DC, U.S. Department of Agriculture, Agricultural Research Service. Available from https://health.gov/dietaryguidelines/2015-scientific-report/. Accessed 25 September 2017

62. Zhang Z, Cogswell ME, Gillespie C, et al. Association between usual sodium and potassium intake and blood pressure and hypertension among U.S. adults: NHANES 2005–2010. *PLoS One* 2013;8:e75289. PMID:24130700

63. Ekinci EI, Clarke S, Thomas MC, et al. Dietary salt intake and mortality in patients with type 2 diabetes. *Diabetes Care* 2011;34:703–709. PMID:21289228

EXERCISE

Perry E. Bickel, MD

Exercise is recommended for most people of all ages to promote physical and mental health, function, and well-being. Some benefits are immediate, and others accrue over time. The list of these benefits is growing with increasing research and include improved sleep, mood, cognitive function, and fall avoidance, as well as reduced risk for chronic diseases, weight gain, dementia, and certain cancers. Physical activity has been termed a "best buy" for public health in a recent detailed critical review of the literature with guidelines for physical activity that was commissioned by the U.S. Department of Health and Human Services.[1] The Physical Activity Guidelines Advisory Committee (PAGAC) rated the scientific evidence of benefit for specific health conditions. Those conditions for which the evidence of benefit was rated as either moderate or strong are listed in Table 3.8.

For people with type 2 diabetes, benefits of even modest physical activity offer significant improvement in cardiovascular mortality over remaining sedentary.[1] The American Diabetes Association published a 2016 Position Statement on physical activity/exercise and diabetes[2] and provides updates to its recommendations in its *Standards of Medical Care in Diabetes*.[3] This chapter relies heavily on these up-to-date guidelines and standards with some references to the primary literature.

Note: This Guide addresses the role of exercise in managing type 2 diabetes. Most studies that address exercise and diabetes do so for either type 1 or type 2. It cannot be assumed that what has been shown for type 1 diabetes applies to type 2. Accordingly, this chapter will limit comments to type 2 diabetes and exercise. The reader may refer to the American Diabetes Association Position Statement or *Standards of Medical Care in Diabetes* for specific information about type 1 diabetes and exercise.

THE BENEFITS OF EXERCISE FOR PEOPLE WITH TYPE 2 DIABETES

Just as the general population, people with diabetes who engage in moderate amounts of physical activity have a lower risk of early death compared with inactive people.[4] For adults with type 2 diabetes, strong evidence demonstrates that more physical activity correlates negatively with the risk of cardiovascular death.[1] Exercise, either aerobic or resistance as defined below, improves glycemic control, as well as cardiovascular risk markers, in people with type 2 diabetes.[5] In one randomized control trial (RCT) in people with type 2 diabetes, a combination of aerobic and resistance training over 9 months improved A1C (–0.34% [–27 mmol/mol]) compared with nonexercising control subjects, but neither aerobic training nor resistance training alone resulted in improvement.[6] Overall, the 2018 PAGAC Scientific Report concluded that there is strong evidence that in people with type 2 diabetes the beneficial effects of physical activity on A1C, blood pressure, BMI, and lipids (LDL and HDL, but not triglycerides) indicate that more physical activity slows the progression of disease severity of type 2 diabetes.[1] There is insufficient data to conclude whether physical activity alters the progression of retinopathy, nephropathy, neuropathy, and complications of the diabetic foot.

Table 3.8–Health Benefits of Exercise

Children	
3 to <6 years of yge	**Improved bone health and weight status**
6 to 17 years of age	**Improved cognitive function (ages 6 to 13 years)** Improved cardiorespiratory and muscular fitness Improved bone health Improved cardiovascular risk factor status Improved weight status or adiposity Fewer symptoms of depression

Adults, all ages	
All-cause mortality	Lower risk
Cardiometabolic conditions	Lower cardiovascular incidence and mortality (including heart disease and stroke) Lower incidence of hypertension Lower incidence of type 2 diabetes
Cancer	Lower incidence of **bladder**, breast, colon, **endometrium, esophagus, kidney, stomach, and lung cancers**
Brain health	**Reduced risk of dementia** Improved cognitive function **Improved cognitive function follows or following bouts of aerobic activity** **Improved quality of life** **Improved sleep** **Reduced feelings of anxiety and depression in healthy people and in people with existing clinical syndromes** Reduced incidence of depression
Weight status	**Reduced risk of excessive weight gain** Weight loss and the prevention of weight regain following initial weight loss when a sufficient dose of moderate-to-vigorous physical activity is attained An additive effect on weight loss when combined with moderate dietary restriction

Older adults	
Falls	Reduced incidence of falls **Reduced incidence of fall-related injuries**
Physical function	**Improved physical function in older adults with and without frailty**

Women who are pregnant or postpartum	
During pregnancy	**Reduced risk of excessive weight gain** **Reduced risk of gestational diabetes** No risk to fetus from moderate-intensity physical activity
During postpartum	**Reduced risk of postpartum depression**

Individuals with preexisting medical conditions	
Breast cancer	**Reduced risk of all-cause and breast cancer mortality**
Colorectal cancer	**Reduced risk of all-cause and colorectal cancer mortality**
Prostate cancer	**Reduced risk of prostate cancer mortality**

(continued)

Table 3.8 *(continued)*

	Children
Osteoarthritis	**Decreased pain** **Improved function and quality of life**
Hypertension	**Reduced risk of cardiovascular mortality** **Reduced risk of increased blood pressure over time**
Type 2 diabetes	**Reduced risk of cardiovascular mortality** **Reduced progression of disease indicators: A1C,** **blood pressure, blood lipids, and BMI**
Multiple sclerosis	**Improved walking** **Improved physical fitness**
Dementia	**Improved cognition**
Some conditions with impaired executive function (attention deficit hyperactivity disorder, schizophrenia, multiple sclerosis, Parkinson's disease, and stroke)	**Improved cognition**

Note: Benefits in **bold font** are those added in 2018; benefits in normal font are those noted in the 2008 Scientific Report.[1] Only outcomes with strong or moderate evidence of effect are included in the table.

AMERICAN DIABETES ASSOCIATION RECOMMENDATIONS FOR EXERCISE

The American Diabetes Association recommends an integrated program of activity that includes aerobic exercise, resistance exercise, flexibility and balance training, and reduction in sedentary behavior, as follows:[3]

- ≥150 min per week of moderate to vigorous aerobic exercise that is spread over at least three days per week, with no more than two consecutive days without activity
- Two to three sessions per week of resistance exercise on nonconsecutive days
- Two to three sessions per week of flexibility and balance training for older adults with diabetes
- Interrupting periods of sedentary behavior every 30 min with short bouts (e.g., 3 min) of walking, standing, or performing other light activities

More detailed recommendations are presented in Table 3.9.

Types of Activity

- **Physical activity** is any movement that results in the increased expenditure of energy above a basal level.
- **Exercise** is physical activity that is structured for the purpose of increasing physical fitness or improving health.
  - **Aerobic exercise** (also known as endurance or cardio) is sustained activity that involves rhythmic, submaximal contractions of large muscle groups (brisk walking, jogging, swimming, biking).

Table 3.9–American Diabetes Association Recommendations for Exercise

	Aerobic	Resistance	Flexibility and balance
Type of exercise	■ Prolonged, rhythmic activities using large muscle groups (e.g., walking, cycling, and swimming) ■ May be done continuously or as HIIT	■ Resistance machines, free weights, resistance bands, and/or body weight as resistance exercises	■ Stretching: static, dynamic, and other stretching; yoga ■ Balance (for older adults): practice standing on one leg, exercises using balance equipment, lower-body and core resistance exercises, tai chi
Intensity	■ Moderate to vigorous (subjectively experienced as "moderate" to "very hard")	■ Moderate (e.g., 15 repetitions of an exercise that can be repeated no more than 15 times) to vigorous (e.g., 6–8 repetitions of an exercise that can be repeated no more than 6–8 times)	■ Stretch to the point of tightness or slight discomfort ■ Balance exercises of light to moderate intensity
Duration	■ At least 150 min/week at moderate to vigorous intensity for most adults with diabetes ■ For adults able to run steadily at 6 miles per h (9.7 km/h) for 25 min, 74 min/week of vigorous activity may provide similar cardioprotective and metabolic benefits	■ At least 8–10 exercises with completion of 1–3 sets of 10–15 repetitions to near fatigue per set on every exercise early in training	■ Hold static or do dynamic stretch for 10–30 sec; 2–4 repetitions of each exercise ■ Balance training can be any duration
Frequency	■ 3–7 days/week, with no more than 2 consecutive days without exercise	■ A minimum of 2 nonconsecutive days/week, but preferably 3	■ Flexibility: ≥2–3 days/week ■ Balance: ≥2–3 days/week

(continued)

Table 3.9 *(continued)*

	Aerobic	Resistance	Flexibility and balance
Progression	■ A greater emphasis should be placed on vigorous-intensity aerobic exercise if fitness is a primary goal of exercise and not contraindicated by complications. ■ Both HIIT and continuous exercise training are appropriate activities for most individuals with diabetes.	■ Beginning training intensity should be moderate, involving 10-15 repetitions per set, with increases in weight or resistance undertaken with a lower number of repetitions (8–10) only after the target number of repetitions per set can consistently be exceeded. ■ Increase in resistance can be followed by a greater number of sets and finally by increased training frequency.	■ Continue to work on flexibility and balance training, increasing duration and/or frequency to progress over time.

Source: Colberg.[2]

- **Resistance exercise** (also known as strength training) involves repeated, short, near maximal contractions against a counteracting force (free weights, weight machines, resistance bands, and/or body weight exercises, such as push-ups or pull-ups).
- **Flexibility exercises** are intended to maintain and increase the range of motion of joints and may include dynamic and static stretching, as well as yoga and tai chi.
- **Balance exercises** are valuable for older adults to improve gait and reduce fall risk and may include activities that promote lower body and core strength (yoga, tai chi, core muscle exercises, balance machines).

■ **Sedentary behavior** is any behavior performed while awake and sitting, reclining, or lying that requires minimal energy expenditure.

Levels of Exercise

A given activity may vary according to intensity, duration, and frequency. One way to categorize aerobic exercise **intensity** is the subjective experience of the individual. A useful description of "moderate-intensity" aerobic exercise is activity that may raise a mild sweat and produces the sensation of working but that can be maintained while having a conversation. A common example of moderate-intensity aerobic exercise is brisk walking. Exercise that exceeds the capacity to maintain conversation would then be "vigorous." Other more objective measures of exercise intensity include heart rate reserve, oxygen uptake reserve, and METs. One MET is the energy required to sit quietly. Moderate-intensity exercise corresponds to 3 to <6 METs, and vigorous exercise requires ≥6 METs. Another simple method of gauging exercise intensity is to calculate a predicted maximum heart rate (220 minus the person's age) and try to achieve between 60% (low intensity) to 90% (high intensity) of that maximum value. The American Diabetes Association Position Statement of 2016 provides recommended intensity, duration, and frequency for the different types of exercise for people with diabetes (Table 3.9), and these recommendations are consistent with those endorsed in the 2020 edition of the *Standards of Medical Care in Diabetes*.[2,3]

High-intensity interval training (HIIT) is a form of aerobic exercise that involves engaging in very intense bursts of activity lasting from seconds to minutes that are interspersed with recovery periods. Interest in HIIT has grown due to the possibility of gaining metabolic and fitness benefits with a shorter time commitment than is required for more traditional, continuous aerobic exercise. In 2011, Little et al. reported that a 2-week course of HIIT was associated with improved average 24-h blood glucose control and 3-h postprandial glycemia in people with type 2 diabetes.[7] A subsequent meta-analysis supported HIIT as a means of "improving metabolic health, particularly in those at risk for or with type 2 diabetes" but concluded that larger RCTs of longer duration were necessary for confirmation.[8] People with diabetes considering HIIT should be clinically stable and able to engage regularly in at least moderate-intensity exercise.[2]

Yoga and **tai chi** are forms of mind-body training that improve flexibility and balance and may have beneficial effects for people with type 2 diabetes. A recent meta-analysis of 12 RCTs favored a yoga intervention versus usual care with significant improvements in the primary outcome of fasting blood glucose (BG) (~ −23 mg/dl mean difference), as well as in secondary outcomes of postprandial BG, A1C, total cholesterol, LDL cholesterol, and HDL cholesterol.[9] A 2015 meta-analysis of 15 RCTs of tai chi for treating type 2 diabetes did not support the effectiveness of tai chi in terms of fasting blood glucose or A1C reduction.[10] However, tai chi may offer other benefits of improved balance, flexibility, and strength that would be of value to people with type 2 diabetes.

Additional Points of Emphasis

- There is no level of moderate-to-vigorous exercise that is too low to reduce risk of death.[11]
- Sedentary behavior increases the risk for all-cause mortality, cardiovascular disease and death, type 2 diabetes, and some cancers (endometrium, lung, and colon). Thus, in addition to engaging in aerobic and resistance training, people with type 2 diabetes should avoid prolonged sitting or other inactivity.[2,3,12] Specific recommendations include the following:[13]
  - Interrupting periods of inactivity every 30 min with 3 min of light walking or mild body-weight resistance exercise.
  - Light walking for 15 min after meals to reduce postprandial hyperglycemia.
  - Performing nonexercise physical activity, such as household chores, gardening, dog walking, etc.
- Gradually increasing exercise intensity and duration may reduce exercise-related injuries and increase exercise compliance.

■ Exercise acutely increases the uptake of glucose into muscle independently of insulin action and also increases insulin sensitivity. The augmented insulin sensitivity dissipates over the ensuing hours but may persist up to 24 h[13] or even 72 h.[14,15] In order to minimize wide variations in insulin sensitivity and glycemia, people with type 2 diabetes should engage in exercise regularly, preferably daily but not less frequently than every other day. The risk of exercise-induced hypoglycemia in type 2 diabetes is low, unless the patient is on insulin or insulin secretagogue therapy, in which case precautions are recommended (see below). Very intense exercise (e.g., sprinting, brief, very vigorous aerobic exercise, heavy weightlifting) may transiently raise blood glucose due to the increased secretion of counterregulatory hormones, thereby leading to hyperglycemia.

■ People with diabetes who engage in supervised training may gain more benefit than those who train on their own.[2]

SAFETY CONSIDERATIONS

Safety considerations for exercise include pre-exercise medical clearance, prevention of exercise-induced hypoglycemia and hyperglycemia, exercise and diabetes medication management, and exercise and microvascular complications.

Pre-exercise Medical Clearance

Unnecessary pre-exercise medical evaluations for clearance represent both a barrier to starting to exercise and a source of potential harm from false positive exams and the ensuing costly diagnostic work-up.[16] Per the American Diabetes Association 2016 Position Statement, asymptomatic people with diabetes who are receiving standard diabetes care do not generally need to undergo medical clearance prior to starting a program of physical activity that does not exceed brisk walking.[2] However, those individuals who contemplate performing vigorous activity (e.g., jogging, singles tennis, soccer) are recommended to be precleared with a medical evaluation, which should include a detailed history, assessment for cardiac risk factors, and attention to nonclassical presentations of cardiovascular disease in people with diabetes.

It should be noted that the American College of Sports Medicine recommends a more conservative approach, whereby sedentary people with diabetes who plan to begin increased activity of any intensity should undergo a medical clearance exam with further testing as clinically indicated.[16] The 2020 edition of *Standards of Medical Care in Diabetes* continues to endorse the less conservative approach, because the risk of adverse events for asymptomatic adults with type 2 diabetes engaging in low- or moderate-intensity exercise is low. This recommendation applies only to asymptomatic adults who are receiving care consistent with established clinical guidelines. Note: Because autonomic neuropathy increases the risk of exercise-related adverse events, the 2020 Standards emphasize that patients with diabetes complicated by autonomic neuropathy undergo cardiac evaluation prior to increasing their current level of physical activity.[3]

Prevention of Exercise-Induced Hypoglycemia

Exercise-induced hypoglycemia is more common in type 1 diabetes than in type 2 diabetes. Nevertheless, for people with type 2 diabetes treated with insulin or with insulin secretagogues (sulfonylureas or glinides), exercise-induced changes in sensitivity to insulin may cause hypoglycemia. Several strategies that help prevent exercise-induced hypoglycemia are available that either adjust insulin dosing or carbohydrate intake or exploit the hyperglycemic effects of specific types and intensities of exercise.[2]

■ Modify insulin dosing/secretagogue dosing/carbohydrate intake as follows:
- Reduce premeal **bolus** insulin if activity is to begin within 90 min of meal (e.g., reduce single bolus dose by 25%–75% depending on exercise intensity and duration).[17]
- Ingest 15–30 g of rapidly metabolized carbohydrate before or during exercise depending on pre-exercise blood glucose, activity type, intensity, and duration.[18]

■ Perform short (10 sec) maximal sprints either just before or after moderate-intensity exercise.[19]

■ Perform bouts of high-intensity (anaerobic) exercise distributed during moderate (aerobic)-intensity exercise.

■ Perform resistance exercises before, during, or after moderate-intensity aerobic activity.

Because the increase in insulin sensitivity that may occur in the hours after exercise may be prolonged, nocturnal hypoglycemia may complicate exercise training in people with type 2 diabetes who are treated with insulin or a secretagogue. Strategies to prevent nocturnal hypoglycemia include reducing the overnight **basal** insulin dose, eating a bedtime snack, and using a continuous glucose monitor to alarm to hypoglycemia while sleeping.

Prevention of Exercise-Induced Hyperglycemia

As noted above, very intense exercise, either aerobic or resistance, may increase blood glucose due to the increased release of counterregulatory hormones. Exercise-induced hyperglycemia is more likely to occur if the individual is hyperglycemic prior to exercise and more insulin deficient. Consuming too much carbohydrate prior to exercise may lead to prolonged hyperglycemia after exercise. Strategies to counteract this effect include taking additional bolus insulin, performing moderate-intensity aerobic exercise between bouts of high-intensity exercise, and following the high-intensity exercise with a low-intensity cooldown.[13] Patients with type 2 diabetes who have very elevated blood glucose levels prior to exercise (>300 mg/dl [>16.6 mmol/L]) can go ahead and exercise if they are feeling well, are adequately hydrated, and do not have evidence of ketones in the urine.[15]

Exercise and Diabetes Medication Management

Some medications frequently prescribed to people with diabetes may increase exercise risk. Table 3.10 summarizes major categories of these drugs, considerations for exercise, and adjustments that may be helpful to limit risk.

Table 3.10–Recommendations for Exercising Safely

Type/class of medication	Exercise considerations	Safety/dose adjustments
Diabetes		
Insulin	■ Deficiency: hyperglycemia, ketoacidosis ■ Excess: hypoglycemia during and after exercise	■ Increase insulin dose pre- and postexercise for deficiency ■ Decrease prandial and/or basal doses for excess insulin
Insulin secretagogues	■ Exercise-induced hypoglycemia	■ If exercise-induced hypoglycemia has occurred, decrease dose on exercise days to reduce hypoglycemia risk
Metformin	■ None	■ Generally safe; no dose adjustment for exercise
Thiazolidinediones	■ Fluid retention	■ Generally safe; no dose adjustment for exercise
Dipeptidyl peptidase-4 inhibitors	■ Slight risk of congestive heart failure with saxagliptin and alogliptin	■ Generally safe; no dose adjustment for exercise
Glucagon-like peptide 1 receptor agonists	■ May increase risk of hypoglycemia when used with insulin or sulfonylureas but not when used alone	■ Generally safe; no dose adjustment for exercise but may need to lower insulin or sulfonylurea dose
Sodium–glucose contransporter 2 inhibitors	■ May increase risk of hypoglycemia when used with insulin or sulfonylureas but not when used alone	■ Generally safe; no dose adjustment
Hypertension		
β-Blockers	■ Hypoglycemia unawareness and unresponsiveness; may reduce maximal exercise capacity	■ Check blood glucose before and after exercise; treat hypoglycemia with glucose
Other agents	■ Regular exercise training may lower blood pressure; some agents increase risk of dehydration	■ Doses may need to be adjusted to accommodate the improvements from training and avoid dehydration
Cholesterol		
Statins	■ Muscle weakness, discomfort, and cramping in a minority of users	■ Generally safe; no dose adjustment for exercise
Fibric acid derivatives	■ Rare myositis or rhabdomyolysis; risk increased with gemfibrozil and statin combination	■ Avoid exercise if these muscle conditions are present

Source: Colberg.[2]

Exercise and Microvascular Complications[2,3]

Proliferative or severe nonproliferative retinopathy increases the risk for vitreous hemorrhage during either aerobic or resistance exercise of vigorous intensity and may be contraindicated. Patients with these findings may benefit from an ophthalmology consultation prior to engaging in vigorous exercise. These patients should also avoid jumping, jarring activities, head-down activities, breath holding (e.g., Valsalva maneuver), or any activity that might increase intracranial pressure (e.g., straining).

Peripheral neuropathy must be addressed with attention to appropriate foot care (daily examination for blisters, sores, and ulcers) and to the use of proper footwear in order to prevent ulceration or podiatric issues. If ulceration develops, early detection and prompt treatment are necessary to lower the risk of amputation. Patients with a loss of protective sensation should be cautioned against high-impact exercises, which may cause injury or trauma (specifically to the lower extremities) and go undetected; this becomes even more critical in patients with a history of foot ulcers or Charcot foot.

Autonomic neuropathy may lead to a number of issues that limit or prevent exercise training: postural hypotension, inability to adjust the heart rate to increased activity, delayed gastric emptying, impaired thermoregulation, and dehydration during exercise. Those with postural hypotension should avoid sudden changes in posture or direction. Those with cardiac dysautonomia may require pre-exercise medical evaluation with or without exercise stress testing.

Diabetic kidney disease does not impose specific exercise restrictions. Exercise may increase microalbuminuria but does not promote the progression of diabetic kidney disease.

SPECIAL POPULATIONS

Special populations that should be considered when discussing exercise and diabetes management include children and adolescents, older adults, and pregnant women.

Children and Adolescents

Children and adolescents with type 2 diabetes should ideally perform moderate or vigorous aerobic activity for 60 min daily, and in addition should engage in muscle- and bone-strengthening activities ≥3 days per week.[20]

Older Adults

Older adults are at increased risk of becoming overheated, especially those who may be dehydrated due to chronic hyperglycemia or who have impaired sweating due to neuropathy. Accordingly, older adults should avoid exercising under hot and/or humid conditions.[13]

Pregnant Women with Diabetes

Pregnant women who engage in regular physical activity are less likely to develop gestational diabetes mellitus. Accordingly, daily 20–30 min of moderate-intensity exercise is recommended for pregnant women who are at risk for or who have gestational diabetes mellitus. Also, pregnant women with a preexisting diagnosis of diabetes are recommended to begin regular exercise before and during pregnancy. Pregnant women who take insulin need to follow the same precautions as nonpregnant women regarding the effects of exercise on insulin sensitivity and peripheral glucose uptake.[2]

JUMPING OVER THE BARRIERS TO EXERCISE

Physicians have the "easy" job of writing the "prescription" of regular exercise. Their patients face the much harder task of overcoming numerous barriers to exercise and of making exercise a habit, whether those barriers be societal, cultural, political, or personal (psychological, physical, metabolic). For people with diabetes, the barriers are that much higher due to the safety considerations that diabetes and its treatment impose. Nevertheless, there is evidence that behavioral interventions may help people with type 2 diabetes increase their participation in physical activity with associated reductions in A1C of 0.21%–0.44%.[21] Successful exercise prescriptions and behavioral strategies for A1C reduction include the following techniques:

- Once a physical activity is performed in one setting, encourage performance of that activity in other settings.
- Use follow-up prompts (e.g., phone calls).
- Prompt review of behavioral goals. (Were goals achieved?)
- Provide information on where and when to be active.
- Plan social support and social change.
- Support goal setting for physical activity by the individual (specific, measurable, achievable, relevant, timely).
- Use time management to allow time for physical activity.
- Prompt focus on past success.
- Identify barriers and problem solve.
- Provide information on the benefits and costs of physical activity to the individual.

The use of pedometers to promote increased physical activity is a promising method to provide measurable feedback, but to this point the literature remains equivocal on their efficacy.[2] In one study of adults with type 2 diabetes, the use of step counters increased daily steps but did not lower the A1C.[22] Another study estimated 7,000 steps per day, 7 days per week (49,000 steps/week) to be a "good proxy" for attaining the recommended goal of 150 min per week of moderate-to-vigorous physical activity.[23] New Internet-based technologies may provide effective feedback and support for people attempting to become physically active.

CONCLUSION

Physical activity and exercise join nutrition and drug therapy as essential aspects of the care of patients with diabetes. In addition to improving glycemic control, reducing cardiovascular disease risk factors, and reducing cardiovascular mortality in people with type 2 diabetes, physical activity and exercise exert many other positive effects on cognition, mood, sleep, well-being, and cancer risk. Key recommendations are that people with type 2 diabetes engage in ≥150 min per week of at least moderate-intensity physical activity, equivalent to brisk walking, and perform two to three sessions per week of resistance exercise. Appropriate precautions must be taken to account for the effects of exercise on glucose uptake into muscle and on insulin sensitivity, to minimize the potential impact on diabetic complications, and to reduce the risk of overheating in older adults. In addition to increasing physical activity, people of all ages should reduce sedentary behaviors, for example by sitting for ≤30 min in one stretch. Technology is one of the forces that may encourage sedentary behaviors, but technology in the form of accelerometers, Internet-based applications, e-mail, social media, and smartphones may also promote effective platforms and strategies that increase compliance and persistence with physical activity/exercise programs.

REFERENCES

1. 2018 Physical Activity Guidelines Advisory Committee. *2018 Physical Activity Guidelines Advisory Committee Scientific Report*. Washington, DC, U.S. Department of Health and Human Services, 2018

2. Colberg SR, Sigal RJ, Yardley JE, Riddell MC, Dunstan DW, Dempsey PC, et al. Physical activity/exercise and diabetes: a position statement of the American Diabetes Association. *Diabetes Care* 2016;39(11):2065–2079. doi: 10.2337/dc16-1728. Epub 2016 Dec 8. PubMed PMID: 27926890

3. American Diabetes Association. 5. Lifestyle management: standards of medical care in diabetes 2019. *Diabetes Care* 2019;42(Suppl. 1):S46–S60. doi: 10.2337/dc19-S005. Epub 2018 Dec 19. PubMed PMID: 30559231

4. Sluik D, Buijsse B, Muckelbauer R, Kaaks R, Teucher B, Johnsen NF, et al. Physical activity and mortality in individuals with diabetes mellitus: a prospective study and meta-analysis. *Arch Intern Med* 2012;172(17):1285–1295. doi: 10.1001/archinternmed.2012.3130. Epub 2012 Aug 8. PubMed PMID: 22868663

5. Yang Z, Scott CA, Mao C, Tang J, Farmer AJ. Resistance exercise versus aerobic exercise for type 2 diabetes: a systematic review and meta-analysis. *Sports Med* 2014;44(4):487–499. doi: 10.1007/s40279-013-0128-8. Epub 2013 Dec 4. PubMed PMID: 24297743

6. Church TS, Blair SN, Cocreham S, Johannsen N, Johnson W, Kramer K, et al. Effects of aerobic and resistance training on hemoglobin A1c levels in patients with type 2 diabetes: a randomized controlled trial. *JAMA*

2010;304(20):2253–2262. doi: 10.1001/jama.2010.1710. Epub 2010 Nov 26. PubMed PMID: 21098771; PubMed Central PMCID: PMCPMC3174102

7. Little JP, Gillen JB, Percival ME, Safdar A, Tarnopolsky MA, Punthakee Z, et al. Low-volume high-intensity interval training reduces hyperglycemia and increases muscle mitochondrial capacity in patients with type 2 diabetes. *J Appl Physiol (1985)* 2011;111(6):1554–1560. doi: 10.1152/japplphysiol.00921.2011. Epub 2011 Aug 27. PubMed PMID: 21868679

8. Jelleyman C, Yates T, O'Donovan G, Gray LJ, King JA, Khunti K, et al. The effects of high-intensity interval training on glucose regulation and insulin resistance: a meta-analysis. *Obes Rev* 2015;16(11):942–961. doi: 10.1111/obr.12317. PubMed PMID: 26481101

9. Cui J, Yan JH, Yan LM, Pan L, Le JJ, Guo YZ. Effects of yoga in adults with type 2 diabetes mellitus: A meta-analysis. *J Diabetes Investig* 2017;8(2):201–209. doi: 10.1111/jdi.12548. Epub 2016 Jul 3. PubMed PMID: 27370357; PubMed Central PMCID: PMCPMC5334310

10. Lee MS, Jun JH, Lim HJ, Lim HS. A systematic review and meta-analysis of tai chi for treating type 2 diabetes. *Maturitas* 2015;80(1):14–23. doi: 10.1016/j.maturitas.2014.09.008. Epub 2014 Dec 3. PubMed PMID: 25449822

11. U.S. Department of Health and Human Services. *Physical Activity Guidelines for Americans.* 2nd ed. Washington, DC, U.S. Goverment Printing, 2018

12. Dempsey PC, Larsen RN, Sethi P, Sacre JW, Straznicky NE, Cohen ND, et al. Benefits for type 2 diabetes of interrupting prolonged sitting with brief bouts of light walking or simple resistance activities. *Diabetes Care* 2016;39(6):964–972. doi: 10.2337/dc15-2336. Epub 2016 May 22.PubMed PMID: 27208318

13. Colberg SR. Key points from the updated guidelines on exercise and diabetes. *Front Endocrinol (Lausanne)* 2017;8:33. doi: 10.3389/fendo.2017.00033. Epub 2017 Mar 8. PubMed PMID: 28265261; PubMed Central PMCID: PMCPMC5317029

14. Colberg SR, Sigal RJ, Fernhall B, Regensteiner JG, Blissmer BJ, Rubin RR, et al. Exercise and type 2 diabetes: the American College of Sports Medicine and the American Diabetes Association: joint position statement executive summary. *Diabetes Care* 2010;33(12):2692–2696. doi: 10.2337/dc10-1548. Epub 2010 Dec 1. PubMed PMID: 21115771; PubMed Central PMCID: PMCPMC2992214

15. Colberg SR, Sigal RJ, Fernhall B, Regensteiner JG, Blissmer BJ, Rubin RR, et al. Exercise and type 2 diabetes: the American College of Sports Medicine and the American Diabetes Association: joint position statement. *Diabetes Care* 2010;33(12):e147–e167. doi: 10.2337/dc10-9990. Epub 2010 Dec 1. PubMed PMID: 21115758; PubMed Central PMCID: PMCPMC2992225

16. Riebe D, Franklin BA, Thompson PD, Garber CE, Whitfield GP, Magal M, et al. Updating ACSM's recommendations for exercise preparticipation health screening. *Med Sci Sports Exerc* 2015;47(11):2473–2479. doi: 10.1249/MSS.0000000000000664. Epub 2015 Oct 17. PubMed PMID: 26473759

17. Rabasa-Lhoret R, Bourque J, Ducros F, Chiasson JL. Guidelines for premeal insulin dose reduction for postprandial exercise of different intensities and durations in type 1 diabetic subjects treated intensively with a basal-bolus insulin regimen (ultralente-lispro). *Diabetes Care* 2001;24(4):625–630. doi: 10.2337/diacare.24.4.625. Epub 2001 Apr 24. PubMed PMID: 11315820

18. Grimm JJ, Ybarra J, Berne C, Muchnick S, Golay A. A new table for prevention of hypoglycaemia during physical activity in type 1 diabetic patients. *Diabetes Metab* 2004;30(5):465–470. Epub 2005 Jan 27. PubMed PMID: 15671916

19. Bussau VA, Ferreira LD, Jones TW, Fournier PA. The 10-s maximal sprint: a novel approach to counter an exercise-mediated fall in glycemia in individuals with type 1 diabetes. *Diabetes Care* 2006;29(3):601–606. doi: 10.2337/diacare.29.03.06.dc05-1764. Epub 2006 Mar 1. PubMed PMID: 16505513

20. Janssen I, Leblanc AG. Systematic review of the health benefits of physical activity and fitness in school-aged children and youth. *Int J Behav Nutr Phys Act* 2010;7:40. doi: 10.1186/1479-5868-7-40. Epub 2010 May 13. PubMed PMID: 20459784; PubMed Central PMCID: PMCPMC2885312

21. Avery L, Flynn D, van Wersch A, Sniehotta FF, Trenell MI. Changing physical activity behavior in type 2 diabetes: a systematic review and meta-analysis of behavioral interventions. *Diabetes Care* 2012;35(12):2681–2689. doi: 10.2337/dc11-2452. Epub 2012 Nov 23. PubMed PMID: 23173137; PubMed Central PMCID: PMCPMC3507564

22. Qiu S, Cai X, Chen X, Yang B, Sun Z. Step counter use in type 2 diabetes: a meta-analysis of randomized controlled trials. *BMC Med* 2014;12:36. doi: 10.1186/1741-7015-12-36. Epub 2014 Feb 28. PubMed PMID: 24571580; PubMed Central PMCID: PMCPMC4016223

23. Tudor-Locke C, Leonardi C, Johnson WD, Katzmarzyk PT, Church TS. Accelerometer steps/day translation of moderate-to-vigorous activity. *Prev Med* 2011;53(1-2):31–33. doi: 10.1016/j.ypmed.2011.01.014. Epub 2011 Feb 8. PubMed PMID: 21295063

PHARMACEUTICAL INTERVENTION

Marconi Abreu, MD
Nicole McNulty, PharmD, BCACP
Ildiko Lingvay, MD, MPH, MSCS

The approach to the pharmacological treatment of type 2 diabetes has changed dramatically over the past decade. This change was driven by two main factors. First, the therapeutic options have increased exponentially. Currently there are >60 individual agents or combinations of agents approved by the U.S. Food and Drug Administration (FDA) for lowering the glucose level in patients with type 2 diabetes, belonging to 12 different therapeutic classes (Table 3.11). Choosing the right option for an individual patient relies on understanding the mechanisms of actions, efficacy, and safety of each of these classes and agents within a class, as well as understanding each patient's goals, motivations, and compelling needs. Second, a new regulatory guidance was introduced in 2008, requiring demonstration of cardiovascular safety as a prerequisite for licensing of agents indicated for the treatment of type 2 diabetes. As a result, a wealth of new data has accumulated regarding the cardiovascular safety and efficacy of the newer agents, and several new drugs have additional cardiovascular indications on the label.

In this chapter, we provide an overview of the various glucose-lowering classes and describe the currently recommended approach to the pharmacological treatment of patients with type 2 diabetes.

OVERVIEW OF PHARMACOLOGIC CLASSES

Medications for the treatment of type 2 diabetes can be categorized into five groups: those enhancing the effectiveness of endogeneous insulin, those increasing the supply of insulin, those acting on noninsulin hormonal systems, those inhibiting the reabsorption of glucose within the kidney, and those with other or unknown mechanisms of action. Metformin, α-glucosidase inhibitors (AGIs), and thiazolidinediones (TZDs) enhance the effectiveness of endogeneous insulin within the liver, gastrointestinal tract, muscle, and/or adipose tissues. Secretagogues, such as sulfonylureas and the glinides, as well as injected insulins increase circulating levels of insulin. Agents acting on hormonal systems include synthetic amylin, glucagon-like peptide 1 receptor agonists (GLP-1 RAs), and dipeptidyl-peptidase-4 (DPP-4) inhibitors, and they affect glucagon, insulin secretion, gastric emptying, and appetite. Sodium–glucose cotransporter 2 (SGLT2) inhibitors reduce reabsorption of filtered glucose from the renal tubular lumen, resulting in increased urinary excretion of glucose and lower plasma glucose concentrations.

The following sections review individual pharmacologic agents, but numerous combination formulations are available that may assist in improving adherence and simplifying treatment plans.

BIGUANIDES

Mechanism of Action and Glycemic Efficacy

Metformin belongs to the biguanide class of drugs and can reduce A1C by ≤1.5% independently of patient age, body weight, duration of diabetes, and insulin

Table 3.11–Clinical Characteristics and Cost of the Available Glucose-Lowering Classes

Therapeutic class	Agents in class	A1C lowering	CV benefits	Weight effects	Hypoglycemia risk	Main side effects	Cost
Biguanides	Metformin Metformin XR	↓↓	↓ MI	Neutral/↓	Low	Bloating, abdominal cramping, diarrhea	$
Sulfonylureas	Glimepiride Chlorpropamide Glyburide Glipizide Tolazamide Tolbutamide	↓↓		↑↑	↑↑		$–$$
Meglitinides	Repaglinide Nateglinide	→		↑	↑		$$
a-Glucosidase inhibitors	Acarbose Miglitol	→		Neutral	Low	Bloating, abdominal cramping, flatulence, diarrhea	$–$$
SGLT2 inhibitors	Dapagliflozin Empagliflozin Canagliflozin Ertugliflozin	→	↓MACE ↓HHF	↓↓	Low	Polyuria Genitourinary infections Normoglycemic diabetic ketoacidosis	$$$
DPP-4 inhibitors	Sitagliptin Saxagliptin Linagliptin Alogliptin	→	CV safety	Neutral/↓	Low		$$$

(continued)

Table 3.11 *(continued)*

Therapeutic class	Agents in class	A1C lowering	CV benefits	Weight effects	Hypoglycemia risk	Main side effects	Cost
GLP-1 receptor agonists	Lixisenatide Exenatide Liraglutide Dulaglutide Albiglutide Exenatide ER Semaglutide	↓↓	↓MACE	↓↓	Low	Nausea, vomiting, constipation, diarrhea, dyspepsia, abdominal cramping	$$$
Thiazolidinediones	Pioglitazone Rosiglitazone	↓↓	↓MACE	↑↑	Low	Lower extremity edema ↑Heart failure risk	$ $$$
Dopamine agonists	Bromocriptine	↓	CV safety	Neutral/↓	Low	Headache, dizziness	$$$
Bile acid sequestrants	Colesevelam	↓		Neutral	Low	Constipation	$$$
Amylin mimetics	Pramlintide	↓		↓	Low	Nausea, vomiting	$$$
Insulin	See Table 3.7	↓↓		↑↑	↑↑		$–$$$

CV, cardiovascular; DPP-4, dipeptidyl-peptidase-4; GLP-1, glucagon-like peptide 1; HHF, hypertensive heart failure; MACE, major cardiovascular event; MI, myocardial infarction; SGLT2, sodium–glucose cotransporter 2.

levels.[1] Metformin induces glucose lowering primarily by reducing hepatic glucose output by suppressing gluconeogenesis and glycogenolysis and increasing insulin-mediated glucose uptake by skeletal muscles and adipocytes.[1] Metformin also improves insulin sensitivity by decreasing oxidation of free fatty acids (FFAs). Metformin is absorbed mostly by the small intestines with negligible absorption from the stomach or large intestines.[2] There is substantial variability in bioavailability of immediate-release metformin (55 +/– 16%), which decreases with multiple dosing. Following single-dose administration of the immediate-release formulation, plasma concentrations are reached ≤3 h and subsequently fall rapidly. Metformin extended-release (XR) is absorbed more slowly, with a maximum plasma concentration reached in 7 h.[3] Absorption of metformin XR is similar whether given once daily or twice daily at the same total daily dosage,[3] and efficacy is similar between the two formulations. Although suggested to be taken with food to reduce gastrointestinal adverse effects, a high-fat meal has been reported to decrease the bioavailability, although this does not appear to be clinically significant.

Renal clearance is the major mode of elimination of metformin. It is readily filtered at the glomerulus secondary to its small molecule size and being non–protein bound. It also has low lipid solubility, preventing passive reabsorption.[2] Renal clearance of metformin decreases in proportion to decreasing renal function, suggesting that maximal dosage should be decreased as well. Because of its rapid clearance, metformin is usually taken two to three times daily with the immediate-release formulation or once or twice daily with the extended-release formulation. Fig. 3.1 describes the dosing recommendations of all glucose-lowering agents, including metformin, according to renal function.

Enthusiasm about the use of metformin as the drug of choice in the treatment of diabetes is expressed in most guidelines as a result of its superior performance in overweight patients in the UK Prospective Diabetes Study (UKPDS). In that subgroup, initial treatment with metformin as opposed to sulfonylureas or insulin was associated with less hypoglycemia and weight gain and a statistically significant reduction in all-cause mortality.[4,5] Metformin has been associated with modest beneficial changes in lipids, blood pressure, weight, and other cardiovascular risk markers associated with insulin resistance in some but not all studies.[4]

Metformin should be started at a low dose and titrated upward slowly. The starting dose of metformin is 500 mg once or twice daily with breakfast and/or the evening meal. After 1–2 weeks, the dose may be increased sequentially until unacceptable adverse effects arise or the patient is taking the maximally effective dose of 1,000 mg twice daily. Metformin immediate-release (IR) and XR, specifically the 500 mg and 750 mg formulations, are readily available as a generic prescription with low copay costs at retail pharmacies. Metformin may also be prescribed as a marketed solution 500 mg/5 mL, available branded or generic. Due to its long-standing support as a first-line agent, metformin has been formulated into several FDA-approved combination therapies along with SGLT2 inhibitors, DPP-4 inhibitors, sulfonylureas, TZDs, and meglitinides.

Adverse Effects and Monitoring

The main concern regarding metformin treatment historically has been lactic acidosis, which had a higher association with phenformin and buformin and ultimately

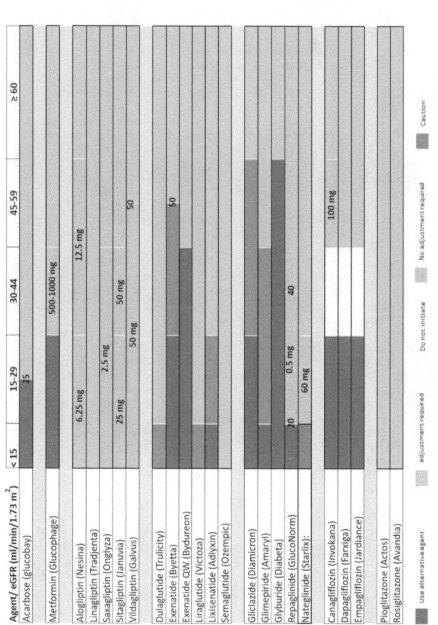

Figure 3.1 Recommended renal dose adjustments for glucose-lowering agents according to Food and Drug Administration labeling.

Source: Adapted from Diabetes Canada Clinical Practice Guidelines Expert Committee. Diabetes Canada 2018 Clinical Practice Guidelines for the Prevention and Management of Diabetes in Canada. Can J Diabetes. 2018;42(Suppl 1):S1–S325.

resulted in their removals from market. Numerous studies have investigated the correlation of lactic acidosis and metformin use and have shown that true metformin-associated lactic acidosis is very rare, and it is unlikely that metformin will induce lactic acidosis as long as the liver and kidneys process lactate. Relying on studies that assessed metabolic acidosis that was or was not related to metformin therapy,[6] the FDA published a drug safety communication in April 2016 updating prescribing information based on renal function as a measure of glomerular filtrate rate (GFR) instead of blood creatinine concentration. Current labeling recommendations are as follows:[7]

1. Metformin is contraindicated in an estimated glomerular filtrate rate (eGFR) <30 mL/min/1.73 m^2.
2. Starting metformin in patients with an eGFR between 30 mL/min/1.73 m^2 and 45 mL/min/1.73 m^2 is not recommended; however, if patients are currently prescribed metformin, therapy may be continued after assessing benefits and risks of treatment. Alternatively, in the absence of active kidney disease and/or conditions that predispose to hypoperfusion, metformin may be initiated at half the usual initial dose with maximum dosage of 1,000 mg daily.
3. Metformin therapy may be initiated in patients with an eGFR >45 mL/min/1.73 m^2.

Metformin's main side effects are gastrointestinal, notably diarrhea, nausea, abdominal pain, dyspepsia, or reduced appetite. The tolerability of the XR formulation is comparable to or increased compared with the IR formulation.[2,3] These side effects are frequent (10%–30%) at dosages >1,750 mg daily, but in ~5% of patients may occur and persist even at lower doses.[3] In many patients, these side effects are transient and can be minimized by slow titration of the dose and can be alleviated by dose reduction when persistent. Chronic metformin use has also been associated with vitamin B12 deficiency. Although there are no established guidelines for proactive testing, periodic measurement of vitamin B12 levels may be considered in metformin-treated patients, especially those with anemia or peripheral neuropathy or in the elderly.[8] A 2014 meta-analysis analyzing the effects of metformin on vitamin B12 concentrations found that the recommended amount of vitamin B12 by the Institute of Medicine (2.4 µg daily) may not be sufficient in patients using metformin.[9] It is reasonable to consider supplementation of vitamin B12, but dosing should be individualized according to different ethnicity and dietary habits.

Cardiovascular Safety and Efficacy

To date, no cardiovascular outcomes trial (CVOT) with metformin has been completed, but cardiovascular benefits of metformin have been demonstrated in a few randomized clinical trials and several large observational studies.[10] A small, prespecified group of 1,700 overweight individuals from the UKPDS study group were randomized to diet alone (n = 411), intensive control with metformin (n = 342), or intensive control with sulfonylurea or insulin (n = 951). Metformin versus dietary therapy demonstrated reduction in myocardial infarction (hazard ratio [HR] 0.61 [95% CI 0.41–0.89]) and all-cause mortality (HR 0.64 [95% CI 0.45–0.91]).[11] Expanded major cardiovascular event (MACE) end points were investigated in the HOME study, in which 390 patients were enrolled to receive metformin versus placebo, and in SPREAD-DIMCAD, in which 304 patients were enrolled to receive metformin versus glipizide.[5] Metformin was associated with a 40% reduction in the secondary macrovascular end point in the HOME study (HR 0.60 [95% CI 0.40–0.92][12] and a 46% reduction in the primary composite cardiovascular end point in SPREAD-DIMCAD (HR 0.54 [95% CI 0.3–0.9]).[13] An ongoing study called VA-IMPACT (**NCT 02915198**) is evaluating the effect of metformin on cardiovascular outcomes in patients with prediabetes and established cardiovascular disease.

Summary

Metformin is an effective, weight-neutral, low-cost, glucose-lowering agent with a low risk of hypoglycemia. With the updated renal dosing recommendations from the FDA, metformin can be prescribed safely to more individuals with mild to moderate renal dysfunction. Its availability as a combination agent may also help increase adherence for patients who need additional glycemic control past metformin monotherapy.

Although no large CVOT trial with metformin has been completed, there is evidence to suggest metformin has macrovascular benefits beyond its well-established glycemic efficacy.

SULFONYLUREAS AND MEGLITINIDES

Mechanism of Action and Glycemic Efficacy

The β-cell secretes insulin in a glucose-dependent fashion. Glucose enters the cell and is metabolized to ATP. A higher ratio of ATP/ADP closes the ATP-dependent potassium channel (sulfonylurea receptor [SUR] receptor), preventing potassium from exiting the cell, consequently depolarizing the β-cell membrane. This change in membrane potential opens the voltage-dependent calcium channel, allowing calcium concentration to rise inside the β-cell and thus triggering insulin release into the circulation.

Sulfonylureas and glinides exert their glucose-lowering effects through binding to the SUR receptor, closure of the potassium channel, and depolarization of the β-cell membrane regardless of ambient glucose concentration. They reduce both fasting and postprandial glucose with a net effect of ~1%–1.5% reduction in A1C from a baseline A1C of 8.5%–9.0% (69–75 mmol/mol). They achieve maximum glycemic effect at half of the maximum allowable dose.

Glinides are nonsulfonylurea insulin secretagogues. Their action is also mediated through the SUR receptor, and they hold some structural homology to the sulfonylureas but do not contain the actual sulfonylurea moiety. Both repaglinide and nateglinide are rapidly absorbed after oral administration and rapidly cleared by hepatic metabolism. They are short acting and therefore require dosing before each meal (up to three times daily). Repaglinide also reduces fasting blood glucose levels, despite its short half-life, and reduces A1C equivalently to sulfonylureas. Nateglinide has the shortest residence time in the SUR receptor and does not affect fasting blood glucose. It has a lower risk for hypoglycemia than repaglinide and sulfonylureas, but its efficacy in lowering A1C is modest.

Adverse Effects and Monitoring

Sulfonylureas have been associated with faster therapeutic failure than any other hyperglycemic agents.[14,15] They are also associated with moderate weight gain and a higher risk of hypoglycemia, sometimes severe. Sulfonylureas and glinides binding to the SUR receptor activate insulin release in a glucose-independent fashion, which explains the high potential for hypoglycemia in susceptible patients. The elderly and those with lower eGFR (due to lower clearance of insulin, sulfonylurea metabolites, and reduced gluconeogenesis) have a higher risk of developing severe and nocturnal hypoglycemia with these drugs. This risk is directly related to the pharmacologic half-life, degree of affinity to the SUR receptor, and degree of renal excretion of the individual drug. The first-generation sulfonylureas (tolbutamide, tolazamide, and chlorpropamide) have more protein binding, have more drug-to-drug interaction, cost more than other available sulfonylureas, and are more likely to cause severe and prolonged hypoglycemia due to their much higher affinity with the SUR receptor. Therefore, their use is not recommended anymore. The second-generation sulfonylureas (glyburide, glipizide, and glimepiride) are largely free of drug-to-drug interactions and have lower total dosage requirements. They are metabolized mainly by the liver and cleared renally. Glyburide has a higher affinity for the SUR receptor than glimepiride and glipizide and has an active metabolite that must be excreted by the kidney. Thus, glyburide should be avoided in patients with even mild renal insufficiency, while glipizide and glimepiride can be used carefully in patients with moderate renal impairment. Nateglinide, on the other hand, is the insulin secretagogue with the lowest risk of hypoglycemia.

Other adverse effects occurring in <5% of patients include gastrointestinal symptoms, such as nausea, heartburn, and vomiting, and skin reactions, including rashes, purpura, and pruritus. Very rare side effects include hematological reactions (leukopenia, thrombocytopenia, or hemolytic anemia) and cholestasis (with or without jaundice). Modest weight gain may occur with treatment.

Cardiovascular Safety and Efficacy

The effects of insulin secretagogues binding to potassium channels in various tissues, including vascular tissue (where they may reduce vasodilation), is still being debated. The clinical importance of this effect is unknown.

The human myocardium has an ATP-dependent potassium channel (KATP channels), which shares some analogy with the pancreatic SUR receptor. During ischemia, when ATP generation decreases, this channel is typically closed. This favors an efflux of potassium, which reduces action potential duration, the duration of calcium influx, and intracellular calcium accumulation. This behavior suggests that the myocardium ATP-dependent potassium channels are involved in the protection against stunning and arrhythmias and in the mechanism of ischemic preconditioning.[16] Different sulfonylureas and glinides can block these channels to different degrees, prolonging myocardium cell depolarization during ischemia, allowing calcium entry and accumulation for longer periods of time, potentially affecting cardiac rhythm in the setting of ischemia. This seems to be less of a concern with glimepiride, glipizide, and glinides than with glyburide and first-generation sulfonylureas. The UKPDS showed no increase in cardiovascular disease events with sulfonylureas compared with other therapies.[15] The CAROLINA trial is the first and only properly designed CVOT evaluating cardiovascular outcomes of a sulfonylurea drug in a population with high cardiovascular risk. It compared glimepiride against linaglipitin, a drug with neutral cardiovascular risk/benefit, and demonstrated comparable cardiovascular safety over a median follow-up of 6 years.[17]

Summary

Despite robust initial lowering in A1C, sulfonylurea use is associated with higher incidence of treatment failure, weight gain, and risk for hypoglycemia. Glinides and sulfonylureas (with the exception of glimepiride) lack data from CVOTs to support cardiovascular safety in high-risk patients. Currently, the most appealing reason to prescribe a sulfonylurea in the U.S. is cost and lack of access to a better alternative. This class of medications has been mostly replaced by safer alternatives. The GRADE trial (NCT01794143) is an ongoing clinical trial comparing the long-term effectiveness of major glycemic-lowering medications. This study will provide guidance to clinicians on which medications are most appropriate for the treatment of type 2 diabetes, including relevant information on the durability of sulfonylureas and their potential future role as second-line agents after metformin for patients with type 2 diabetes. When prescribing a sulfonylurea, providers should use the lowest dose required to achieve desirable glycemic control and pay special attention to hypoglycemia, especially in the elderly and patients with kidney disease.

TZDs

Mechanism of Action and Glycemic Efficacy

TZDs, also called glitazones, improve insulin action in muscle, adipose cells, and liver. They activate the nuclear peroxisome proliferator–activated receptor (PPAR) g, which is expressed abundantly in adipose tissue but is also found in pancreatic β-cells, endothelium, and macrophages. The net results of its activation is a reduction in plasma FFA levels and mobilization of fat out of muscle, liver, and β-cells with redistribution to the subcutaneous compartment. Pioglitazone, but not rosiglitazone, also activates PPAR-a receptors. PPAR-a is expressed predominantly in the liver, heart, and muscle. Its activation results in an increased uptake of glucose and FFA in those tissues, increased fatty acid oxidation, decreased inflammation, and slowing of atherosclerosis.[18]

TZDs augment β-cell secretory dynamics. The long-term use of pioglitazone and rosiglitazone preserves and improves β-cell function, slowing down the progression of impaired glucose tolerance to overt diabetes, and in some cases reverting impaired glucose tolerance to normal glucose tolerance. Patients using this class of medication have a lower risk of therapeutic failure compared with metformin or sulfonylureas.[14,19]

Glitazones improve both fasting and postprandial glucose in patients with type 2 diabetes and reduce A1C to an extent similar to as sulfonylureas and metformin. Their metabolic effects take 8–12 weeks to reach full potential.

Pioglitazone therapy should be considered fourth-line for most patients, after metformin, SGLT2, and GLP-1 RAs or DPP-4 inhibitors.[20] It should be typically started at 15 mg and can be titrated to 30 mg after 1 month if no significant adverse events are noted. The 45-mg dose provides only modest additional benefit over the 30-mg dose and therefore should be avoided in most patients given the additional risk for weight gain, fluid retention, and other adverse events without a commensurate additional efficacy.

Pioglitazone is now generic, and its cost is reasonable and attainable for those who do not have access to the newer agents. Therefore, in such situations, it is the preferred second-line agent.

Additional Effects

Different TZDs have different effects on circulating lipids. Rosiglitazone (PPAR-g only) elevates serum HDL and LDL and moderately increases apolipoprotein B (ApoB). Pioglitazone (PPAR-g and a) increases HDL but reduces LDL, ApoB, and triglycerides. Both agents improve a number of inflammatory and cellular markers associated with excess cardiovascular risk. Glitazones also improve transaminitis and histologic changes related to nonalcoholic steatohepatitis, including improvement in fibrosis.[21]

Adverse Effects and Monitoring

Weight gain and fluid retention are the most common adverse events experienced with these agents. The weight gain observed with pioglitazone is variable from patient to patient and mostly due to an increase in subcutaneous fat. In the IRIS study using 45 mg of pioglitazone, the mean weight gain observed was 2.6 kg vs. 0.5 kg with placebo. In the pioglitazone group, 52.2% of patients gained >4.5 kg and 11.4% gained >13.6 kg.[22] The weight gain with TZDs is dose dependent and greater when used in combination with insulin or sulfonylureas. It can be mitigated by using TZDs in combination with diet, exercise, or glucose-lowering agents that promote weight loss (metformin, SGLT2 inhibitors, or GLP-1 RA).

Fluid retention seen with TZDs typically manifests as peripheral edema and occurs in 4%–6% of patients. Fluid retention is more likely to occur in patients with baseline peripheral edema, those with left ventricular dysfunction, or those treated with insulin.[23,24] To minimize this adverse effect, TZDs should be initiated at the lowest dose and titrated over months while monitoring the development of peripheral edema, dyspnea, and exertional fatigue. Interestingly, TZD-related edema responds better to treatment with thiazide diuretic and spironolactone than to furosemide.[25] In the PROActive trial, pioglitazone use was also associated with higher rates of heart failure (11% vs. 8% in the placebo group), but a similar number of hospitalization and deaths from heart failure.[24]

Because another agent in this class was removed from the market due to liver failure, the package insert recommends obtaining liver function test prior to initiating TZDs. TZDs should not be initiated if alanine aminotransferase is more than three times the upper limit, or they should be held while definitive evaluation is ongoing. If no alternative etiology is found, TZDs should not be restarted.[26]

The use of both pioglitazone and rosiglitazone increases the fracture risk in postmenopausal women.[24,27] The fractures observed in clinical trials evaluating TZDs have been mostly in distal extremities (hands and feet) rather than in more classic osteoporotic fractures sites such as the hip and spine. Providers should consider ordering a baseline bone mineral density before starting glitazone therapy in postmenopausal woman or in those with a higher fracture risk.

Pioglitazone, but not rosiglitazone, was associated with a numeric imbalance in new cases of bladder cancer in the pioglitazone group compared with placebo.[24] Due to bladder cancer concerns, health regulatory agencies in France and Germany suspended pioglitazone use. Several cohort and meta-analysis studies have been conducted at the request of the FDA to further evaluate these risks, and results have been conflicting. An observational follow-up of the PROactive clinical trial showed a trend in the risk of bladder cancer related to the duration of use and cumulative dose of pioglitazone. In 2016, the FDA updated its prescribing information, stating that "Pioglitazone may increase the risk of bladder cancer. Do not use in patients with active bladder cancer. Use caution when using in patients with a prior history of bladder cancer."[28,29]

Cardiovascular Safety and Efficacy

The PROactive trial randomized 5,238 patients with type 2 diabetes and clinical cardiovascular disease to 45 mg/day of pioglitazone or placebo. The primary end point, a composite of all-cause mortality, nonfatal myocardial infarction (including silent myocardial infarction), stroke, acute coronary syndrome, endovascular or surgical intervention in the coronary or leg arteries, and amputation above the ankle, fell short of statistical significance (HR 0.90 [CI 0.80–1.02], $P = 0.095$). It is important to note, though, that the main secondary outcome—which has now been established as the standard primary outcome for most cardiovascular outcome studies—was the composite of cardiovascular death, nonfatal myocardial infarction, or nonfatal stroke (three-point MACE). In the trial, MACE was significantly reduced (HR 0.84 [CI 0.72–0.98], $P = 0.027$) with an effect size similar to that seen with SGLT2 inhibitors and GLP-1 RA.[30-32] Additionally, in participants with a prior history of myocardial infarction or stroke, pioglitazone therapy reduced the recurrence of myocardial infarction and stroke by 28% and 47%, respectively. A subsequent trial, IRIS, randomized patients with insulin resistance, but without diabetes, who had a recent ischemic stroke or transient ischemic attack to receive either pioglitazone (target dose, 45 mg daily) or placebo. After a median follow-up of 4.8 years, a statistically significant 24% reduction in fatal and nonfatal myocardial infarction or stroke (HR 0.76 [95% CI 0.62–0.93], $P = 0.007$) was observed. The number needed to treat >4.8 years to prevent one event was estimated at 35.[22]

The RECORD study evaluated the cardiovascular safety of rosiglitazone in patients with type 2 diabetes. The primary outcome was the time to the first occurrence of cardiovascular hospitalization or cardiovascular death. After a mean 5.5 years follow-up, rosiglitazone showed no increase in the primary outcome (HR 0.99 [95% CI 0.85–1.16], $P = 0.93$). Those receiving rosiglitazone had higher rates of heart failure than active comparator (HR 2.1 [95% CI 1.35–3.27], $P = 0.001$); however, there was no statistical difference in the rates of myocardial infarction (HR 1.14 [95% CI 0.80–1.63], $P = 0.47$),[27] putting to rest concerns raised from a previous meta-analysis.[33]

Summary

Glitazones are the only true insulin sensitizers currently available for the treatment of diabetes. They have a robust effect on A1C reduction and lower risk for secondary failure than any other agent used to treat type 2 diabetes; yet the benefits should be weighed against the risks of fluid retention, weight gain, fractures, and the potential (albeit very low) risk of bladder cancer.

SGLT2 INHIBITORS

Mechanism of Action and Glycemic Efficacy

The human kidney filters ~180 g of glucose/day. The amount of glucose reabsorbed in the proximal tubules is directly proportional to the GFR and plasma glucose levels.[34] In the individual without diabetes, the rate at which glucose is filtered is typically lower than the maximum reabsorption capacity of the kidney. As a result, all filtered glucose is reabsorbed in the proximal tubules and no glucose is excreted in the urine.[35] The SGLT2 transporter, which is located in the S1 segment of the proximal tubules, absorbs roughly 80%–90% of the filtered glucose; the remaining glucose is absorbed by the SGLT1 transporter (10%–20%). The SGLT1 transporter is also found in the small intestines and plays a major role in absorption of dietary glucose and galactose.

Individuals with diabetes have an increased ability to reabsorb glucose due to a chronic elevation of plasma glucose that leads to an overexpression of SGLT2 transporters. Consequently, in a maladaptive manner, patients with diabetes reabsorb more glucose than healthy individuals at any level of glycemia.[36] SGLT2 inhibitors block the reabsorption of both glucose and sodium from the proximal tubule of the kidney, thus inducing glycosuria and natriuresis, which ultimately results in a decrease in plasma glucose and sodium.

To date, there are four selective SGLT2 inhibitors approved in the U.S.: empagliflozin, dapagliflozin, canagliflozin, and ertugliflozin. While full inhibition of SGLT1 transport is associated with severe diarrhea, partial intestinal SGLT1 transport blockage translates clinically into slower glucose absorption, modestly increased GLP-1 secretion, and improvement in postprandial hyperglycemia. Sotagliflozin is the first dual inhibitor of SGLT1 and SGLT2, but it currently is still undergoing preapproval evaluation.[37,38]

Treatment with SGLT2 inhibitors typically produces a dose-dependent increase in urinary glucose excretion of ~40–80 g/day. SGLT2 inhibitors reduce A1C by ~0.5%–1.0%. Within the class, canagliflozin 300 mg is regarded as having the most potent glucose-lowering effect; yet there are no head-to-head trials comparing the different SGLT2 inhibitors. In patients with normal renal function, SGLT2 inhibitors improved A1C similarly to metformin[39,40] and similarly or superior to sulfonylurea[41-44] and DPP-4 inhibitors.[45-48] Since the mechanism of action of these drugs does not depend on the degree of insulin resistance or β-cell function, they effectively lower blood glucose in all individuals with type 2 diabetes as long as renal function is preserved. The addition of an SGLT2 inhibitor to insulin-treated patients typically reduces the/an insulin dose by ~50% while still reducing A1C by ~0.8%.[49,50] Of note, glucose lowering with these agents is highly dependent on the baseline A1C as well as renal function; thus, minimal to no glycemic effect is noted in patients with near-normal glycemia or eGFR<45.[51]

Additional Effects

Since gliflozins improve fasting blood glucose, one would expect that SGLT2 inhibition would lead to a reduction in hepatic glucose production; yet chronic use leads to the opposite effect. The blockage of SGLT2 transport, also present in the pancreatic α-cells, leads to a paradoxical rise in glucagon and an increase in endogenous hepatic glucose production. This undesirable effect on the α-cells partially offsets the increase in urinary excretion observed with these drugs.[52] One hypothesis to be explored is whether the concomitant use of a GLP-1 RA, which reduces glucagon levels, can ameliorate this problem and thus enhance the efficacy of these drugs.

Sodium and glucose reabsorption are coupled in the proximal tubule. SGLT2 inhibition causes a natriuresis resulting in a negative salt and water balance, reducing plasma volume and decreasing systolic blood pressure by ≤5 mmHg. This effect is observed within 1–2 weeks of initiation of therapy. The modest reduction in plasma volume following initiation of these drugs results in a small decline in GFR of ~4–5 ml/min/1.73m², which typically returns to baseline over a matter of weeks. There is a growing body of evidence that SGLT2 inhibition protects the kidneys and slows the progression of diabetic nephropathy; it is hypothesized that vasoconstriction of the afferent arteriole decreases intraglomerular pressure, resulting in renoprotection. Angiotensin-converting enzyme inhibitors also reduce intraglomerular pressure and hyperfiltration by inducing vasodilation of efferent renal arterioles. With a complementary mechanism of action, the combination of angiotensin-converting enzyme inhibitors and SGLT inhibitors will likely become the standard of care in treating diabetic nephropathy. This hypothesis has been further validated by several large outcome trials using SGLT2 inhibitors in high-risk populations.[30,32,53–54]

The glycosuria induced by SGLT2 inhibition results in the loss of ~160–320 calories/day, leading to weight loss of ~2.5–3.0 kg. Despite continued glycosuria, the weight loss plateaus because of a paradoxical increase in appetite and caloric intake.[55] Hypothetically, the co-administration with GLP-1 RA might offset the hyperphagia observed with the chronic administration of gliflozins.

SGLT2 inhibitors modestly increase both LDL and HDL cholesterol by 3%–5% and 5%–8%, respectively, without any changes in the HDL/LDL ratio. These changes in lipids are not associated with any adverse outcome.[30,32,56]

Cardiovascular Safety and Efficacy

While tight glycemic control reduced and prevented microvascular complications in patients with type 2 diabetes,[15] its effect on macrovascular disease has been typically modest and took >10 years to become evident.[57] The EMPA-REG Outcome trial was the first large CVOT to show a statistically significant reduction of macrovascular events of a glucose-lowering agent[30] (Table 3.12), a result achieved despite a minimal difference in A1C between treatment groups. This finding suggested that the cardiovascular protective effect of empagliflozin is not mediated through glucose lowering; yet the exact mechanism(s) through which cardioprotection occurs is still not elucidated. Interestingly and then unexpectedly, this trial found that empagliflozin greatly reduced the occurrence of hospitalizations for heart failure and improvement in renal outcomes.

Subsequent cardiovascular outcome studies have largely confirmed these findings (Table 3.12). Interestingly, the macrovascular benefit seen with gliflozins are observed ≥3 months after the initiation of therapy. This finding is in contrast with studies using statins and anti-hypertensive drugs, which showed beneficial effects >1 year on therapy. Several hypotheses suggest that early onset of the beneficial effect of SGLT2 inhibitors on cardiovascular outcomes is not related to the slowing of the atherosclerotic process, but rather due to death related to heart failure (reduction in sudden death due to ventricular arrhythmias). The EMPEROR trials are evaluating the use of empagliflozin in patients with and without diabetes with heart failure and reduced ejection fraction (NCT03057977) and with preserved ejection fraction (NCT03057951) and should provide more information on the

Table 3.12–Cardiovascular and Renal Outcomes Studies Evaluating SGLT2 Inhibitors

Study	EMPA-REG[30,53]	CANVAS[32,58]	DECLARE-TIMI[5856]	CRE-DENCE[‡54]
Drug	Empagliflozin	Canagliflozin	Dapagliflozin	Canagliflozin
n	7,020	10,142	17,160	4,401
A1C (%)	8.1	8.2	8.3	8.3
Age (years)	63	63.3	63.9	63
BMI (kg/m²)	30	32	32	31
Diabetes duration (years)	57% >10 years	13.5	11	15.8
Prior CVD/CHF (%)	99/10	65.6/14.4	40.5/9.9	50.4/14.4
Median follow-up (years)	3.1	2.4	4.2	2.62
Three-point MACE	0.86 (0.74–0.99)†	0.86 (0.75–0.97)†	0.93 (0.84–1.03)†	0.80 (0.67–0.95)
Cardiovascular death	0.62 (0.49–0.77)	0.87 (0.72–1.06)	0.98 (0.82–1.17)	0.78 (0.61–1.0)
Myocardial infarction	0.87 (0.70–1.09)	0.85 (0.69–1.05)	0.89 (0.77–1.01)	NR
Stroke	1.18 (0.89–1.56)	0.90 (0.71–1.15)	1.01 (0.84–1.21)	NR
HF hospitalization	0.65 (0.50–085)	0.67 (0.52–0.87)	0.73 (0.61–0.88)†	0.61 (0.47–0.80)
All-cause mortality	0.68 (0.57–0.82)	0.87 (0.74–1.01)	0.93 (0.82–1.04)	0.83 (0.68–1.02)
Renal composite outcome*	0.54 (0.4–0.75)	0.60 (0.47–0.77)	0.76 (0.67–0.87)	0.70 (0.59–0.82)†

CVD, cardiovascular disease; CHF, chronic heart failure; HF, heart failure; MACE, major cardiovascular events; NR, not reported.

*Renal composite outcomes were as follows: EMPA-REG (post-hoc): doubling of the serum creatinine, initiation of renal-replacement therapy, or death from renal disease; CANVAS: sustained 40% reduction in the eGFR, need for renal-replacement therapy, or death from renal causes; DECLARE-TIMI 58: ≥40% decrease in eGFR to <60 ml/min/1.73 m2, end-stage renal disease, or death from renal or cardiovascular cause; CREDENCE: end-stage kidney disease, a doubling of serum creatinine level, or death from renal or cardiovascular causes.

‡CREDENCE enrolled patients with type 2 diabetes and eGFR 30–90 ml/min/1.73 m² and albumin-to-creatinine ratio of 300–5,000.

†Primary outcome.

issue. With these fairly consistent results among trials, it is safe to conclude that the use of SGLT inhibitors, as a class, can reduce cardiovascular mortality, reduce hospitalization for heart failure, and prevent the progression of kidney disease.

Adverse Effects and Monitoring

SGLT2 inhibitors are generally well-tolerated drugs. In fact, in studies comparing SGLT2 inhibitors with placebo, the proportions of patients who reported adverse events, serious adverse events, and adverse events leading to the discontinuation were similar between groups.[30,32] Genital infection is the most frequently reported adverse effect of gliflozins. About 10% of females and uncircumcised males reported a genital mycotic infection, typically ≤6 months of the initiation of therapy. Those events are typically mild and easy to treat with over-the-counter medications or oral fluconazole, although rare occurrences of necrotizing fasciitis of the perineum (Fournier's gangrene) have been reported post marketing (not different from placebo in the large CVOTs using SGLT2 inhibitors). Urosepsis was rarely seen with gliflozins and was slightly more frequent compared with placebo in the regulatory trials, but not in subsequent CVOTs, nor in a large, real-world study.[59] Overall rates of urinary tract infection, complicated urinary tract infection, or pyelonephritis are similar to placebo. The rates of hypoglycemia, acute renal failure, thromboembolic events, bone fracture, and events consistent with volume depletion were also similar to placebo.

The increase in glucagon in conjunction with the mild hypovolemia induced by these agents creates a proketogenic environment. The incidence of diabetic ketoacidosis (DKA) in patients with type 2 diabetes is rare (1 case for every 500–700 treated patients), but increases two- to fivefold when these agents are used. Most patients who developed DKA while taking an SGLT2 inhibitor had an atypical presentation, often presenting with euglycemic or with only slightly elevated blood glucose levels (mostly <250 mg/dL [<13.9 mmol/l]), resulting in delayed diagnosis and treatment. Many cases have been associated with a missed diagnosis of latent autoimmune diabetes in adults, initiation of ketogenic diet, infection, or a hypovolemic state. This risk of euglycemic DKA, albeit rare, if not promptly recognized can result in severe complications, prolonged hospitalizations, and even death. Therefore, when prescribing an SGLT2 inhibitor, providers should advise patients against initiations of ketogenic diets, discuss symptoms of DKA, ask patients to hold the SGLT2 inhibitor during acute illness, and encourage maintenance of good hydration. We recommend holding SGLT2 inhibitors 2 days prior to planned surgery, to minimize the risk of peri-operative DKA. A recent publication proposes a neumonic (STOP DKA) for the management of SGLT2-induced ketosis, outlining practical steps patients and physicians can take to prevent deterioration into metabolic acidosis.[60]

Currently, the FDA recommends using SGLT2 inhibitors only if eGFR is >45 mL/min/1.73 m² due to their reduced effect on glycemic control at lower eGFR (Fig. 3.1). But in light of the recent evidence of renal and cardiovascular efficacy at even lower eGFR states, it is anticipated that the approved eGFR cutoff will decrease to >30 mL/min/1.73 m², at least when primarily used for treatment of chronic kidney disease or prevention of macrovascular events, especially those related to heart failure.

SGLT2 inhibitors should be started cautiously in frail patients with severe hyperglycemia, those with impaired renal function, or those on high-dose diuretics or drugs acting on the renin-angiotensin-aldosterone pathway. These patients might be at higher risk for acute adverse events related to the osmotic diuresis associated with these drugs. In such patients, clinicians can start the gliflozins at a lower dose, reduce the dose of diuretic and/or angiotensin receptor blocker/ angiotensin-converting enzyme inhibitors, instruct patients to monitor for symptoms of hypovolemia (reduced urine output/dizziness), and consider measuring renal function in 1–2 weeks after initiation. As previously stated, the initial drop in eGFR commonly seen with the initiation of an SGLT2 inhibitor corrects by itself over the course of several weeks. In CREDENCE, which enrolled patients with diabetic nephropathy, use of canagliflozin was not associated with an increase in acute kidney injury.[54]

An increased risk of fracture and amputation was observed with canagliflozin in the CANVAS program. This risk was not confirmed in the subsequent CREDENCE trial and was not observed in any other SGLT2 inhibitor trials. Until more clarification is available in the possible risk for amputation, providers should consider factors that may increase the risk of amputation, such as a history of neuropathy, peripheral vascular disease, diabetic foot ulcers, and prior amputation before the initiation of canagliflozin.[32,54,61]

Summary

SGLT2 inhibitors' glucose-lowering effect is comparable to that of DPP-4 inhibitors. Their glucose-lowering efficacy is related to renal function and is uniquely independent of the duration of diabetes and β-cell function. SGLT2 inhibitors induce weight loss, decrease blood pressure, and have beneficial effects on renal and cardiovascular outcomes. They are well tolerated, dosed orally once daily, and do not cause hypoglycemia. They are approved for use as monotherapy and add on to any other antihyperglycemic agent, including insulin. The American College of Clinical Endocrinology positions SGLT2 inhibitors and/or GLP-1 as the preferred second-line therapy, after metformin, for most patients with type 2 diabetes who can afford these agents. The American Diabetes Association recommends SGLT2 inhibitors as the preferred second-line agent (after metformin) in those with heart failure or chronic kidney disease (Fig. 3.2). It also positions an SGLT2i and/or GLP-1RA as the preferred second-line agent in those with established atherosclerotic cardiovascular disease.[8,20]

GLP-1 RAs

Mechanism of Action and Glycemic Efficacy

GLP-1 is an incretin hormone secreted in response to food intake in the intestinal enteroendocrine L-cells as well as neurons within the nucleus of the solitary tract in the brainstem. GLP-1 exerts its action by binding to the GLP-1 receptors, and it's rapidly degraded by the DPP-4 enzyme. GLP-1 exerts pleiotropic effects across multiple organs, including stimulation of insulin secretion in a glucose-dependent manner, suppression of glucagon secretion, delay in gastric emptying, reduction in appetite, and increase in satiety, all of which improve glucose metabolism.[63] DPP-4 activity is thought to be increased in obese patients with type 2 diabetes, attenuating the response of native GLP-1 and GIP.[63]

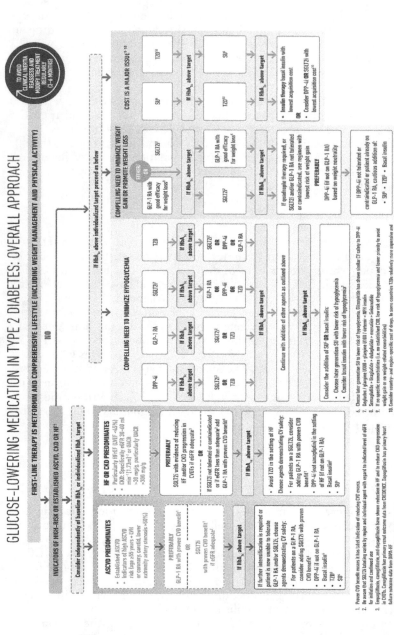

Figure 3.2 American Diabetes Association recommendations regarding initiating and advancing pharmacologic therapy for type 2 diabetes.

ASCVD, atherosclerotic cardiovascular disease; CKD, chronic kidney disease; CVD, cardiovascular disease; DPP-4, dipeptidyl-peptidase-4; eGFR, estimated glomerular filtrate rate; GLP-1 RAs, glucagon-like peptide 1 receptor agonists; HF, heart failure; SGLT2i, sodium–glucose cotransporter 2 inhibitor; SU, sulfonylurea ;TZD, thiazolidinedione.

Source: Adapted from Buse 62.

Two pharmacologic approaches have been developed to harness the incretin pathway for the treatment of type 2 diabetes: DPP-4 inhibitors, which slow the degradation of the native active GLP-1 and therefore lead to a physiologic increase in the GLP-1 level, and GLP-1 RAs, which directly activate the GLP-1 receptors and therefore lead to pharmacologic levels of GLP-1 action.

The first agent within the GLP-1 RA class, approved by FDA in 2005, was exenatide, and since then six additional agents were brought to market (Table 3.11). The GLP-1 RAs are considered the most heterogeneous of the glucose-lowering classes from several standpoints. Structurally, some are extendin based (i.e., exenatide, lixisenatide), while others are based on the native GLP-1 molecule (liraglutide, semaglutide, albiglutide, dulaglutide); some have a small molecular weight (exenatide, liraglutide, lixisenatide, semaglutide), while others have a much larger molecular weight (dulaglutide, albiglutide). Their duration of action, and therefore frequency of administration, also varies greatly, from exenatide and lixisenatide (which only last for a few hours) to liraglutide (which is administered daily) and dulaglutide, albiglutide, exenatide ER, and semaglutide (which are all administered weekly). Most importantly, their clinical efficacy to lower glucose also varies significantly from product to product as demonstrated by head-to-head trials.[64-66] Liraglutide led to greater A1C reduction compared with exenatide, exenatide ER, and albiglutide, and it was similar to dulaglutide,[64] while semaglutide was superior to both exenatide ER[66] and dulaglutide.[65] The average A1C lowering expected with these agents ranged from 0.8% to 1.8%, making the GLP-1 RAs the most effective glucose-lowering class next to insulin.

Table 3.13 contains practical information regarding the clinical use of GLP-1 RAs. Currently most agents in this class are administered subcutaneously in the abdomen, thigh, or upper arm. The two short-acting agents (exenatide and lixisenatide) are to be administered 60 min prior to meals, while all other agents are administered independent of mealtime. Several oral GLP-1 RAs are currently under investigation, with one of them—semaglutide—approved in 2019 and available in tablet form for prescription.

Of note, the combination of DPP-4 inhibitors and GLP-1 RAs has been shown to be safe[67]; their combination is not recommended since GLP-1 RAs are resistant to degradation by DPP-4 inhibitors. Therefore, there is little, if any, added value to using this expensive combination.

Additional Effects

There are several advantages to the GLP-1 RA class. First, the insulin stimulation caused by GLP-1 RAs is glucose dependent, which means that the risk of hypoglycemia is minimal and mainly occurs in settings where these agents are combined with either insulin or sulfonylureas—which increase insulin levels irrespective of prevailing glucose.

Second, they promote weight loss. The mechanisms through which these agents promote weight loss is not fully understood, but it is thought to be primarily through direct central effects that promote satiety.[63] Other mechanisms, including delayed gastric emptying and the associated nausea, have a minimal contribution. Weight loss is also highly variable with the various agents in this class. Agents like exenatide and albiglutide have shown modest effects of ≤1–3 kg weight

Table 3.13–Practical Consideration for the Clinical Use of GLP-1 Receptor Agonists

Generic name/ Brand name	Approved doses	Administration frequency	Titration scheme	Device
Exenatide/ Byetta	10 µg	Twice daily	5 µg × 1 month → 10 µg	Multidose pen
Lixisenatide‡/ Adlyxin*	20 µg	Daily	10 µg × 2 weeks → 20 µg	Multidose pens 150 µg/3 ml and 300 µg/3 ml
Liraglutide/ Victoza	1.8 mg	Daily	0.6 mg × 1 week → 1.2 mg × 1 week → 1.8 mg	Multidose pen 18 mg/3 ml
Albiglutide/ Tanzeum*	30 mg 50 mg	Weekly	None	Single-dose pens 30 mg and 50 mg
Exenatide ER/ Bydureon	2 mg	Weekly	None	Single-dose pens 2 mg
Dulaglutide/ Trulicity	0.75 mg 1.5 mg	Weekly	None	Single-dose pens 0.75 mg and 1.5 mg
Semaglutide/ Ozempic	0.5 mg 1.0 mg	Weekly	0.25 mg × 4 → 0.5 mg × 4 → 1 mg	Multidose pens 2 mg/1.5 ml
Semaglutide/ Rybelsus	3 mg 7 mg 14 mg	Daily	3 mg × 1 month → 7 mg × 1 month → 14 mg	None (tablet taken by mouth)

*No longer marketed.

‡At this time, only marketed as fixed-dose combination with lantus insulin (lantus 100 units/lixisenatide 33 µg = Soliqua 100/33).

loss, while liraglutide and semaglutide have a more pronounced effect with observed weight loss ranging from 3 kg to 6.5 kg in various clinical trials. In fact, liraglutide (at a dose of 3.0 mg/day) is also licensed for the treatment of obesity, and semaglutide (at a dose of 2.4 mg/week) is currently undergoing preapproval evaluation for an obesity indication. In SUSTAIN 7, a 40-week head-to-head trial comparing semaglutide 0.5 mg/week and 1.0 mg/week to dulaglutide 0.75 mg/week and 1.5 mg/week, weight decreased by an average of 4.6 kg with semaglutide 0.5 mg/week compared with 2.3 kg with dulaglutide 0.75 mg/week and by 6.5 kg with semaglutide 1.0 mg/week compared with 3.0 kg with dulaglutide 1.5 mg/week.[65]

These agents also have a modest beneficial effect on total cholesterol and LDL and have been shown to reduce blood pressure by 1–5 mmHg.

Liraglutide may improve nonalcoholic steatohepatitis, probably driven by weight loss, insulin sparing effects, and its anti-inflammatory effects; semaglutide is currently under investigation seeking a label indication for nonalcoholic steatohepatitis.[68]

Side-Effect Profile

The most common adverse events associated with these agents are gastrointestinal in nature. Nausea is the most frequent of these, having been reported in 10%–40% of individuals; followed by vomiting (5%–20%); and less commonly diarrhea, constipation, abdominal discomfort, and dyspepsia. These symptoms usually occur upon initiation and titration of therapy, tend to be mild or moderate in severity, but most importantly improve with continuous use. Several agents have a recommended titration schedule (Table 3.13) intended to minimize the gastrointestinal side effects. Decreasing food intake may decrease the risk of gastrointestinal symptoms or hasten their resolution.

Other side effects are much less common or only theoretical. Personal or family history of medullary thyroid carcinoma or multiple endocrine neoplasia syndrome type 2 are contraindications because medullary thyroid carcinoma has occurred during preclinical testing in rodents. An excess risk of medullary thyroid carcinoma has not been observed in any clinical trials to date, nor in ≥14 years of clinical experience since the first agent in this class has been approved.

Whether these agents increase the risk of pancreatitis has been highly debated, but recent evidence from large placebo-controlled clinical trials which blindly adjudicated each suspicious event has not supported the initial concern.[69] Nevertheless, should pancreatitis occur while taking these agents, they should be promptly discontinued.

Acute kidney injury has been reported in a few cases, usually in the setting of severe adverse gastrointestinal reactions with dehydration. Prompt treatment of severe gastrointestinal symptoms and associated dehydration should prevent such events.

No dose adjustment is recommended for any GLP-1 RA for patients with renal impairment (Fig. 3.1). Liraglutide, dulaglutide, and semaglutide can be used in end-stage renal disease, with close monitoring for adverse events. Exenatide and exenatide ER are not recommended in individuals with eGFR <30 mL/min/1.73 m^2, and lixisenatide is not recommended in individuals with eGFR <15 mL/min/1.73 m^2 (Fig. 3.1).

Injection site reactions are rare, except for exenatide ER, which can cause subcutaneous nodules at the injection site that tend to resolve over a course of 4–8 weeks.

A small increase in heart rate (1–6 bpm) has been noted with all GLP-1 RAs, but this has not been associated with a deleterious cardiovascular effect.

Cardiovascular Safety

The cardiovascular safety of this class has been unequivocally established based on seven cardiovascular outcome studies which have been completed to date (Table 3.14). In fact, several of these agents (liraglutide, albiglutide, dulaglutide, and semaglutide) were able to demonstrate a beneficial effect by significantly lowering the occurrence of MACE, including myocardial infarction, stroke, and cardiovascular death. Based on the findings in these studies, the current treatment guidelines recommend using GLP-1 RAs with a proven cardiovascular benefit as a second-line glucose-lowering agent (after metformin) in patients with type 2 diabetes and preexistent cardiovascular disease.

Summary

GLP-1 RAs are the most effective glucose-lowering agents, have the most potent weight-loss effect amongst glucose-lowering agents, and have a low risk of hypoglycemia. In addition, several agents in this class have shown significant reduction in cardiovascular disease. Thus, GLP-1 RAs are currently recommended as second-line agents (after metformin) for patients with atherosclerotic cardiovascular disease, as well as those in whom weight loss and hypoglycemia prevention are desirable.

DPP-4 INHIBITORS

Mechanism of Action and Glycemic Efficacy

The incretin hormones, glucose-dependent insulinotropic polypeptide (GIP) and glucagon-like peptide (GLP-1), are released by the gut in response to food and are rapidly inactivated by the enzyme DPP-4. GLP-1, which is released from the ileum and colon, stimulates insulin release in a glucose-dependent manner, inhibits glucagon in a glucose-dependent manner, delays gastric emptying, reduces appetite, and promotes satiety. GIP, released by the duodenum, is also responsible for stimulation of insulin release from pancreatic β-cells and may promote β-cell proliferation and survival. DPP-4 activity is thought to be increased in obese patients with type 2 diabetes, attenuating the response of native GLP-1 and GIP.[75]

DPP-4 inhibitors block degradation of native GLP-1, thus increasing its bioavailability and lowering A1C by ~0.4%–0.8%; sitagliptin, saxagliptin, linagliptin, and alogliptin have all been FDA approved.

Side-Effect Profile

DPP-4 inhibitors are well tolerated with only occasional or rare reports of nausea, vomiting, diarrhea, flu-like symptoms, arthralgias, and skin reactions.[75] DPP-4 inhibitors have substantially fewer gastrointestinal issues compared with GLP-1 RAs.[76] They have low hypoglycemic risk, although this does increase when used in combination with insulin or secretagogues, and they do not induce weight gain. There have been some concerns of pancreatitis induced by DPP-4 inhibitor use; however, a meta-analysis including 134 trials showed no significant increase of pancreatitis with DPP-4 inhibitor use.[76] Bullous pemphigoid is an acquired autoimmune blistering disease and has been associated with several DPP-4 inhibitors.[77] Annual, estimated incidence of bullous pemphigoid ranges between 2.4 and 21.7 new cases per million population.[78] Bullous pemphigoid has been reported a median of 2.25 years (range 9 months to 5 years) after initiating DPP-4 inhibitor therapy and is primarily seen in elderly, male patients. More reports have been associated with vildagliptin, but cases have also been linked with linagliptin and sitagliptin. If patients present with a blistering skin disease while taking DPP-4 inhibitors, the DPP-4 inhibitor should be stopped and patients referred to dermatology. In more recent years, several clinical cases have reported possible associations with DPP-4 inhibitor use and the onset of arthritis/arthralgias. In a systematic review and meta-analysis of >79,000 patients, DPP-4 inhibitors were associated with a slightly but significantly increased risk of overall arthralgia (relative ratio [RR] 1.13 [95% CI 1.04–1.22]) and a nonsignificant increased risk of serious arthralgia.[78]

Table 3.14–Cardiovascular Outcome Studies Evaluating GLP-1 RAs

Study	ELIXA[70]	LEADER[31]	SUSTAIN 6[71]	EXSCEL[67]	Harmony[72]	PIONEER 6[73]	REWIND[74]
Drug	Lixisenatide	Liraglutide	Semaglutide sq	Exenatide ER	Albiglutide	Semaglutide oral	Dulaglutide
n	6,068	9,340	3,297	14,752	9,463	3,183	9,901
Age (years)	60	64	65	63 (median)	64	66	66
Duration of diabetes (years)		12.8	13.9			14.9	10.5
BMI (kg/m^2)	30	33	33	32 (median)	32	32.3	32
A1C (%)	7.7	8.7	8.7	8.0 (median)	8.7	8.2	7.3
Prior CVD (%)	100	72.4	72.2	73	100	84.7	31
Median follow-up (years)	2.1	3.8	2.1	3.2	1.6	1.4	5.4
Event rate* (%/year) Active/placebo	6.4/6.3‡	3.4/3.9	3.1/4.2	3.7/4.0	4.6/5.9	3.8/4.8	2.35/2.66
HR (95% CI)*	1.02 (0.89–1.17)	0.87 (0.78–0.97)	0.74 (0.58–0.95)	0.91 (0.83–1.0)	0.78 (0.68–0.90)	0.79 (0.57–1.11)	0.88 (0.79–0.99)

CVD, cardiovascular disease; HR, hazard ratio.

*Primary outcome was three-point MACE (major cardiovascular events = first occurrence of myocardial infarction, stroke, or cardiovascular death), except for ELIXA, where it was ‡four-point MACE (three-point MACE plus unstable angina).

DPP-4 inhibitors are dosed once daily, independent of meals. The renal dosing for agents in this class varies and is summarized in Fig. 3.1. Linagliptin is the only DPP-4 inhibitor that does not require dose adjustment for patients with low renal function. Sitagliptin may be used at the lowest dosage in hemodialysis or peritoneal dialysis without regard to timing of dialysis. Neither saxagliptin nor alogliptin have been studied in peritoneal dialysis but may be used at the lowest dosage in hemodialysis. It is recommended to administer saxagliptin postdialysis and alogliptin without regard to timing of dialysis.

Sitagliptin and linagliptin are not extensively metabolized by the liver, and no dosage adjustments are necessary for mild to moderate liver impairment. Saxagliptin is metabolized by the liver, mainly through the isoenzyme CYP3A4, and the dose should be reduced when used with concomitant strong CYP3A4 inhibitors. Alogliptin has minimal hepatic metabolism via CYP2D6 and CYP3A4 and may be used in mild to moderate hepatic impairment. If clinically significant liver enzyme elevation occurs postalogliptin initiation, therapy should be suspended and a cause investigated, but if no cause is found, the DPP-4 inhibitor should not be resumed.

Cardiovascular Safety

To date four cardiovascular outcome studies have established the cardiovascular safety of these agents (Table 3.15). These randomized, double-blinded, placebo-controlled trials enrolled a total of ~50,000 patients, evaluating cardiovascular safety in patients with type 2 diabetes at high risk for or with a prior cardiovascular event.[79] The key results are summarized in Table 3.15. An unexpected safety signal regarding an increase in the risk of heart failure hospitalization was observed in the SAVOR-TIMI 53 study with saxagliptin, but not in the other studies. These findings did result in an FDA drug safety communication issued for saxagliptin and alogliptin for their potential to increase the risk of heart failure, especially in patients with underlying heart and kidney disease.

Summary

DPP-4 inhibitors are reasonable adjunctive therapy options when minimizing hypoglycemia risk and weight gain are important considerations. Robust cardiovascular outcomes studies have proven the safety of these agents but have not demonstrated any superiority in MACE outcomes.

OTHER GLUCOSE-LOWERING CLASSES

Centrally Acting Agents

The circadian rhythm of dopamine release is believed to play a role in the regulation of peripheral insulin sensitivity, and glucose and lipid metabolism.[84] Bromocriptine quick-release (QR) is a dopamine D_2 receptor agonist which has been associated with a reduction in fasting and postprandial glucose levels through a dampening of sympathetic tone. It has minimal effect on A1C, lowering levels ~0.3%. It is extensively metabolized by the liver, mainly through CYP3A4 isoenzymes, and should be administered with food to increase the bioavailability.[85] It is minimally excreted via the kidneys.

Table 3.15—Cardiovascular Outcomes Studies Evaluating DPP-4 Inhibitors

	SAVOR-TIMI 53[80]	EXAMINE[81]	TECOS[82]	CARMELINA[83]	CAROLINA[17]
Drug§	Saxagliptin	Alogliptin	Sitagliptin	Linagliptin	Linagliptin
n	16,492	5,380	14,617	6,979	6033
Age (years)	65.1	61	65.5	65.9	64.0
BMI (kg/m^2)	31.2	28.7	30.2	31.4	30.1
A1C (%)	8.0	8.0	7.2	8.0	7.2
Prior CVD (%)	78.6	100	74	58.5†	42
Median follow-up (years)	2.1	1.5	3.0	2.2	6.3
Event rate* (%/year) Active/placebo	3.48/3.43	7.53/7.87	4.06/4.17	5.64/5.50	1.87/1.90
HR (95% CI)*	1.00 (0.89–1.12)	0.96 (≤1.16)	0.98 (0.89–1.08)	1.02 (0.89–1.17)	0.98 (0.84–1.14)
Heart failure hospitalization HR (95% CI)	1.27 (1.07–1.51)	1.19 (0.89–1.59)	1.00 (0.83–1.20)	0.90 (0.74–1.08)	1.21(0.92–1.59)

CVD, cardiovascular disease; HR, hazard ratio.

*Primary end point three-point MACE (cardiovascular death, nonfatal myocardial infarction, or nonfatal stroke) for all studies except TECOS, where the primary end point was four-point MACE (three-point MACE or unstable angina requiring hospitalization).

‡EXAMINE—only enrolled patients 15–90 days after an acute coronary event.

†CARMELINA - prior CVD not reported, instead ischemic heart disease is provided.

§All comparators were placebo except for CAROLINA where it was glimepiride.

Bromocriptine-QR should be initiated at 0.8 mg in the morning upon awakening with food and increased weekly, in order to mitigate potential side effects, until a maximal tolerated dose is achieved (≤4.8 mg daily). No renal or hepatic adjustments are required; however, caution should be exercised in patients with severe hepatic dysfunction due to bromocriptine's extensive hepatic metabolism. It is contraindicated in women who are breastfeeding and should be avoided in patients with psychiatric disorders due to its effects on dopamine. Nausea, vomiting, headache, dizziness, hypotension, and fatigue are the most commonly reported adverse effects in clinical trials, and occur in up to one-third of patients in clinical practice.[85]

The impact of bromocriptine-QR on major adverse cardiovascular outcomes (MACE) was evaluated in a 52-week study in which 3,070 patients were randomized 2:1 to bromocriptine-QR or placebo. A total of 14 MACE events occurred in the bromocriptine-QR arm compared with 15 events in the placebo arm, resulting in a 52% relative risk reduction (HR 0.48 [95% CI 0.23–1.00]).[86] While these results are reassuring regarding cardiovascular safety, there were very few events observed, thus precluding any definitive conclusions regarding the cardiovascular efficacy of this agent. Bromocriptine-QR has also been associated with a mild decrease in triglycerides, blood pressure, and heart rate.[87]

Bile Acid Sequestrant

Colesevelam is a second-generation, nonabsorbed bile acid sequestrant that was approved in January 2008 as adjunctive therapy to diet and exercise in patients with type 2 diabetes; however, the mechanism for improving glycemic control is not well understood. It provides an A1C reduction of ~0.5% in addition to a dose-dependent reduction of LDL-C of ~15%. Triglyceride elevations are also seen in a dose-dependent manner and increase ~5%–10% from baseline.[88] HDL changes are negligible.

Colesevelam is administered at a dose of 1,875 mg twice daily with meals or 3,750 mg once daily with a meal. It does not require dosage adjustments in renal or hepatic insufficiency. The most common adverse effects are gastrointestinal in nature and include constipation, flatulence, and dyspepsia.[89] It should not be used in patients with gastrointestinal obstruction or severe motility disorders and is contraindicated in patients with triglyceride levels >500 mg/dl or in patients with a history of pancreatitis.[89]

Amylin Agonist

Amylin is a neuroendocrine hormone synthesized and co-secreted with insulin by pancreatic β-cells, although it can be found in several other tissues. Like insulin, amylin plasma concentrations are lower in the fasting state and rise in response to caloric intake.[90] Fasting amylin concentrations are low in patients with insulin deficiency (e.g., type 1 diabetes) and have no significant response after carbohydrate ingestion. On the other hand, in patients with impaired glucose control, amylin levels rise and remain elevated 2 h post ingestion of carbohydrate, an abnormal response compared with healthy adult patients with normal glycemic control.[90] Amylin's role in glucose homeostasis is thought to occur through suppression of glucagon secretion via a glucose-dependent mechanism, slowing gastric emptying and increasing satiety.[91,92]

Pramlintide was developed as a soluble, stable synthetic analog of human amylin. It is indicated for use in type 1 diabetes and insulin-treated patients with type 2 diabetes for mealtime subcutaneous injection. In patients with type 1 diabetes on basal-bolus therapy, the use of pramlintide compared with placebo resulted in an A1C reduction of 0.4%–0.6% and mean body weight reduction of 0.8–1.3 kg.[90] In a single study, pramlintide also resulted in decreased postprandial glucose excursions and a reduction in prandial insulin doses compared with placebo.[90] Pramlintide is initiated at 15 µg subcutaneously immediately before each main carbohydrate-containing meal. The dose may be titrated every 3 days ≤60 µg.

In patients with type 2 diabetes, pramlintide has been evaluated in conjunction with basal-bolus insulin and premix insulin therapies. Similar to studies in type 1 diabetes, the amylin analog resulted in A1C reductions of 0.7%–0.8% and mean body weight reductions of 1.4–1.6 kg.[90] Initial starting doses in type 2 diabetes treatment are 60 µg immediately before each carbohydrate-containing meal and can be titrated, no sooner than every 3 days, to a maximal dose of 120 µg three times daily before meals.

Nausea, vomiting, reduced appetite, and headache are the most common adverse effects and increase in severity with increasing dosage. To minimize adverse effects, doses should be titrated slowly or may be introduced sequentially with one meal and increased to three meals daily. In patients experiencing continued adverse effects, doses should be decreased to the maximally tolerated dose. The risk of hypoglycemia is increased when pramlintide is used concurrently with insulin and is more common in patients with type 1 diabetes. Insulin doses should be reduced by 50% when initiating pramlintide with subsequent insulin titration based on blood glucose values (ideally postprandial readings). Patients should be educated to use glucose tablets or gel for hypoglycemia treatment rather than a carbohydrate source that is absorbed by the gut. Pramlintide will not affect counterregulatory hormones or symptomatic responses to insulin-induced hypoglycemia. Due to its effect on gastric emptying, patients should be aware that delayed absorption of oral medications can occur, including antibiotics and oral contraceptives. Administration of these medications should be given 1 h prior or 2 h post injection of pramlintide.

AGIs

AGIs such as acarbose and miglitol delay carbohydrate absorption from the small intestine by competitively inhibiting α-glucosidase, an enzyme found in the brush border of the small intestine.[93,94] Delaying the absorption of complex carbohydrate results in reduced postprandial glucose and serum insulin levels. The hydrolysis of oligosaccharides and disaccharides to glucose and fructose is reduced, but there is no effect on lactose. AGIs reduce A1C ~0.5%–0.8% and are indicated for treatment in combination with diet or other antidiabetic agents but are not generally viewed as first-line agents unless other pharmacologic agents are contraindicated.[93]

There are a few dissimilarities between acarbose and miglitol. Miglitol is almost completely absorbed in the upper small intestine and is associated with a dose-dependent decrease in A1C lowering, whereas acarbose is not.[93] To achieve their glucose-lowering effects, AGIs must be taken immediately before meals. A program analogous to that described with metformin should be initiated starting with the smallest available dosage once daily with the first bite of the largest meal.

Every 2–4 weeks, an additional tablet can be added until the drug is taken three times daily before meals. Maximal effective doses are generally one-half of the maximal indicated dosage. There are no recommendation for dosage adjustment in renal impairment; however, if serum creatinine is >2 mg/dL or creatinine clearance is <25 mL/min, use is not recommended.

The major adverse effects are flatulence, abdominal distress, or distension and diarrhea.[94,95] Adverse effects are dose dependent and, similarly to metformin, are present at the onset of treatment but decline with continued use or reduction in dosage. These adverse symptoms result from the excessive blockade of carbohydrate absorption in the small bowel, leading to fermentation and gas production in the colon. Intestinal distension or diarrhea may be harmful in the presence of inflammatory bowel disease or other major intestinal disorders, and use in this patient population should be avoided. Hypoglycemia in patients on AGIs should be treated with glucose gel or tablets.

Acarbose has been evaluated in patients with coronary heart disease; however, a large study of >6,500 Chinese patients did not find reduction in the primary five-point MACE end point (HR 0.98 [CI 0.86–1.11]).[79]

INSULINS

Mechanism of Action and Glycemic Efficacy

Insulin has been used therapeutically for nearly one century. Insulin works by suppressing hepatic glucose production and increasing glucose uptake by insulin-sensitive tissues, notably muscle and adipose tissue. The improved glycemic control achieved with insulin therapy also increases the responsiveness of tissues to insulin. Insulin should have unlimited efficacy to reduce plasma glucose. If taken properly in sufficient amounts, it should normalize blood glucose from any baseline level.

Insulin preparations are generally categorized as basal insulin types, prandial or corrective insulin formulations, or mixed (i.e., premix or fixed-ratio combination [FRC]) insulin preparations. Basal insulins are meant to suppress hepatic glucose production and control glycemia during periods of fasting and in-between meals; available preparations include NPH (neutral protamine hagedorn), glargine U100 and detemir U100 (first-generation basal analogs), and degludec U100 or U200 and glargine U300 (second-generation basal analogs). The overarching characteristic of these preparations is the slowing of absorption from the subcutaneous depot, which prolongs biologic action, flattens peak action of the insulin, and results in a more consistent pharmacodynamic profile. NPH insulin is considered an intermediate-acting insulin, while second-generation basal analogs have an extended biologic profile compared with first-generation basal analogs (Table 3.16).

Prandial or corrective insulin preparations are designed to control postprandial glycemia and "correct" or lower blood glucose levels when they exceed target values. Available preparations in order of slowest to fastest preparations are regular insulin U100, first-generation prandial analogs such as aspart U100, lispro U100 or U200, and glulisine U100, Faster Insulin Aspart (FIASP), and inhaled insulin (Technosphere insulin). Modifications to the regular insulin molecule, eccipients, or delivery method result in faster absorption, earlier biologic peak, and shorter duration of action (Table 3.16).

Table 3.16–Insulin Products: Pharmacokinetics and Pharmacodynamics

Insulin	Onset	Peak	Duration (h)
Inhaled insulin			
Technosphere	12 min	35–55 min	1.5–4.5
Ultra rapid-acting insulin			
Fast-acting aspart	2.5 min	50–70 min	3–5
Rapid-acting insulin			
Lispro Aspart Glulisine	5–20 min	30–90 min	3–5
Short-acting insulin			
Regular U100	30 min	2–4 h	5–8
Intermediate-acting insulin			
NPH	1–3 h	4–12 h	18–24
Long-acting insulin			
Detemir Glargine	1h	Relative flat	≤24
Ultra long-acting insulin			
Glargine (U300) Degludec (U100, U200)	1–6 h	Relative flat	36–42
Mixed insulin			
NPH/regular mix 70/30	30–60 min	3–6 h	12–24
Analog mixed insulin			
Lispro mix 50/50 Lispro mix 75/25 Aspart mix 70/30	5–20 min	2–4 h	16–24
Concentrated insulin			
U500 regular	30 min	4–8 h	≤24, depending on amount

There is high interindividual variability, and patient-specific onset, peak, and duration may vary from times listed in table. Peak and duration are dose dependent, with longer duration of actions typically seen with large doses.

Source: Adapted from 2019 Consumer Guide. *Diabetes Forecast* March/April 2019.

Insulins used today are no longer extracted from the pancreases of cattle and pigs. Instead they are produced by genetically altered bacteria or yeast and are structurally identical to human insulin. Several insulin analogs are also available, in which amino acid substitutions and/or additions produce insulins with altered pharmacokinetics upon subcutaneous injection. The three rapid-acting insulin analogs—lispro, aspart, and glulisine—have undergone modifications to the insulin molecule that reduce the tendency to form dimers and hexamers, resulting in more rapid absorption after subcutaneous injection compared with regular insulin. Once injected, they start working within 15 min, peak in 60–90 min, and are effective for ~4–6 h. Of note is that all subcutaneously injected insulin preparations (whether basal or prandial) have a dose-dependent pharmacokinetic and pharmacodynamic profile, where larger insulin doses result in higher peaks of biologic activity and a longer duration of action. These rapid-acting insulin analogs are associated with a somewhat lower risk of hypoglycemia with similar or slightly greater improvements in A1C compared with regular insulin. Two additional and even faster-acting preparations have been approved in the U.S.: FIASP and inhaled Technosphere insulin (Afrezza) (Table 3.16 and 3.17). FIASP is actually aspart insulin with the addition of nicotinamide and L-arginine hydrochloride, which accelerates insulin absorption and results in greater insulin action within the first 1–2 h after the meal injection. FIASP has FDA indications for administration either at the start of a meal or within 20 min after starting a meal. Afrezza is by far the insulin with the fastest onset and shortest duration of action, capitalizing on the rapid absorption of the insulin powder into the alveolar circulation. Using a small whistle-like inhaler device to deliver insulin to the pulmonary tree, patients administer one or more prefilled 4-unit, 8-unit, and 12-unit cartridges to match their prandial and corrective insulin needs. Afrezza should not be used in patients with chronic lung disease, such as asthma or chronic obstructive pulmonary disease, or in smokers; furthermore, it requires pulmonary function test monitoring prior to starting therapy and periodically thereafter.

The evolution of longer-acting basal insulin analogs has produced insulin preparations that have efficacy in lowering A1C and fasting plasma glucose similar to immediate predecessors. Their advantage is due to their flatter, more prolonged, and more consistent biologic action that translates into a lower risk of overall and nocturnal hypoglycemia. For example, glargine U100 and detemir insulin are associated with less hypoglycemia (especially nocturnal) than NPH insulin, while glargine U300 and degludec have an even safer hypoglycemia profile than glargine U100 itself.[96] In most patients with type 2 diabetes, all basal insulin preparations can be dosed once daily in the evening; on the other hand, for patients with type 1 diabetes (or other insulin-sensitive patients with insulin deficiency) some of the basal preparations are safer and more effective when dosed twice daily (b.i.d.); these include NPH insulin, detemir insulin, and to some extent glargine U100 insulin. There are other subtle differences between basal insulin preparations that should be noted. Insulin detemir has been associated with less weight gain (1–2 kg difference) compared with glargine U100 or NPH insulin.[97] Detemir and glargine U300 require ~10%–15% higher dose (in units) achieve glycemic efficacy similar to that of other insulin preparations. While most basal insulins are interchangeable on a 1:1 ratio when switching between preparations, most product inserts recommend reducing the basal dose by 20% when switching from a b.i.d. formulation to

Table 3.17–Practical Information Regarding Categories of Insulin, Brands, and Packaging

Category/name of insulin	Brand name (manufacturer)	Units/ vials	# Pens/ box × # units/ pen	Observation
		Rapid acting		
Technosphere	Afrezza (Mannkind)		N/A	Inhaled 4-, 8-, and 12-unit cartridges 1 unit of insulin = ~1.5 units of Afrezza
Fast-acting Aspart (U100)	FIASP (Novo Nordisk)	1,000	5 × 300	1-unit increments and max 80-unit dose
Aspart (U100)	Novolog (Novo Nordisk)	1,000	5 × 300	1-unit increments and max 60-unit dose
Lispro (U100)	Admelog (Sanofi-Aventis)	1,000	5 × 300	1-unit increments and max 60-unit dose
Lispro (U100)	Humalog (Lilly)	1,000	5 × 300	1-unit increments and max 60-unit dose
Lispro (U200)	Humalog (Lilly)	2,000	2 × 600	1-unit increments and max 60-unit dose
		Short acting		
Regular human	Humulin R (Lilly)	1,000	N/A	
Regular human	Novolin R (Novo Nordisk) ReliOn Novolin R	1,000	N/A	ReliOn brand sold only at Walmart
		Intermediate acting		
NPH Human (U100)	Humulin N (Lilly)	1,000	5 × 300	1-unit increments and max 60-unit dose
NPH Human (U100)	Novolin N (Novo Nordisk) ReliOn Novolin N	1,000	N/A	ReliOn sold only at Walmart
		Long acting		
Detemir (U100)	Levemir (Novo Nordisk)	1,000	5 × 300	1-unit increments and max 80-unit dose
Glargine (U100)	Lantus (Sanofi-Aventis)	1,000	5 × 300	1-unit increments and max 80-unit dose
Glargine (U100)	Basaglar (Lilly)	1,000	5 × 300	1-unit increments and max 80-unit dose
Glargine (U300)	Toujeo (Sanofi-Aventis)	N/A	3 × 450	2-unit increments and max 80-unit dose

(continued)

Table 3.17 *(continued)*

Category/name of insulin	Brand name (manufacturer)	Units/ vials	# Pens/ box × # units/ pen	Observation
Glargine (U300)	Toujeo max (Sanofi-Aventis)	N/A	2 × 900	2-unit increments and max 160-unit dose
Degludec (U100)	Tresiba (Novo Nordisk)	N/A	5 × 300	1-unit increments and max 80-unit dose
Degludec (U200)	Tresiba (Novo Nordisk)	N/A	3 × 600	2-unit increments and max 160-unit dose
Insulin mixtures				
NPH/regular (70%/30%) (U100)	Humulin 70/30 (Lilly)	1,000	5 × 300	1-unit increments and max 60-unit dose
NPH/regular (70%/30%) (U100)	Novolin 70/30 (Novo Nordisk) ReliOn Novolin 70/30	1,000	N/A	1-unit increments and max 60-unit dose ReliOn brand sold only at Walmart
Protamine/lispro (50%/50%) (U100)	Humalog Mix 50/50 (Lilly)	1,000	5 × 300	1-unit increments and max 60-unit dose
Protamine/ lispro (75%25%) (U100)	Humalog Mix 75/25 (Lilly)	1,000	5 × 300	1-unit increments and max 60-unit dose
Protamine/ aspart (70%/30%) (U100)	Novolog Mix 70/30 (Novo Nordisk)	1,000	5 × 300	1-unit increments and max 60-unit dose
Ultra-concentrated insulin				
Regular (U500)	Humulin R U500 (Lilly)	5,000	2 × 1,500	5-unit increments and max 300-unit dose for pen use Special syringe available (for vial use)
Insulin/GLP-1 fixed combinations				
Insulin degludec/ liraglutide	Xultophy 100/3.6 (Novo Nordisk)	N/A	5 × 300	1-unit insulin increment and max 50 units insulin/1.8 mg liraglutide per dose
Insulin glargine/ lixisenatide	Soliqua 100/33 (Sanofi)	N/A	5 × 300	1-unit increment and max 60 units insulin and 20 units lixisenatide

once-daily administration. In pregnancy, the only basal preparations approved for use are NPH and detemir insulin, although in type 1 diabetes glargine U100 has been used without reported deleterious issues. For more information on insulin use in pregnancy, see Chapter 4.

Several premix insulin combinations are available in the U.S. They combine an intermediate-acting protamine insulin with a prandial insulin (regular insulin or rapid-acting analog). Outside the U.S., a combination of insulin degludec U100 and aspart insulin is available and has the advantage of a lower risk of hypoglycemia compared with traditional premix formulations. Premix formulations come in a variety of combinations of protaminated to nonprotaminated insulin, including 70/30, 75/25, and 50/50. Advantages of using a premix formulation include a single co-pay and only one insulin preparation to cover both basal and prandial needs. In addition, NPH/regular premix insulin is available over the counter (except in Indiana) and at a much-reduced cost compared with other insulins (at Walmart or other stores when using discount coupons or apps like GoodRx). Premix insulin use, however, is associated with more weight gain and hypoglycemia when compared with basal insulin alone or basal plus one injection of rapid-acting insulin analog. Moreover, patients must adjust their eating schedule to accommodate the NPH peak in order to avoid hypoglycemia. This means ensuring a consistent meal intake at lunch and frequently a small snack at bedtime, which can contribute to additional caloric intake and weight gain.

There are several concentrated insulins on the market which have slightly altered pharmacokinetics compared with the normal (U100) concentration; they are used mainly to facilitate administration and reduce the potential discomfort of patients requiring large insulin doses. For example, in patients requiring >200 units of insulin per day, an option might be to switch them to regular insulin U500, which is associated in many nonrandomized studies with improvement in glycemic control thought to be driven mostly by improved insulin adherence.[98] Regular U500 has a slightly delayed onset, peak, and duration of action compared with regular U100.[99] It is typically administered 45 min prior to a meal and is typically dosed twice daily (50% before breakfast and 50% before dinner) or in patients with the highest insulin dose requirements, three times daily (40% before breakfast, 30% before lunch, and 30% before dinner).

Degludec U200 and lispro U200 have similar insulin pharmacokinetics compared with their U100 counterparts. They are used in patients requiring a higher dose of basal bolus insulin to decrease discomfort associated with high-volume injection.

Insulin/GLP-1 FRCs

There are currently two fixed-ratio insulin/GLP-1 RA combination injectable products approved in the U.S.: insulin degludec/liraglutide (IDegLira or brand name Xultophy) and insulin glargine/lixisenatide (IGlarLixi or brand name Soliqua) (see Table 3.17). Both are only available in a prefilled pen form. There are several studies comparing insulin/GLP-1 fixed combinations against basal insulin, basal plus one, or more prandial insulin doses.[100-103] These studies have shown better glycemic control of FRC compared with basal insulin or GLP-1 RA monotherapy, and similar glycemic control to basal plus one or more prandial insulin injections; the consistent finding has been a mitigation of weight gain from the combination of GLP-1 RA and basal insulin, a lower incidence of gastrointestinal side effects due to the slower uptitration of the FRC dose, and either similar or less hypoglycemia associated with the improvement in A1C. These agents are simple to use, requiring only one shot/day, with doses simply titrated to a fasting blood glucose target. While IGlarLixi (Soliqua) needs to be administered before breakfast, IDegLira (Xultophy) can be given at any time of the day, independent of meal intake. There is currently no head-to-head study comparing the two available FRCs.

The FDA has approved the use of FRC products in patients failing oral agent therapy, or those not well controlled on basal insulin or GLP-1 RA treatment. Insulin degludec/liraglutide (IDegLira) should be started at 10 units for insulin-naïve patients and 16 units (equivalent to 16 units of insulin degludec and 0.6 mg of liraglutide) for those previously on basal insulin. The dose should be titrated biweekly by 2 units based on fasting blood glucose until desirable fasting blood glucose is reached or the maximum deliverable dose is reached (50 units, corresponding to 1.8 mg of liraglutide). Insulin glargine/lixisenatide should be started at 15 units (15 units of glargine and 5 µg of lixisenatide) in those who are insulin naïve or currently taking <30 units of basal insulin and 30 units in those taking >30 units of insulin. The dose should be titrated weekly by 2 units until desirable fasting blood glucose is reached or the maximum deliverable dose is reached (60 units, corresponding to 20 mg of lixisenatide).

Finally, there is no evidence that the FRC are any more effective than the loose (or separate) use of basal insulin with a GLP-1 RA preparation.

Cardiovascular Safety and Efficacy

Despite its undeniable association with hypoglycemia, randomized controlled trials support the cardiovascular safety of insulin therapy.[96,104] UKPDS 33 demonstrated similar cardiovascular disease outcomes in patients treated with insulin versus conventional therapy with the metformin and/or sulfonylurea.[15] The ORIGIN study showed no increased risk of cardiovascular events when insulin glargine U100 was compared with standard of care in patients with prediabetes or newly diagnosed diabetes; similarly the DEVOTE trial showed a comparable cardiovascular safety profile for degludec and glargine.[96,105] While liraglutide (but not lixisenatide) has demonstrated benefits in reducing cardiovascular events in high-risk patients, it is unknown whether these benefits would translate to the FRC of IDegLira.

Adverse Effects and Monitoring

Insulin therapy is associated with weight gain and hypoglycemia. Weight gain with basal insulin is typically between 1 kg and 3 kg, but can be more substantial when prandial therapy is also added. Weight gain is greater when insulin is used in combination with TZDs and/or sulfonylureas. Of note, in basal insulin replacement, exceeding 0.5 units/kg/day results in more weight gain than glycemic benefit.[106]

Risk for hypoglycemia is typically low when basal insulin only is used in combination with GLP-1 RA or agents other than sulfonylureas or glinides. Hypoglycemia with basal insulin can be minimized by using a basal analog instead of NPH, with glargine U300 and degludec insulin carrying the lowest risk of hypoglycemia. Other rare, and quite uncommon, adverse side effects of insulin therapy include skin reactions at injection sites (itching, redness, and swelling) or persistent lumps or swelling at these sites that may represent delayed hypersensitivity reactions. Allergy to insulin is rare, typically mild, usually related to an excipient as opposed to the insulin molecule itself, and can be managed by trying a different insulin product and/or taking an H2 blocker; systemic hypersensitivity to insulin is extremely rare and should be immediately referred to a specialist.

While weight gain and hypoglycemia risk are greater with FRC than with GLP-1 RA use without insulin, the combination product is consistently associated with less weight gain, and the same or lower risk of a hypoglycemic event, than continued uptitration of basal insulin alone. In general, patients using an FRC experience very little to no weight gain when adding the FRC to noninjectable agents, lose weight when switching from a basal insulin to an FRC, or gain a modest amount of weight (1–2 kg) when switching from GLP-1 RA treatment to an FRC preparation.

Summary

Insulin therapy is a safe and effective option to improve glycemic control in patients with type 2 diabetes who failed oral therapy or those with symptomatic and severe hyperglycemia. Challenges to insulin-replacement therapy include hypoglycemia risk, weight gain, increased need for blood glucose monitoring, and reduced adherence with multiple daily injections. Combining insulin with GLP-1 RA treatment is an effective and safe manner to improve glycemic control. A practical approach to insulin initiation and intensification is discussed the Advancement of Pharmacological Therapy section.

INITIATION OF PHARMACOLOGICAL THERAPY

Metformin has been regarded as first-line therapy, in eligible patients, for the management of type 2 diabetes by the *Standards of Medical Care in Diabetes* since its FDA approval in 1994. The recommendation of metformin as first-line therapy is also supported by the American Association of Clinical Endocrinologists, the European Association for the Study of Diabetes (EASD), and the International Diabetes Federation guidelines. The support for metformin is based upon decades of clinical evidence for its use, affordability, tolerability, low risk for hypoglycemia, and weight-neutral impact.

Metformin's mechanism of action lends to its first-line recommendation as well. It is well established that metformin reduces hepatic gluconeogenesis and hepatic glucose production, but there is also evidence that some of metformin's metabolic effects may involve the release of GLP-1 and peptide YY.[10] Both mechanisms of action would be beneficial in patients with type 2 diabetes who experience increased hepatic glucose production and impairments in the incretin system.

Although metformin has not undergone the same cardiovascular scrutiny as other more recently approved anti-diabetic therapies, cardiovascular benefit has been noted in the UKPDS substudy and some large observational studies.[10,107] Benefits demonstrated include modification of cardiovascular risk factors such as weight, blood pressure, lipids, inflammatory markers, hypercoagulability, platelet dysfunction, and microvascular reactivity.[10]

At this time, metformin remains a cornerstone therapy in the management of type 2 diabetes based on its longstanding use, demonstrated efficacy, low cost, and safety profile.

ADVANCEMENT OF PHARMACOLOGICAL THERAPY

Next Steps (Second- and Third-Line Therapies)

It is critical that each patient's glycemic control is monitored on a regular basis (every 3–6 months) and treatment intensified without delay when glycemia remains above target. Therapeutic inertia—representing the delay in initiating or intensifying therapy when disease targets are not being met—is significant in the field and unnecessarily exposes the patient to the deleterious long-term effects of chronic hyperglycemia.

The EASD/American Diabetes Association consensus statement[8,108] provides helpful guidance on how to intensify therapy, taking into consideration each patient's co-morbidities and compelling needs (Fig. 3.2; also see Fig. 9.2 in the 2020 edition of *Standards of Medical Care in Diabetes*[8]). In fact, consideration may be given to using dual therapy from the start in appropriate patients in order to sustain glycemic control more effectively.[109] The first consideration in selecting the second-line agent is the presence of cardiovascular disease or chronic kidney disease. If atherosclerotic cardiovascular disease prevails, then a GLP-1 RA or an SGLT2 inhibitor is recommended. Of note, the use of these agents in this population should be irrespective of prevailing A1C or A1C goals, as these have been shown to reduce the risk irrespective of glycemia. Should a third-line agent be needed to achieve glycemic targets, the drug from the other class (GLP-1 RA or SGLT2 inhibitor) should be added. These recommendations were based on the findings from various cardiovascular outcome studies, which showed that most GLP-1 RAs (Table 3.14) and most SGLT2 inhibitors (Table 3.12) decrease major cardiovascular events in patients with preexistent cardiovascular disease. Of note, the cardiovascular effect of the combination of these two classes has not been studied to date.

Should prevention of hospitalization for heart failure be of major concern (e.g., if the patient has preexistent heart failure), then SGLT2 inhibitors are the treatment of choice, followed by GLP-1 RAs as third-line agents if additional glucose lowering is needed. SGLT2 inhibitor CVOTs (Table 3.12) consistently showed a dramatic lowering in the risk of hospitalization for heart failure in high-risk patients, while GLP-1 RAs have had a neutral effect on heart failure.

In patients with coexistent chronic kidney disease and/or diabetic nephropathy, an SGLT2 inhibitor is preferable, followed by a GLP-1 RA as a third-line agent if needed. These recommendations are also based on findings from the CVOTs, where SGLT2 inhibitors reduced renal microvascular composite outcomes and slowed the fall eGFR over time (Table 3.12). In fact, the first dedicated renal study (CREDENCE) using SGLT2 inhibitors was stopped prematurely due to overwhelming efficacy; in this study, patients taking canagliflozin experienced a significant reduction in the occurrence of end-stage renal disease, doubling of serum creatinine, initiation of hemodialysis, or renal or cardiovascular death. The CVOTs with GLP-1 RAs have also shown a significant reduction in the progression of albuminuria in patients with diabetic nephropathy. Of note, there is an ongoing study called FLOW (**NCT 03819153**) specifically evaluating the effect of semaglutide on renal outcomes in patients with type 2 diabetes and albuminuric diabetic kidney disease.

It is notable that despite their known benefits in preventing the progression of kidney disease, and the fact that the cardiovascular benefits observed with SGLT2 inhibitors are independent of baseline eGFR values (down to 30 ml/min/1.73 m2), they all carry a label restriction for eGFR levels <45 ml/min/1/73 m^2 or <60 ml/min/1/73 m^2 (depending on the agent; see Fig. 3.1). Several manufacturers have submitted, or plan to submit, a request to the regulatory bodies to change this label restriction. In patients with eGFR<30 ml/min/m^2 a GLP-1 RA is relatively safe to use (exenatide-based products recommend against use in eGFR <30 ml/min/m^2), does not require a dose alteration, and should be the preferred second agent.

In lower-risk patients without prevalent cardiovascular disease or chronic kidney disease, treatment should be decided based on the individual patient's compelling needs (for both glycemic reduction and secondary factors). Should weight loss be desirable, a glucose-lowering agent that also promotes weight loss should be the second-line therapy. Currently the two common classes of glucose-lowering agents, other than metformin, that are known to promote weight loss are GLP-1 RAs and SGLT2 inhibitors. As noted earlier, there is significant heterogeneity in the weight response to the various agents within the GLP-1 RA class, with semaglutide being the most effective, followed by liraglutide and dulaglutide.[65,109] SGLT2 inhibitor agents are associated with a more consistent and modest weight loss compared with certain GLP-1 RAs.[110,111]

Should hypoglycemia be a main consideration for an individual patient, then agents with a low risk for hypoglycemia can be considered. These include DPP-4 inhibitors, GLP-1 RAs, SGLT2 inhibitors, or TZDs, as second-line agents or in combination. Of note, when these agents are combined with either a, not an sulfonylurea or insulin, the risk of hypoglycemia is higher, and therefore sulfonylureas and insulin should be used with caution in patients at high risk for hypoglycemia or its complications. Acarbose and miglitol, which are more common options in Asia, might also be appropriate options given their low risk of hypoglycemia.

Lastly, the cost of prescription medications remains a major consideration for individuals with type 2 diabetes, who require lifelong treatment, usually with multiple agents. With the exception of metformin, sulfonylureas, TZDs, acarbose and human insulin preparations (regular, NPH, and premix 70/30), all other glucose-lowering agents carry very high list prices, which represent a barrier, especially for patients paying out of pocket for their medications. For patients who cannot afford the cost of newer agents, less expensive options and combinations thereof are available.

It is important to note that the use of insulin is recommended as a second- or third-line therapy in type 2 diabetes only in those with severe and symptomatic hyperglycemia. GLP-1 RAs should be the first injectable therapy, initiated before insulin, in most patients (Fig. 3.3).

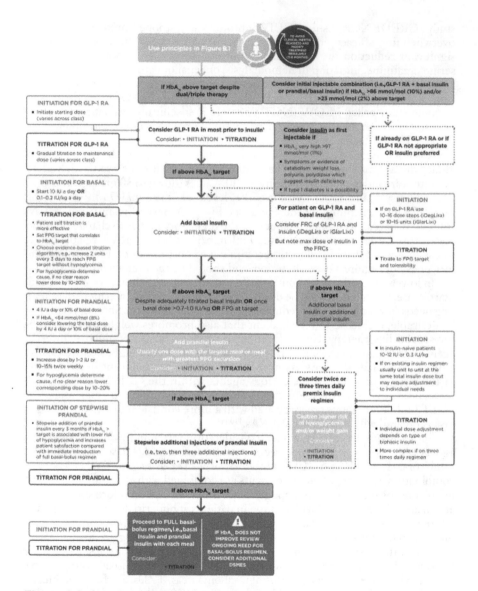

Figure 3.3 American Diabetes Association recommendations regarding initiating injectable therapy, including insulin.

FPG, fasting plasma glucose; FRC, fixed-ratio combination; GLP-1 RA, glucagon-like peptide 1 receptor agonist; PPG, postprandial plasma glucose.

Source: Adapted from Davies et al.[108]

Initiating Insulin

Although initiation of injectable therapies (GLP-1 RA or insulin) can be done at any stage of diabetes, it is particularly encouraged in some special circumstances (Fig. 3.3). A GLP-1 RA is the preferred first injectable over insulin for most patients with type 2 diabetes. When initiating a GLP-1 RA, the lowest recommended dose should be started and titrated according to label to minimize the risk of side effects. Should additional glucose lowering be necessary after reaching the maximum dose of a GLP-1 RA, basal insulin should be added as the second injectable therapy.

Basal insulin should be considered the first injectable only in cases where symptoms of ongoing catabolism are present (weight loss, polyuria, and polydipsia) and A1C >11% (97 mmol/mol), blood glucose levels are >300 mg/dL (>16.7 mmol/L), or type 1 diabetes is a possibility. Basal insulin should be initiated at 10 units or 0.1–0.2 u/kg, and titrated by 2 units twice weekly to reach the fasting blood glucose target established for the individual patient, typically 80–130 mg/dl (4.4–7.2 mmol/L), without hypoglycemia.[112] In situations where cost is a major decision factor, bedtime intermediate human insulin NPH can be used instead. If basal insulin is not sufficient to achieve the A1C goal, or if the dose is much higher than 0.5 units/kg/day, then a GLP-1 RA should be considered as an add-on therapy.

If the target glycemic control is not achieved with either basal insulin or GLP-1 RA therapy alone, changing to a fixed-dose combination therapy with GLP-1 RA plus basal insulin can be an easier alternative. Information regarding the titration of these fixed-dose insulin/GLP-1 RA combinations is provided in the Insulin/GLP-1 FRCs section above.

Intensifying Insulin Therapy

If glycemic goals are not reached despite having titrated to the "optimal" dose of basal insulin (i.e., ~0.5–0.7 units/kg/day) and GLP-1 RA, the next step is the addition of mealtime insulin coverage. This can be accomplished either by *1*) adding one injection of prandial insulin to the largest daily meal, followed by the addition of mealtime insulin coverage to the remaining meals if needed, or *2*) substituting the basal insulin to premix insulin, which can be administered twice (sometimes even three times) daily prior to meals. Upon initiation of prandial or premix insulin, sulfonylurea products should be discontinued (if applicable). Prandial insulin can be initiated at 4 units daily or 10% of the basal dose, administered before the largest meal of the day.[113] In those with A1C <8% (<64 mmol/mol) a reduction of the basal dose by 4 units or 10% should be considered to reduce the risk of hypoglycemia. The prandial insulin dose can then be increased by 1–2 units twice weekly to achieve desirable glycemic targets (<130–150 mg/dl [7.2–8.3 mmol/L] before the next meal or at bedtime, or <180 mg/dl [<10.0 mmol/L] 2 h after eating) without hypoglycemia. Additional prandial insulin doses can be added every 3 months in a stepwise fashion if the A1C remains above target. The use of basal bolus insulin allows for a flexible meal schedule over premix insulin.

If choosing to intensify therapy with premix insulin instead of prandial insulin, convert the total daily dose of basal insulin to premix (unit to unit) and split the dose to be administered before breakfast and before dinner. Each dose is intended to cover two meals or a meal and a snack. A split a.m./p.m. dose of 50%/50% works well in most obese, insulin-resistant patients, while a 66%/33% might be more appropriate in leaner patients, those who have smaller evening meals, or those at higher risk for nocturnal hypoglycemia. The morning dose can be further titrated based on the predinner blood glucose level, while the predinner dose is adjusted based on the fasting blood glucose value.

CONCLUSION

The pharmacologic treatment of type 2 diabetes has seen a tremendous transformation in the past decade. While a healthy diet and lifestyle, along with metformin, remain the cornerstone of treatment for type 2 diabetes, the next step in pharmacologic therapy now takes into consideration the major cardiorenal co-morbidities as well as key patient-centric considerations like weight loss, risk of hypoglycemia, or cost constraints. The use of agents with a proven cardio-protective effect is now recommended in patients at high cardiovascular risk, while in low-risk patients it is preferable to use agents which do not promote weight gain. Insulin remains the most effective glucose-lowering class, but it has now taken a step back in the treatment algorithm given its associated risk of weight gain and hypoglycemia, and high associated treatment burden.

In response to the rapid changes in this field, the American Diabetes Association has changed the format of the *Standards of Medical Care in Diabetes* publication to a living document,[114] which is now updated every time new evidence that impacts clinical practice becomes available. This will contain the most up-to-date information in the field, along with pharmacologic treatment recommendations.

REFERENCES

1. Jabbour S, Ziring B. Advantages of extended-release metformin in patients with type 2 diabetes mellitus. *Postgrad Med J* 2011;123(1):15–23

2. Graham GG, Punt J, Arora M, et al. Clinical pharmacokinetics of metformin. *Clin Pharmacokinet* 2011;50(2):81–98

3. Fujita Y, Inagaki N. Metformin: New preparations and nonglycemic benefits. *Curr Diabetes Rep* 2017;17(1):5

4. Bailey CJ. Metformin: historical overview. *Diabetologia* 2017;60(9):1566–1576

5. DeFronzo RA, Goodman AM. Efficacy of metformin in patients with non-insulin-dependent diabetes mellitus. The Multicenter Metformin Study Group. *N Engl J Med* 1995;333(9):541–549

6. Lalau JD, Kajbaf F, Protti A, Christensen MM, De Broe ME, Wiernsperger N. Metformin-associated lactic acidosis (MALA): moving towards a new paradigm. *Diabetes, Obes Metab* 2017;19(11):1502–1512

7. U.S. Food and Drug Administration. Drug safety communication: FDA revises warnings regarding use of the diabetes medicine metformin in certain patients with reduced kidney function [Internet], 2016. Available from https://www.fda.gov/media/96771/download. Accessed 8 April 2016

8. American Diabetes Association. Pharmacologic approaches to glycemic treatment: standards of medical care in diabetes 2020. *Diabetes Care* 2020;43(Suppl. 1):S98–S110

9. Liu Q, Li S, Quan H, Li J. Vitamin B12 status in metformin treated patients: systematic review. *PloS One* 2014;9(6):e100379

10. Inzucchi SE. Is it time to change the type 2 diabetes treatment paradigm? no! metformin should remain the foundation therapy for type 2 diabetes. *Diabetes Care* 2017;40(8):1128–1132

11. UK Prospective Diabetes Study (UKPDS) Group. Effect of intensive blood-glucose control with metformin on complications in overweight patients with type 2 diabetes (UKPDS 34). *Lancet* 1998;352(9131):854–865

12. Kooy A, de Jager J, Lehert P, et al. Long-term effects of metformin on metabolism and microvascular and macrovascular disease in patients with type 2 diabetes mellitus. *Arch Intern Med* 2009;169(6):616–625

13. Hong J, Zhang Y, Lai S, et al. Effects of metformin versus glipizide on cardiovascular outcomes in patients with type 2 diabetes and coronary artery disease. *Diabetes Care* 2013;36(5):1304–1311

14. Viberti G, Kahn SE, Greene DA, et al. A diabetes outcome progression trial (ADOPT): an international multicenter study of the comparative efficacy of rosiglitazone, glyburide, and metformin in recently diagnosed type 2 diabetes. *Diabetes Care* 2002;25(10):1737–1743

15. UK Prospective Diabetes Study (UKPDS) Group. Intensive blood-glucose control with sulphonylureas or insulin compared with conventional treatment and risk of complications in patients with type 2 diabetes (UKPDS 33). *Lancet* 1998;352(9131):837–853

16. Negroni JA, Lascano EC, del Valle HF. Glibenclamide action on myocardial function and arrhythmia incidence in the healthy and diabetic heart. *Cardiovasc Hematol Agents Med Chem* 2007;5(1):43–53

17. Rosenstock J, Kahn SE, Johansen OE, et al. Effect of linagliptin vs glimepiride on major adverse cardiovascular outcomes in patients with type 2 diabetes: the CAROLINA randomized clinical trial. *JAMA* 2019;322(12):1155–1166

18. Yki-Järvinen H. Thiazolidinediones. *N Engl J Med* 2004;351(11):1106–1118

19. DeFronzo RA, Tripathy D, Schwenke DC, et al. Prevention of diabetes with pioglitazone in ACT NOW: physiologic correlates. *Diabetes* 2013;62(11):3920–3926

20. Garber AJ, Abrahamson MJ, Barzilay JI, et al. Consensus statement by the American Association of Clinical Endocrinologists and American College of Endocrinology on the Comprehensive Type 2 Diabetes Management Algorithm—2019 executive summary. *Endocrine Practice: official journal of the American College of Endocrinology and the American Association of Clinical Endocrinologists* 2019;25(1):69–100

21. Cusi K, Orsak B, Bril F, et al. Long-term pioglitazone treatment for patients with nonalcoholic steatohepatitis and prediabetes or type 2 diabetes mellitus: a randomized trial. *Ann Intern Med* 2016;165(5):305–315

22. Kernan WN, Viscoli CM, Furie KL, et al. Pioglitazone after ischemic stroke or transient ischemic attack. *N Engl J Med* 2016;374(14):1321–1331

23. Erdmann E, Charbonnel B, Wilcox RG, et al. Pioglitazone use and heart failure in patients with type 2 diabetes and preexisting cardiovascular disease: data from the PROactive study (PROactive 08). *Diabetes Care* 2007;30(11):2773–2778

24. Dormandy JA, Charbonnel B, Eckland DJ, et al. Secondary prevention of macrovascular events in patients with type 2 diabetes in the PROactive Study (PROspective pioglitAzone Clinical Trial In macroVascular Events): a randomised controlled trial. *Lancet* 2005;366(9493):1279–1289

25. Karalliedde J, Buckingham R, Starkie M, et al. Effect of various diuretic treatments on rosiglitazone-induced fluid retention. *J Am Soc Nephrol* 2006;17(12):3482–3490

26. Pioglitazone prescribing information [Internet], c2009-2017. Available from https://general.takedapharm.com/actospi. Accessed 24 May 2019

27. Home PD, Pocock SJ, Beck-Nielsen H, et al. Rosiglitazone evaluated for cardiovascular outcomes in oral agent combination therapy for type 2 diabetes (RECORD): a multicentre, randomised, open-label trial. *Lancet* 2009;373(9681):2125–2135

28. Lewis JD, Habel LA, Quesenberry CP, et al. Pioglitazone use and risk of bladder cancer and other common cancers in persons with diabetes. *JAMA* 2015;314(3):265–277

29. Erdmann E, Harding S, Lam H, Perez A. Ten-year observational follow-up of PROactive: a randomized cardiovascular outcomes trial evaluating pioglitazone in type 2 diabetes. *Diabetes Obes Metab* 2016;18(3):266–273

30. Zinman B, Wanner C, Lachin JM, et al. Empagliflozin, cardiovascular outcomes, and mortality in type 2 diabetes. *N Engl J Med* 2015;373(22):2117–2128

31. Marso SP, Daniels GH, Brown-Frandsen K, et al. Liraglutide and cardiovascular outcomes in type 2 diabetes. *N Engl J Med* 2016;375(4):311–322

32. Neal B, Perkovic V, Mahaffey KW, et al. Canagliflozin and cardiovascular and renal events in type 2 diabetes. *N Engl J Med* 2017;377(7):644–657

33. Nissen S, Wolski K. Effect of Rosiglitazone on the Risk of Myocardial Infarction and Death from Cardiovascular Causes. *N Engl J Med* 2007;356:2457–2471

34. Gerich JE. Role of the kidney in normal glucose homeostasis and in the hyperglycaemia of diabetes mellitus: therapeutic implications. *Diabet Med* 2010;27(2):136–142

35. Valtin H. *Renal Function: Mechanisms Preserving Fluid and Solute Balance in Health.* 2nd ed. Boston, Little Brown and Company, 1983, p. 65–68

36. Farber SJ, Berger EY, Earle DP. Effect of diabetes and insulin of the maximum capacity of the renal tubules to reabsorb glucose. *J Clin Invest* 1951;30(2):125–129

37. Zambrowicz B, Freiman J, Brown PM, et al. LX4211, a dual SGLT1/SGLT2 inhibitor, improved glycemic control in patients with type 2 diabetes in a randomized, placebo-controlled trial. *Clin Pharmacol Ther* 2012;92(2):158–169

38. Powell DR, Zambrowicz B, Morrow L, et al. Sotagliflozin decreases postprandial glucose and insulin concentrations by delaying intestinal glucose absorption. *J Clin Endocrinol Metab* 2020;105(4):e1235–e1249

39. Rosenstock J, Chuck L, Gonzalez-Ortiz M, et al. Initial combination therapy with canagliflozin plus metformin versus each component as monotherapy for drug-naive type 2 diabetes. *Diabetes Care* 2016;39(3):353–362

40. Henry RR, Murray AV, Marmolejo MH, Hennicken D, Ptaszynska A, List JF. Dapagliflozin, metformin XR, or both: initial pharmacotherapy for type 2 diabetes, a randomised controlled trial. *Int J Clin Pract* 2012;66(5):446–456

41. Del Prato S, Nauck M, Duran-Garcia S, et al. Long-term glycaemic response and tolerability of dapagliflozin versus a sulphonylurea as add-on therapy to metformin in patients with type 2 diabetes: 4-year data. *Diabetes Obes Metab* 2015;17(6):581–590

42. Cefalu WT, Leiter LA, Yoon KH, et al. Efficacy and safety of canagliflozin versus glimepiride in patients with type 2 diabetes inadequately controlled with metformin (CANTATA-SU): 52 week results from a randomised, double-blind, phase 3 non-inferiority trial. *Lancet* 2013;382(9896):941–950

43. Leiter LA, Yoon KH, Arias P, et al. Canagliflozin provides durable glycemic improvements and body weight reduction over 104 weeks versus glimepiride in patients with type 2 diabetes on metformin: a randomized, double-blind, phase 3 study. *Diabetes Care* 2015;38(3):355–364

44. Ridderstrale M, Andersen KR, Zeller C, et al. Comparison of empagliflozin and glimepiride as add-on to metformin in patients with type 2 diabetes: a 104-week randomised, active-controlled, double-blind, phase 3 trial. *Lancet Diabetes Endocrinol* 2014;2(9):691–700

45. Schernthaner G, Gross JL, Rosenstock J, et al. Canagliflozin compared with sitagliptin for patients with type 2 diabetes who do not have adequate glycemic control with metformin plus sulfonylurea: a 52-week randomized trial. *Diabetes Care* 2013;36(9):2508–2515

46. Lavalle-Gonzalez FJ, Januszewicz A, Davidson J, et al. Efficacy and safety of canagliflozin compared with placebo and sitagliptin in patients with type 2 diabetes on background metformin monotherapy: a randomised trial. *Diabetologia* 2013;56(12):2582–2592

47. Rosenstock J, Hansen L, Zee P, et al. Dual add-on therapy in type 2 diabetes poorly controlled with metformin monotherapy: a randomized double-blind trial of saxagliptin plus dapagliflozin addition versus single addition of saxagliptin or dapagliflozin to metformin. *Diabetes Care* 2015;38(3):376–383

48. Roden M, Weng J, Eilbracht J, et al. Empagliflozin monotherapy with sitagliptin as an active comparator in patients with type 2 diabetes: a randomised, double-blind, placebo-controlled, phase 3 trial. *Lancet Diabetes Endocrinol* 2013;1(3):208–219

49. Wilding JP, Norwood P, T'Joen C, Bastien A, List JF, Fiedorek FT. A study of dapagliflozin in patients with type 2 diabetes receiving high doses of insulin plus insulin sensitizers: applicability of a novel insulin-independent treatment. *Diabetes Care* 2009;32(9):1656–1662

50. Rosenstock J, Jelaska A, Frappin G, et al. Improved glucose control with weight loss, lower insulin doses, and no increased hypoglycemia with empagliflozin added to titrated multiple daily injections of insulin in obese inadequately controlled type 2 diabetes. *Diabetes Care* 2014;37(7):1815–1823

51. Cho YK, Lee J, Kang YM, et al. Clinical parameters affecting the therapeutic efficacy of empagliflozin in patients with type 2 diabetes. *PloS One* 2019;14(8):e0220667

52. Bonner C, Kerr-Conte J, Gmyr V, et al. Inhibition of the glucose transporter SGLT2 with dapagliflozin in pancreatic alpha cells triggers glucagon secretion. *Nat Med* 2015;21(5):512–517

53. Wanner C, Inzucchi SE, Lachin JM, et al. Empagliflozin and progression of kidney disease in type 2 diabetes. *N Engl J Med* 2016;375(4):323–334

54. Perkovic V, Jardine MJ, Neal B, et al. Canagliflozin and renal outcomes in type 2 diabetes and nephropathy. *N Engl J Med* 2019;380(24):2295–2306

55. Ferrannini G, Hach T, Crowe S, Sanghvi A, Hall KD, Ferrannini E. Energy balance after sodium-glucose cotransporter 2 inhibition. *Diabetes Care* 2015;38(9):1730–1735

56. Wiviott SD, Raz I, Bonaca MP, et al. Dapagliflozin and cardiovascular outcomes in type 2 diabetes. *N Engl J Med* 2019;380(4):347–357

57. Holman RR, Paul SK, Bethel MA, Matthews DR, Neil HA. 10-year followup of intensive glucose control in type 2 diabetes. *N Engl J Med* 2008;359(15):1577–1589

58. Neal B, Perkovic V, de Zeeuw D, et al. Rationale, design, and baseline characteristics of the Canagliflozin Cardiovascular Assessment Study (CANVAS)—a randomized placebo-controlled trial. *Am Heart J* 2013;166(2):217–223 e211

59. Filion KB, Yu OH. Sodium-glucose cotransporter-2 inhibitors and severe urinary tract infections: reassuring real-world evidence. *Ann Intern Med* 2019;171(4):289–290

60. Goldenberg RM, Gilbert JD, Hramiak IM, Woo VC, Zinman B. Sodium-glucose co-transporter inhibitors, their role in type 1 diabetes treatment and a risk mitigation strategy for preventing diabetic ketoacidosis: the STOP DKA protocol. *Diabetes Obes Metab* 2019;21(10):2192–2202

61. Perkovic V, de Zeeuw D, Mahaffey KW, et al. Canagliflozin and renal outcomes in type 2 diabetes: results from the CANVAS Program randomised clinical trials. *Lancet Diabetes Endocrinol* 2018;6(9):691–704

62. Buse JB, Wexler DJ, Tsapas A, et al. Update to: management of hyperglycemia in type 2 diabetes, 2018. a consensus report by the American Diabetes Association (ADA) and the European Association for the Study of Diabetes (EASD). *Diabetes Care* 2019:dci190066

63. Drucker DJ. Mechanisms of action and therapeutic application of glucagon-like peptide-1. *Cell Metab* 2018;27(4):740–756

64. Madsbad S. Review of head-to-head comparisons of glucagon-like peptide-1 receptor agonists. *Diabetes Obes Metab* 2016;18(4):317–332

65. Pratley RE, Aroda VR, Lingvay I, et al. Semaglutide versus dulaglutide once weekly in patients with type 2 diabetes (SUSTAIN 7): a randomised, open-label, phase 3b trial. *Lancet Diabetes Endocrinol* 2018;6(4):275–286

66. Ahmann AJ, Capehorn M, Charpentier G, et al. Efficacy and safety of once-weekly semaglutide versus exenatide ER in subjects with type 2 diabetes (sustain 3): a 56-week, open-label, randomized clinical trial. *Diabetes Care* 2018;41(2):258–266

67. Holman RR, Bethel MA, Mentz RJ, et al. Effects of once-weekly exenatide on cardiovascular outcomes in type 2 diabetes. *N Engl J Med* 2017;377(13):1228–1239

68. Armstrong MJ, Gaunt P, Aithal GP, et al. Liraglutide safety and efficacy in patients with non-alcoholic steatohepatitis (LEAN): a multicentre, double-blind, randomised, placebo-controlled phase 2 study. *Lancet* 2016;387(10019):679–690

69. Storgaard H, Cold F, Gluud LL, Vilsboll T, Knop FK. Glucagon-like peptide-1 receptor agonists and risk of acute pancreatitis in patients with type 2 diabetes. *Diabetes Obes Metab* 2017;19(6):906–908

70. Pfeffer MA, Claggett B, Diaz R, et al. Lixisenatide in patients with type 2 diabetes and acute coronary syndrome. *N Engl J Med* 2015;373(23):2247–2257

71. Marso SP, Bain SC, Consoli A, et al. Semaglutide and cardiovascular outcomes in patients with type 2 diabetes. *N Engl J Med* 2016;375(19):1834–1844

72. Hernandez AF, Green JB, Janmohamed S, et al. Albiglutide and cardiovascular outcomes in patients with type 2 diabetes and cardiovascular disease (Harmony Outcomes): a double-blind, randomised placebo-controlled trial. *Lancet* 2018;392(10157):1519–1529

73. Husain M, Birkenfeld AL, Donsmark M, et al. Oral semaglutide and cardiovascular outcomes in patients with type 2 diabetes. *N Engl J Med* 2019;381(9):841–851

74. Gerstein HC, Colhoun HM, Dagenais GR, et al. Dulaglutide and cardiovascular outcomes in type 2 diabetes (REWIND): a double-blind, randomised placebo-controlled trial. *Lancet* 2019;394(10193):121–130

75. Zhong J, Gong Q, Goud A, Srinivasamaharaj S, Rajagopalan S. Recent advances in dipeptidyl-peptidase-4 inhibition therapy: lessons from the bench and clinical trials. *J Diabetes Res* 2015;2015:606031

76. Ling J, Ge L, Zhang DH, et al. DPP-4 inhibitors for the treatment of type 2 diabetes: a methodology overview of systematic reviews. *Acta Diabetologica* 2019;56(1):7–27

77. Kridin K, Bergman R. Association of bullous pemphigoid with dipeptidyl-peptidase 4 inhibitors in patients with diabetes: estimating the risk of the new agents and characterizing the patients. *JAMA Dermatology* 2018;154(10):1152–1158

78. Kridin K, Ludwig RJ. The growing incidence of bullous pemphigoid: overview and potential explanations. *Front Med (Lausanne)* 2018;5:220

79. Cefalu WT, Kaul S, Gerstein HC, et al. Cardiovascular outcomes trials in type 2 diabetes: where do we go from here? reflections from a diabetes care editors' expert forum. *Diabetes Care* 2018;41(1):14–31

80. Scirica BM, Bhatt DL, Braunwald E, et al. Saxagliptin and cardiovascular outcomes in patients with type 2 diabetes mellitus. *N Engl J Med* 2013;369(14):1317–1326

81. White WB, Cannon CP, Heller SR, et al. Alogliptin after acute coronary syndrome in patients with type 2 diabetes. *N Engl J Med* 2013;369(14):1327–1335

82. Green JB, Bethel MA, Armstrong PW, et al. Effect of sitagliptin on cardiovascular outcomes in type 2 diabetes. *N Engl J Med* 2015;373(3):232–242

83. Rosenstock J, Perkovic V, Johansen OE, et al. Effect of linagliptin vs placebo on major cardiovascular events in adults with type 2 diabetes and high cardiovascular and renal risk: the CARMELINA randomized clinical trial. *JAMA* 2019;321(1):69–79

84. Schwartz SS, Zangeneh F. Evidence-based practice use of quick-release bromocriptine across the natural history of type 2 diabetes mellitus. *Postgrad Med* 2016;128(8):828–838

85. Kerr JL, Timpe EM, Petkewicz KA. Bromocriptine mesylate for glycemic management in type 2 diabetes mellitus. *Ann Pharmacother* 2010;44(11):1777–1785

86. Gaziano JM, Cincotta AH, Vinik A, Blonde L, Bohannon N, Scranton R. Effect of bromocriptine-QR (a quick-release formulation of bromocriptine mesylate) on major adverse cardiovascular events in type 2 diabetes subjects. *JAHA* 2012;1(5):e002279

87. Lamos EM, Levitt DL, Munir KM. A review of dopamine agonist therapy in type 2 diabetes and effects on cardio-metabolic parameters. *Primary Care Diabetes* 2016;10(1):60–65

88. Avitabile N, Banka A, Fonseca VA. Safety evaluation of colesevelam therapy to achieve glycemic and lipid goals in type 2 diabetes. *Expert Opin Drug Saf* 2011;10(2):305–310

89. Brunetti L, Campbell RK. Clinical efficacy of colesevelam in type 2 diabetes mellitus. *J Pharm Pract* 2011;24(4):417–425

90. Singh-Franco D, Robles G, Gazze D. Pramlintide acetate injection for the treatment of type 1 and type 2 diabetes mellitus. *Clin Ther* 2007;29(4):535–562

91. Hieronymus L, Griffin S. Role of amylin in type 1 and type 2 diabetes. *Diabetes Educator* 2015;41(Suppl. 1):S47–S56

92. Qiao YC, Ling W, Pan YH, et al. Efficacy and safety of pramlintide injection adjunct to insulin therapy in patients with type 1 diabetes mellitus: a systematic review and meta-analysis. *Oncotarget* 2017;8(39):66504–66515

93. van de Laar FA, Lucassen PL, Akkermans RP, van de Lisdonk EH, Rutten GE, van Weel C. Alpha-glucosidase inhibitors for patients with type 2 diabetes: results from a Cochrane systematic review and meta-analysis. *Diabetes Care* 2005;28(1):154–163

94. Scheen AJ. Is there a role for alpha-glucosidase inhibitors in the prevention of type 2 diabetes mellitus? *Drugs* 2003;63(10):933–951

95. Scott LJ, Spencer CM. Miglitol: a review of its therapeutic potential in type 2 diabetes mellitus. *Drugs* 2000;59(3):521–549

96. Marso SP, McGuire DK, Zinman B, et al. Efficacy and safety of degludec versus glargine in type 2 diabetes. *N Engl J Med* 2017;377(8):723–732

97. Swinnen SG, Simon AC, Holleman F, Hoekstra JB, Devries JH. Insulin detemir versus insulin glargine for type 2 diabetes mellitus. *Cochrane Database Syst Rev* 2011(7):CD006383

98. Reutrakul S, Wroblewski K, Brown RL. Clinical use of U-500 regular insulin: review and meta-analysis. *J Diabetes Sci Techol* 2012;6(2):412–420

99. de la Pena A, Riddle M, Morrow LA, et al. Pharmacokinetics and pharmacodynamics of high-dose human regular U-500 insulin versus human regular U-100 insulin in healthy obese subjects. *Diabetes Care* 2011;34(12):2496–2501

100. Aroda VR, Rosenstock J, Wysham C, et al. Efficacy and safety of LixiLan, a titratable fixed-ratio combination of insulin glargine plus lixisenatide in type 2 diabetes inadequately controlled on basal insulin and metformin: the Lixi-Lan-L randomized trial. *Diabetes Care* 2016;39(11):1972–1980

101. Billings LK, Doshi A, Gouet D, et al. Efficacy and safety of IDegLira versus basal-bolus insulin therapy in patients with type 2 diabetes uncontrolled on metformin and basal insulin: the DUAL VII randomized clinical trial. *Diabetes Care* 2018;41(5):1009–1016

102. Mathieu C, Rodbard HW, Cariou B, et al. A comparison of adding liraglutide versus a single daily dose of insulin aspart to insulin degludec in subjects with type 2 diabetes. *Diabetes Obes Metab* 2014;16(7):636–644

103. Rosenstock J, Guerci B, Hanefeld M, et al. Prandial options to advance basal insulin glargine therapy: testing lixisenatide plus basal insulin versus insulin glulisine either as basal-plus or basal-bolus in type 2 diabetes: the GetGoal Duo-2 trial. *Diabetes Care* 2016;39(8):1318–1328

104. Gerstein HC, Bosch J, Dagenais GR, et al. Basal insulin and cardiovascular and other outcomes in dysglycemia. *N Engl J Med* 2012;367(4):319–328

105. Investigators OT, Gerstein HC, Bosch J, et al. Basal insulin and cardiovascular and other outcomes in dysglycemia. *N Engl J Med* 2012;367(4):319–328

106. Reid T, Gao L, Gill J, et al. How much is too much? outcomes in patients using high-dose insulin glargine. *Int J Clin Pract* 2016;70(1):56–65

107. Abdul-Ghani M, DeFronzo RA. Is it time to change the type 2 diabetes treatment paradigm? yes! GLP-1 RAs should replace metformin in the type 2 diabetes algorithm. *Diabetes Care* 2017;40(8):1121–1127

108. Davies MJ, D'Alessio DA, Fradkin J, et al. Management of hyperglycaemia in type 2 diabetes, 2018. A consensus report by the American Diabetes Association (ADA) and the European Association for the Study of Diabetes (EASD). *Diabetologia* 2018;61(12):2461–2498

109. Dungan KM, Povedano ST, Forst T, et al. Once-weekly dulaglutide versus once-daily liraglutide in metformin-treated patients with type 2 diabetes (AWARD-6): a randomised, open-label, phase 3, non-inferiority trial. *Lancet* 2014;384(9951):1349–1357

110. Rodbard HW, Rosenstock J, Canani LH, et al. Oral semaglutide versus empagliflozin in patients with type 2 diabetes uncontrolled on metformin: the PIONEER 2 trial. *Diabetes Care* 2019;42(12):2272–2281

111. Lingvay I, Catarig AM, Frias JP, et al. Efficacy and safety of once-weekly semaglutide versus daily canagliflozin as add-on to metformin in patients with type 2 diabetes (SUSTAIN 8): a double-blind, phase 3b, randomised controlled trial. *Lancet Diabetes Endocrinol* 2019;7(11):834–844

112. American Diabetes Association. 6. Glycemic targets: standards of medical care in diabetes 2020. *Diabetes Care* 2020;43(Suppl. 1):S66–S76

113. Meneghini L, Mersebach H, Kumar S, Svendsen AL, Hermansen K. Comparison of 2 intensification regimens with rapid-acting insulin aspart in type 2 diabetes mellitus inadequately controlled by once-daily insulin detemir and oral antidiabetes drugs: the step-wise randomized study. *Endocr Pract* 2011;17(5):727–736

114. American Diabetes Association. The living standards of medical care in diabetes [Internet], c2020. Available from http://care.diabetesjournals.org/living-standards. Accessed 1 May 2019

ASSESSMENT OF TREATMENT EFFICACY

Asra Kermani, MD
Marconi Abreu, MD

Several parameters are used to assess treatment efficacy. Of these, meeting glycemic targets (Table 3.18) is unique in that it allows both the person with diabetes and the healthcare team to assess the response to therapy. This section will focus on assessment of treatment efficacy as reflected in glycemic targets. A1C, in the absence of confounders, is the primary measure of glycemia as it correlates best with macro- and microvascular disease. However, measurements of fasting, preprandial, and postprandial plasma glucose levels are useful for more detailed medication and lifestyle adjustments. Real-time and intermittently scanned continuous glucose monitor (isCGM) use has rapidly grown over the years, thanks to improvements in sensor accuracy, device size, and cost. Continuous glucose monitoring (CGM) has been progressively replacing self-monitoring of blood glucose (SMBG). It provides a more panoramic view of a patient's glucose results and allows patients and providers to identify trends and modify therapy.

HEMOGLOBIN A1C

Hemoglobin A_{1c} (A1C) is the most commonly utilized test to assess glycemia. It is a form of hemoglobin that is chemically linked to glucose. A1C reflects the average glycemia over 2–3 months (the average life span of red blood cells), but it is more time weighted to glycemic exposure over the previous 30 days. In randomized control trials, an elevation in A1C has the strongest predictive value for development of diabetes-related microvascular complications.[1-3] In the ADAG study, there were not significant differences among racial and ethnic groups between A1C and mean glucose; however, there was a trend showing higher A1C values in Africans/African Americans compared with non-Hispanic whites for a given mean glucose. Additionally, a small study in children showed a lower correlation between A1C and mean glucose. Therefore, in these groups one needs to be attentive to SMBG results in addition to the A1C.

Table 3.18–Glycemic Targets for Patients with Type 2 Diabetes*

A1C	<7.0% (53 mmol/mol)*
Preprandial plasma glucose	80–130 mg/dL (4.4–7.2 mmol/L)
Postprandial plasma glucose†	<180 mg/dL (<10.0 mmol/L)
Time in range (CGM)	>70% between 70–180 mg/dL (3.9–10 mmol/L)

*Referenced to a nondiabetic range of 4.0%–6.0% (20–42 mmol/mol) using National Glycohemoglobin Standardization Program (NGSP) assay.

†Postprandial glucose measurements should be made 1–2 h after the beginning of the meal, generally peak levels in patients with diabetes.

An estimated average glucose (eAG) calculated from the A1C result is typically included in the report. The eAG is often more understandable from the patient's perspective[4] (Table 3.19).

Other glycated serum proteins can be measured in the laboratory but are not as well validated to predict the risk of complications.[5] Each reflects the level of glycemia over shorter periods of time proportional to their circulating half-life. For example, a fructosamine level is a measure of glycated serum proteins, which correlates to the glycemic exposure over the preceding 2–3 weeks.

Circumstances such as anemias and hemoglobinopathies as well as interfering substances can affect A1C results, depending on the assay method used, and should be considered when SMBG results and the A1C are discrepant. Conditions that increase erythrocyte turnover (e.g., bleeding, pregnancy, hemolysis) will spuriously lower A1C concentration in all assays. Additionally, hemoglobinopathies, such as sickle cell trait or disease or hemoglobin C or D, can falsely lower A1C results, when hemoglobin is separated by nonspecific methods based on charge, solubility, and size.[6] In contrast, uremia, high concentrations of fetal hemoglobin as seen in genetic mutations, sickle cell anemia, and thalassemia use of high doses of aspirin (usually >10 g/day), or chronic ingestion of ethanol or opioids, may falsely increase A1C levels. These artifacts do not occur in all methods, and specific reference to the manufacturer's package insert for the test assay used is the best guide to a particular assay's performance in various clinical situations.

A1C should be performed routinely in all people with diabetes at the initial assessment and then 2–4 times per year as part of the American Diabetes Association's *Standards of Medical Care in Diabetes*. This is generally every three months for those with A1C above target or with a recent therapy change, and every 6 months in those who have an A1C at target (<7% or 53 mmol/mol for most) on stable treatment.[7] For pregnant women with diabetes, the A1C may also be assessed more frequently as red cell turnover is faster in pregnancy, and tighter glycemic control is recommended to prevent macrosomia and neonatal hypoglycemia. Point-of-care

Table 3.19–Estimated Average Glucose

A1C (%)	A1C (mmol/mol)	mg/dL*	mmol/L
5	31	97	5.4
6	42	126	7.0
7	53	154	8.5
8	64	183	10.2
9	75	212	11.8
10	86	240	13.3
11	97	269	14.9
12	108	298	16.5

*Linear regression eAG (mg/dL) = 28.7 ´ A1C - 46.7[4]

Source: Nathan.[4]

testing for A1C has become readily available in most clinics, and it correlates well with serum A1C. While point-of-care assays may be National Glycohemoglobin Standardization Program (NGSP) certified or U.S. Food and Drug Administration approved for diagnosis, proficiency testing is not always mandated for performing the test. Therefore, it may be wiser to use these assays for assessing glycemic control in the clinic in patients with existing diabetes. Having the A1C results promptly available at the time of the clinic visit facilitates intensification of therapy, reduces therapeutic inertia, and improves glycemic control.[8]

A target A1C of <7% (<53 mmol/mol) is desirable for most patients, as demonstrated by large randomized controlled trials targeting microvascular complications.[1] However, more or less stringent A1C goals may be customized to individual patients.[7,9] Individualized A1C targets should factor in age, average life expectancy, and other co-morbidities as well as the duration of diabetes and pregnancy. For selected patients with a recent diagnosis of type 2 diabetes with long life expectancy and no known cardiovascular disease, an A1C value <7% might be a reasonable goal (i.e., A1C = 6.5%; <42–48 mmol/mol), as long as the risk for hypoglycemia is low.[7,9] In theory, this may improve microvascular outcomes and possibly macrovascular outcomes if implemented soon after the diagnosis of diabetes. In contrast, those with advanced coronary or renal disease, lower life expectancy, and a high risk of hypoglycemia can have less stringent A1C goals, that is, <7.5%–8% (<58–64 mmol/mol) or higher, if difficult to attain despite maximal efforts, especially if using drugs that can cause hypoglycemia (i.e., insulin and sulfonylureas).

Patients with type 2 diabetes who are planning to get pregnant should have intensification of A1C to <5% (48 mmol/mol) prior to conception.[10] Tight control in this range or lower should be maintained throughout pregnancy to prevent complications to the fetus. If locally available, the primary care provider should refer such patients to a diabetes management program or an endocrinologist experienced in the care of pregnant patients with diabetes.

SELF-MONITORING OF BLOOD GLUCOSE

While A1C is still recognized as the best surrogate marker for the development of long-term diabetes complications, it is limited by the lack of information about intra- and interday glucose variation. A1C does not capture the magnitude of glycemic excursions, frequency of hypo- and hyperglycemia, and its impact on patients' quality of life. For instance, two patients can have the very same A1C value yet completely different blood glucose profiles. Hence, for day-to-day or hour-to-hour glycemic assessment, capillary blood glucose levels using SMBG and CGM are essential tools.

SMBG allows patients to assess the degree of glycemic control between visits. Patients can also more readily visualize patterns of glycemic control and share them it with their providers at the clinic visit. Recording oral intake, activity, symptoms, stressors, and doses of diabetes medications enhances the quality of the blood glucose log and provides greater insights into the multiple factors that can influence glycemic control. However, healthcare providers cannot entirely rely on patients' glucose logs, as SMBG results might be subject to errors in technique, inaccurate record entry into the patient's log, and infrequent glucose capillary glucose measurements.

The frequency and timing of SMBG should be individualized to each patient. It should take into account the nature of his or her diabetes, treatment goals, risk for hypoglycemia, choices of therapy, and affordability. A clear outline of specific glycemic targets and an action plan should be discussed with the patient for out-of-range capillary blood glucose values.[7,11]

Most randomized clinical trials show no improved clinical outcomes associated with SMBG testing in type 2 diabetes patients not using insulin. Notwithstanding, the authors believe that SMBG combined with robust patient education can motivate patients to adjust diet, increase exercise activity, and improve compliance with medications, ultimately resulting in better control. In the absence of periodic SMBG, it is almost impossible for patients to assess their response to lifestyle and medication changes.

SMBG may provide valuable feedback for patients with early type 2 diabetes treated with lifestyle management (nutrition and activity), regarding day-to-day glycemia in response to their efforts. Testing, especially if patients experience symptoms suspicious for hyper- or hypoglycemia, gives patients the opportunity to assess glycemic excursions and contact the healthcare team early, to effectively address challenges with glycemic control during periods of stress, such as those caused by infection or trauma.

SMBG is particularly important for all patients taking insulin or sulfonylureas, as it allows for the identification of both symptomatic and asymptomatic hypoglycemia.[3] Recurrent hypoglycemia can lead to hypoglycemia unawareness and is the most important predictor of severe hypoglycemia. This can lead to trauma, confusion, seizures, loss of consciousness, and death.[12] Patients may not know if they are hyper- or hypoglycemic, and they may consume additional calories and carbohydrate-rich foods when feeling hungry, sweaty, nervous, or upset, regardless of their glucose levels. This can contribute to high glucose variability and marked weight gain. It is very important to educate patients how to check blood glucose to confirm hypoglycemia, how to properly treat hypoglycemia, and when to contact providers for advice on treatment adjustments. Modifying therapy and/or prescribing a continuous glucose monitor with alarms may be necessary, particularly in those with hypoglycemia unawareness.

The frequency of SMBG needs to match individual patient needs and treatment. Useful times to monitor include before meals and at bedtime (to assess the risk of hypoglycemia). Evaluation of blood glucose before and 1–2 h after meals helps to assess the maximal excursion in glucose after a meal and is particularly useful in pregnancy when postprandial hyperglycemia is highly correlated with worse pregnancy outcomes and fetal macrosomia. Checking glucose in the middle of the sleep cycle can assess for nocturnal hypoglycemia, Dawn phenomenon, and Somogyi effect (nocturnal hypoglycemia followed by rebound fasting hyperglycemia).

It is important to recommend SMBG testing frequency and timing that maximize the effectiveness of the data for both patients and providers; patients not using insulin may derive limited value from routine glucose monitoring. For example, patients on oral or injectable medications not associated with hypoglycemia might use SMBG to collect data in preparation to a visit with their healthcare professional, to assess glycemic excursions during periods of stress or illness, or to test when they are concerned about hypoglycemia. SMBG can also be useful when there might be discrepancies between measured blood glucose and A1C levels. For patients on basal insulin, a fasting blood glucose check can be of value in assessing the adequacy of basal insulin replacement[13]; this can be done daily when insulin doses are being actively titrated and less often once the appropriate basal insulin dose has been determined. When using premix insulin preparations twice daily, the fasting blood glucose is used to titrate the evening premix dose, and vice versa the predinner blood glucose informs on changes needed to the morning premix insulin dose. For those actively adjusting a full basal/bolus regimen (multiple daily injections or insulin pump therapy), it is ideal to test blood glucose before meals and bedtime and discuss results and patterns with a healthcare professional in order to make appropriate treatment changes. For more sophisticated patients attempting to optimize glycemic targets on basal/bolus insulin therapy, a useful initial strategy is to have patients concentrate on premeal glucose. Once they achieve premeal glucose levels between 80 mg/dL and 130 mg/dL (4.4–7.2 mmol/L), they can then focus on targeting the 1- to 2-h postprandial glucose levels to <180 mg/dL (<10 mmol/L). Evaluation of both preprandial and postprandial hyperglycemia provides insight into dietary intake, activity, and medications, allowing providers and patients to make appropriate changes to the treatment plan.

Clearly, for those patients who use a correction (supplemental) dose of insulin to correct hyperglycemia before meals, more frequent SMBG is of value. Patients testing 1–2 times daily can alternate SMBG at various times of day in order to obtain a more complete picture of glycemic patterns and excursions. In type 2 diabetes, testing frequency needs to be higher during active insulin dose adjustments and can be reduced once blood glucose levels achieve targets and remain stable.

The patient's glucose logbook has been largely replaced by meter downloads or smartphone apps. If patients are using a logbook, they should be encouraged to keep a record of SMBG in tabular form (columns for each premeal time period as well as bedtime), so glycemic levels at various times of the day can be scanned visually with ease. These logs should always be correlated with the glucose meter results for veracity. Most current meters can be downloaded into a computer at the clinic to generate glucose logs. Some meters allow for patients to input if the glucose was taken pre- or postprandial or during a physical activity, while others are integrated with a smartphone app, allowing for food input and other annotations.

REAL-TIME AND INTERMITTENTLY SCANNED CONTINUOUS GLUCOSE MONITORING

Real-time CGM and isCGM use has rapidly grown over the years, thanks to improvements in sensor accuracy, device size, cost, and insurance reimbursement. Since A1C is the only prospectively evaluated tool for assessing the risk for diabetes complications, it has been used as the primary end point for many CGM studies. Data obtained from CGM use should not be viewed as a replacement to A1C, but rather as a complement to glucose monitoring.

Numerous studies have demonstrated the clinical benefits of CGM in patients with diabetes. In contrast to A1C, CGM captures more effectively the time spent at various blood glucose ranges. It allows patients to directly observe their glycemic excursions in real time and modify their lifestyle. The continuous nature of the glycemic information provides not only a glucose value, but also the direction and speed of glucose change, which can add further value to real-time insulin dosing decisions. CGM data also help healthcare professionals identify patterns of hypo- and hyperglycemia and correlate them with patients' eating habits, daily activities, and medication timing. However, CGM accuracy can be limited by inadequate skin insertion, insufficient capillary blood glucose calibration (required by some brands), and delays in identifying blood glucose changes in dynamic situations.

Time in range (TIR) is the most important CGM metric for assessing overall glycemic exposure. It is the percentage of time that glucose readings fall within a predefined target range. The range will vary depending on the patient population and the individualized glycemic targets for that patient. In February 2019, experts agreed on CGM targets to guide clinicians in using, interpreting, and reporting CGM data in clinical care and research.[14] They recommended specific percentages for time spent in range, above range, or below range for patients needing tighter or less tight glycemic control (see Fig. 3.4). For clarification, the TIR of 70–180 mg/dL (3.9–10.0mmol/L) should be 70% or more of the time in most individuals with type 1 diabetes and type 2 diabetes, while older and higher-risk individuals can aim for 50% or more of their readings to be within that range. It should be noted that the CGM TIR targets for overall glycemia are an, not is in addition and not a replacement to the premeal and postprandial SMBG targets in pregnancy.

Fig. 3.4 displays and compares the targets for TIR (green), time below range (TBR, red), and time above range (TAR, yellow and orange). The image shows different expectations for the various time ranges relating to safety concerns and efficacy based on currently available therapies and medical practice. Most patients with type 2 diabetes should aim for TIR >70%. More aggressive targets of TIR >80% between 63–140 mg/dL (3.5–7.8 mmol/L) have been established for pregnancy, and less stringent targets for the elderly and higher-risk patients with type 2 diabetes.[14]

In order to fundamentally change clinical care with the use of these new metrics, it is important to demonstrate that they can also predict clinical outcomes. TIR has been validated and strongly associated with the risk of microvascular complications, demonstrated a strong relationship with A1C, and should be an acceptable end point for clinical trials.[15–17] Evidence regarding TIR for older and/or high-risk individuals is lacking, and therefore a less rigorous target is recommended, based on expert opinion, for patients more vulnerable to hypoglycemia.

In summary, CGM devices continue to become smaller, more accurate, and less expensive. They should largely replace capillary blood glucose monitoring over the next decade. Long-term cardiovascular studies should prospectively validate this modality of glucose monitoring as a surrogate of clinical outcome.

URINE AND BLOOD KETONE DETERMINATIONS

Patients with type 2 diabetes rarely have ketosis. However, some experts recommend home ketone testing in the presence of serious illness, which can stress a subset of these patients to the point of developing diabetic ketoacidosis. The presence of nonfasting urine ketones in a patient with type 2 diabetes is a worrisome finding that requires further evaluation. This condition can occur in patients using sodium–glucose cotransporter 2 inhibitors who may develop euglycemic diabetic ketoacidosis.[18] Blood glucose meters that also can test for ketones may help such patients detect ketosis more effectively than urine ketone strips.

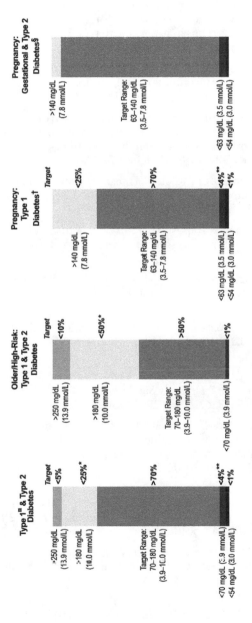

¤ For age <25 yr., if the A1C goal is 7.5%, then set TIR target to approximately 60%. (See *Clinical Applications of Time in Ranges* section in the text for additional information regarding target goal setting in pediatric management.)

† Percentages of time in ranges are based on limited evidence. More research is needed.

§ Percentages of time in ranges have not been included because there is very limited evidence in this area. More research is needed. Please see *Pregnancy* section in text for more considerations on targets for these groups.

* Includes percentage of values >250 mg/dL (13.9 mmol/L).

** Includes percentage of values <54 mg/dL (3.0 mmol/L).

Figure 3.4 CGM-based targets for different diabetes populations.

Source: Battelino.[14]

REFERENCES

1. UK Prospective Diabetes Study (UKPDS) Group. Intensive blood-glucose control with sulphonylureas or insulin compared with conventional treatment and risk of complications in patients with type 2 diabetes (UKPDS 33). *Lancet* 1998;352(9131):837–853

2. UK Prospective Diabetes Study (UKPDS) Group. Effect of intensive blood-glucose control with metformin on complications in overweight patients with type 2 diabetes (UKPDS 34). *Lancet* 1998;352(9131):854–865

3. Diabetes Control Complications Trial Research Group, Nathan DM, Genuth S, et al. The effect of intensive treatment of diabetes on the development and progression of long-term complications in insulin-dependent diabetes mellitus. *N Engl J Med* 1993;329(14):977–986

4. Nathan DM, Kuenen J, Borg R, et al. Translating the A1C assay into estimated average glucose values. *Diabetes Care* 2008;31(8):1473–1478. doi: 10.2337/dc08-0545. Epub 2008 Jun 7

5. Ribeiro RT, Macedo MP, Raposo JF. HbA1c, fructosamine, and glycated albumin in the detection of dysglycaemic conditions. *Curr Diabetes Rev* 2016;12(1):14–19

6. Klonoff DC. Hemoglobinopathies and hemoglobin A1c in diabetes mellitus. *J Diabetes Sci Technol* 2020;14(1)3–7. doi: 10.1177/1932296819841698. Epub 2019 Mar 22

7. American Diabetes Association. 6. Glycemic targets: standards of medical care in diabetes 2020. *Diabetes Care* 2020;43(Suppl. 1):S66–S76. doi: 10.2337/dc20-S00

8. Schnell O, Crocker JB, Weng J. Impact of HbA1c testing at point of care on diabetes management. *J Diabetes Sci Technol* 2017;11(3):611–617. doi: 10.1177/1932296816678263. Epub 2016 Nov 27

9. Garber AJ, Abrahamson MJ, Barzilay JI, et al. Consensus statement by the American Association of Clinical Endocrinologists and American College of Endocrinology on the comprehensive type 2 diabetes management algorithm: 2019 executive summary. *Endocr Pract* 2019;25(1):69–100. https://doi.org/10.4158/CS-2018-0535

10. American Diabetes Association. 14. Management of diabetes in pregnancy: standards of medical care in diabetes 2020. *Diabetes Care* 2020;43(Suppl. 1):S183–S192. doi: 10.2337/dc20-S014

11. American Diabetes Association. 7. Diabetes technology: standards of medical care in diabetes 2020. *Diabetes Care* 2020;43(Suppl. 1):S77–S88. doi: 10.2337/dc20-S007

12. Zoungas S, Patel A, Chalmers J, et al. Severe hypoglycemia and risks of vascular events and death. *N Engl J Med* 2010;363(15):1410–1418. doi: 10.1056/NEJMoa1003795

13. Garber AJ. Treat-to-target trials: uses, interpretation and review of concepts. *Diabetes Obes Metab* 2014;16(3):193–205. doi: 10.1111/dom.12129. Epub 2013 Jun 14

14. Battelino T, Danne T, Bergenstal RM, et al. Clinical targets for continuous glucose monitoring data interpretation: recommendations from the International Consensus on Time in Range. *Diabetes Care* 2019;42(8):1593–1603. doi: 10.2337/dci19-0028. Epub 2019 Jun 8

15. Lu J, Ma X, Zhou J, et al. Association of time in range, as assessed by continuous glucose monitoring, with diabetic retinopathy in type 2 diabetes. *Diabetes Care* 2018;41(11):2370–2376. doi: 10.2337/dc18-1131. Epub 2018 Sep 10

16. Beck RW, Bergenstal RM, Cheng P, et al. The relationships between time in range, hyperglycemia metrics, and HbA1c. *J Diabetes Sci Technol* 2019;13(4):614–626. doi: 10.1177/1932296818822496. Epub 2019 Jan 13

17. Beck RW, Bergenstal RM, Riddlesworth TD, et al. Validation of time in range as an outcome measure for diabetes clinical trials. *Diabetes Care* 2019;42(3):400–405. doi: 10.2337/dc18-1444. Epub 2018 Oct 23

18. Rafey MF, Butt A, Coffey B, et al. Prolonged acidosis is a feature of SGLT2i-induced euglycaemic diabetic ketoacidosis. *Endocrinol Diabetes Metab Case Rep* 2019;2019. doi: 10.1530/EDM-19-0087. [Epub ahead of print]

POPULATION HEALTH AND COST EFFECTIVENESS

Asra Kermani, MD

The prevalence of diabetes and obesity has increased dramatically.[1] The Centers for Disease Control and Prevention estimated in 2017 that the prevalence of diagnosed diabetes is ~30 million people. Per-capita healthcare expense (regardless of diabetes status) in general has continued to increase in the U.S. without a corresponding improvement in outcomes—the 2019 estimate is $10,209 per capita, which is far in excess of other developed nations (Fig. 3.5). Total healthcare spending is expected to be 19% of gross domestic product by 2025 (Fig. 3.6). As a consequence of these changes, addressing diabetes has become a population health concern in the U.S.

Population health is defined as "the health outcomes of a group of individuals, including the distribution of such outcomes within the group."[2] Other factors impacting diabetes care at the level of population health include the high cost and limited access to diabetes self-management education and lack of access to specialty care. Diabetes self-management education has been shown to reduce hospital admissions and readmissions as well as estimated lifetime healthcare costs related to a lower risk for complications.[3,4] Additionally, diabetes outcomes are commonly viewed from a medical context rather than psychosocial context. Thus, diabetes outcomes are greatly influenced by healthcare disparities.[5] Finally, payment reform is changing as reimbursements are increasingly value based, focused on achieving quality measures and reducing unnecessary utilization.

 United States per capita healthcare spending is more than twice the average of other developed countries

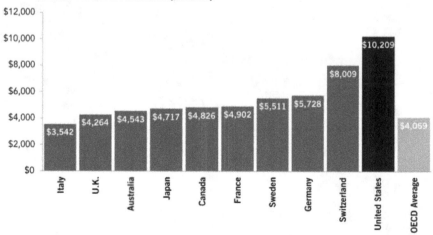

HEALTHCARE COSTS PER CAPITA (DOLLARS)

Figure 3.5 U.S. per capita health spending. Note: Data are for 2017 or latest available. Chart uses purchasing power parities to convert data into U.S. dollars.

Source: Organization for Economic Cooperation and Development, OECD Health Statistics 2018, June 2018. Compiled by PGPF. © 2018 Peter G. Peterson Foundation.

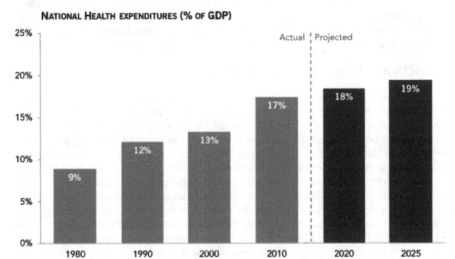

Figure 3.6 U.S. health spending relative to economy. Source: Centers for Medi-care and Medicaid Services, National Health Expenditures, February 2019. Compiled by PGPF. © 2019 Peter G. Peterson Foundation.

STATUS OF DIABETES IN THE U.S. POPULATION

According to the Centers for Disease Control and Prevention, in 2017 there were 30.3 million people with diabetes in the U.S, comprising 9.4% of the pou-lation. People with diagnosed diabetes incur average medical expenditures of ~$13,700 per year, of which ~$7,000 is attributed to diabetes.[1]

The largest components of medical expenditures for patients with diabetes are attributed to inpatient hospital care (see Table 3.20).[6] The American Diabetes Association in 2019 reported that 33%–49% of patients with diabetes still did not

Table 3.20–Medical Expenditures for Patients with Diabetes

Medical expenditures for patients with diabetes	Total medical cost (%)
Hospital inpatient care	43
Prescription medications to treat complications	18
Medications for diabetes and supplies	12
Physician office visits	9
In-home nursing/nonhospital residential stays	8

Source: American Diabetes Association.[6]

meet individual targets for A1C, blood pressure, or lipids, and only 14% met the combined targets for A1C, blood pressure, lipids, and nonsmoking status.[7] While there have been gains in reducing vascular complications of diabetes,[8] progress in cardiovascular risk factor control has recently slowed down.[9] Part of the challenge in addressing population health comes from a fragmented delivery system, which lacks clinical information capabilities, duplicates services, and is poorly designed.

CHRONIC DISEASE MANAGEMENT

There is a gap between the care patients receive and their clinical outcomes, despite the best technology and medical care. This gap, addressed in *Crossing the Quality Chasm*, published by the Institute of Medicine in 2001, outlined a series of problems to be addressed in order to better serve the needs of an aging population with a high burden of chronic diseases—a need that the acute care model fails to serve.[10] An overly complex and uncoordinated healthcare system can lead to delays in care, reduced patient safety, wasteful and duplicative processes, and gaps in coverage and information loss. Providers also need to be incentivized to meet quality measures by payment reform, through value-based payment models as opposed to the traditional fee-for-service system. In addition to fragmented health care, patients often face other obstacles such as access to food, transportation, safe environments, and literacy (often termed social determinants of health), as well as the presence of concomitant depression and the increasingly high cost of medications.

A seminal model to address this chasm is the Chronic Care Model, developed by Ed Wagner as early as 1992.[11] He noted that the requisite elements to effect a systems change for patients with chronic disease are as follows:

■ Changing to a care delivery system that is proactive versus reactive, using a team-based approach.
■ Supporting self-management in patients that strengthens their skills and confidence in becoming managers of their illness.
■ Using decision support based on evidence-based guidelines.
■ Effectively using clinical information systems such as registries that can provide patient- and population-specific data to care teams.
■ Using community resources to enhance patient care.
■ Changing the focus of health systems to shift toward quality-based care.

SHIFT TO POPULATION HEALTH: VALUE-BASED PAYMENTS

In the U.S., the physician reimbursement structure is still largely a fee-for-service model, with some patients belonging to a fee-for-value payment model. However, as hospitals and organizations respond to government-driven value-based incentive and risk models by acquiring medical practices and establishing larger health networks, more payments will be expected to derive from fee-for-value payment models.

The Affordable Care Act of 2010 (ACA) refocused diabetes care from the individual patient level to that of population health, with new value payment models as an incentive to drive a Chronic Care Model approach. The ACA defined a triple aim for population health: to improve the health of a given population, to provide a positive patient experience, and to do so at an affordable cost of care.

To achieve these goals, the Centers for Medicare and Medicaid Services created alternative payment models (APMs) to incentivize medical providers. One such payment model is the Accountable Care Organization (ACO), which comprises groups of doctors, hospitals, and other healthcare providers who come together voluntarily to deliver coordinated, high-quality care to the Medicare patients they serve. This model also applies to non-Medicare commercially insured populations that participate in an ACO. The ACO model focuses on shifting payment to medical providers from fee for service to fee for value.

Value in health care is defined as outcomes divided by cost. However, the prerequisite in this equation is that outcomes must incorporate improved quality of care.[12] Therefore, value does not necessarily improve with cost reduction alone. For example, using an inexpensive medication such as sulfonylurea in elderly patients with type 2 diabetes results in an increased risk of dangerous hypoglycemia, leading to falls, motor vehicle accidents, cognitive loss, seizures, and death. To improve quality of care is part of the value proposition; hence, reimbursements are part of the process of shifting from fee for service to fee for value.

In a value-based model, the performance of medical providers is increasingly based on quality metrics and utilization. Quality metrics are a variety of predefined, evidence-based, preventive health measures that need to be met in order for providers or organizations to receive financial benefits or avoid financial penalty. For diabetes, these may include A1C screening, reducing A1C to <9%, statin use, hypertension control, nephropathy, and retinopathy screening. Utilization refers to frequency of emergency department visits, hospital admissions and readmissions, medication utilization, imaging, procedures, and postacute care costs such as home health and long-term care. Payers benchmark payments to populations of patients based on their risk score, which is defined by disease-related features (e.g., the presence of co-morbidities like neuropathy, retinopathy, or nephropathy). These risk scores are based in part on the disease-specific diagnosis codes. Providers need to accurately code for their patients' disease states as payments are based on patients' anticipated expenses contingent upon added complexities. For example, the expected cost of care for a patient with a diagnosis code of uncontrolled type 2 diabetes in a patient with known diabetic nephropathy might be considerably lower than the expected cost of care for the same patient with a diagnosis code of type 2 diabetes uncontrolled with nephropathy. Therefore, imprecise coding may underestimate the co-morbidities of a patient population, risking a financial penalty to the provider or organization. If providers are able to manage the care for their patients below the projected expense, then shared savings to the medical group can occur.

Savings as high as $1.84 billion were generated over three years in one of the Medicare ACOs named the Medicare Shared Savings Program.[13] The majority of large commercial insurers have also adopted the ACO value-based model for their own patient populations. As of 2017, 34% of total U.S. healthcare payments were tied to APMs. In contrast, 41% of payments were based on fee for service without quality and value measures. The remaining 25% of payments were linked to a modified fee-for-service model linked to quality and value. Within the APMs, commercial insurances consisted of 28.3% of healthcare dollars.[14]

Incorporating Population Health Elements in Clinical Practice

While the size and structure of a medical practice can vary considerably, the following activities can help focus care toward value-based patient outcomes. To begin, clinic providers and clinic staff need to know the quality measures they are responsible for. Work duties should be restructured to allow the office to operate as a team. For example, office staff can check to see if A1C or nephropathy screening was completed in the past year or if the patient received an influenza vaccination; they can alert the providers or order such screenings through a standing delegation order structure if they are due. A simple checklist of the metrics can be used in small offices, whereas larger offices may have integrated alerts in their electronic medical records. If the latter is available, a patient-specific list of missing care elements can be generated and used prior to a clinic appointment to ensure that all quality care gaps are addressed. Using standing orders for staff could minimize barriers and streamline this process. Monitoring performance reports regularly—weekly or biweekly—will keep the volume of work manageable, allow for rapid identification of barriers, and provide the opportunity to devise new solutions to workflow or process challenges. Reorganizing team function and clinic schedules to meet the needs of chronically ill patients, such as ensuring access for urgent work-ins, may prevent costly emergency department visits for hyperglycemia. Finally, reorganizing the staffing schedule can help accommodate added data entry time for preventive health measures.

At a patient level, providers can implement value-based thinking by incorporating current guidelines and best practices in the care of their patients. Before prescribing, the practitioner should discuss medication costs and available alternatives with patients. For labs and/or procedures, the practitioner should consider which are needed to effect change in medical management and which might be redundant.

Accurate coding for diseases allows payers to risk-stratify cases, estimate actual cost of care, and benchmark payments to account for more complex care delivery. As this is a new field, it is useful for providers to share their experiences with colleagues.

Finally, it is vital to include patients in shared decision making and goal setting; mutually understood and agreed-upon objectives, as well as focused and more attainable goals, can be empowering and can allow patients to build upon their successes. Goals may need to be modified or prioritized for those with multiple co-morbidities or those with a limited life span.

Ancillary Patient Support

Providers that are part of Medicare ACOs have access to care coordination services. Care coordination teams use community health workers, licensed vocational nurses, registered nurses, social workers, and/or pharmacists to assist patients with many complex needs. They can assist with medication review and reconciliation, prescription financial assistance, and assessment of resource needs, such as food, housing, transportation, and durable medical equipment—all of which can impact diabetes outcomes. Additionally, they provide home visits for safety assessments.

CURRENT CHALLENGES

Diabetes self-management education and support (DSMES) is not consistently available to patients,[15] and even when it is provided at the time of diagnosis, it may be overwhelming for the patient. Hence, focused and periodic updates are helpful. Diabetes self-management empowers people to take ownership of their health and be more actively involved in their care. Cost and access to self-management education are also barriers, as is the inaccurate perception by some patients and providers that such education is of little value. Using diverse educational modalities can broaden educational access, such as online training, smartphone applications, community-based education, as well as access to information in a culturally and language-appropriate manner.

Access to medical care and diabetes education can be enhanced with the use of telemedicine. Telemedicine has become an alternative vehicle for patient care that can augment care delivery over larger geographic areas, both urban and rural.[16] Numerous studies show a positive impact on glycemic control, lipid lowering, and improved diabetes education with the use of telemedicine services, with concurrent shifts in reimbursements to support telemedicine services.

It is becoming increasingly more challenging for medical professionals to keep up with and assimilate the rapidly changing standards of care and meeting guidelines, as well as the rapid development in new medications and technology. Access to diabetes specialty care is very limited. There is an increased need for decision support systems to be integrated with the electronic medical record.

Incorporating population health at the clinic level is challenging and requires a shift from provider-based care to team-based care. Clinic staff education is a vital part of functioning as a healthcare team. Education around clinical and other process metrics and how to help meet quality outcomes is a team goal, not an individual provider mandate, and requires substantial clinic flow redesign.

CONCLUSION

Population health has become the current focus of both best practice for chronic disease management and also physician payment. APMs continue to evolve and comprise an increasing proportion of payments for both Medicare and commercial insurances. Clinicians and their staff will need to employ new strategies to meet quality measures and to improve patient experience and outcomes.

REFERENCES

1. Centers for Disease Control and Prevention. *Estimates of Diabetes and Its Burden in the United States* Published 2017. Available from https://www.cdc.gov/diabetes/pdfs/data/statistics/national-diabetes-statistics-report.pdf

2. Kindig D, Stoddart G. What is population health? *Am J Public Health* 2003;93(3):380–383. doi: 10.2105/ajph.93.3.380

3. Healy SJ, Black D, Harris C, Lorenz A, Dungan KM. Inpatient diabetes education is associated with less frequent hospital readmission among patients with poor glycemic control. *Diabetes Care* 2013;36(10):2960–2967. doi: 10.2337/dc13-0108. Epub 2013 Jul 8

4. Robbins JM, Thatcher GE, Webb DA, Valdmanis VG. Nutritionist visits, diabetes classes, and hospitalization rates and charges: the Urban Diabetes Study. *Diabetes Care* 2008;31(4):655–660. doi: 10.2337/dc07-1871. Epub 2008 Jan 9

5. White RO, Beech BM, Miller S. Health care disparities and diabetes care: practical considerations for primary care providers. *Clin Diabetes* 2009;27(3):105–112. doi: 10.2337/diaclin.27.3.105

6. American Diabetes Association. Economic costs of diabetes in the U.S. in 2012. *Diabetes Care* 2013;36(4):1033–1046. doi: 10.2337/dc12-2625. Epub 2013 Mar 6

7. American Diabetes Association. Professional Practice Committee: Standards of Medical Care in Diabetes-2019. *Diabetes Care* 2019;42(Suppl. 1):S3

8. Gregg EW, Li Y, Wang J, et al. Changes in diabetes-related complications in the United States, 1990–2010. *N Engl J Med* 2014;370(16):1514–1523. doi: 10.1056/NEJMoa1310799

9. Gregg EW, Hora I, Benoit SR. Resurgence in diabetes-related complications. *JAMA* 2019;321(19):1867–1868. doi: 10.1001/jama.2019.3471

10. Insititute of Medicine. *Crossing the Quality Chasm: A New Health System for the 21st Century.* Washington, DC, National Academies Press, 2001

11. Wagner EH. Chronic disease management: what will it take to improve care for chronic illness? *Eff Clin Pract* 1998;1(1):2–4.

12. Porter ME. What is value in health care? *N Engl J Med* 2010;363(26):2477–2481. doi: 10.1056/NEJMp1011024. Epub 2010 Dec 8

13. Dobson A. *Estimates of Savings by Medicare Shared Savings Program Accountable Care Organizations.* Published 2018. Available from https://www.naacos.com/assets/docs/pdf/Study_of_MSSP_Savings_2012-2015.pdf

14. Peiris D, Phipps-Taylor MC, Stachowski CA, et al. ACOs holding commercial contracts are larger and more efficient than noncommercial ACOs. *Health Aff (Millwood)* 2016;35(10):1849–1856. doi: 10.1377/hlthaff.2016.0387

15. Beck J, Greenwood DA, Blanton L, et al. 2017 National standards for diabetes self-management education and support. *Diabetes Care* 2017;40(10):1409–1419. doi: 10.1177/0145721719897952. Epub 2019 Dec 24

16. Siminerio L, Ruppert K, Huber K, Toledo FG. Telemedicine for Reach, Education, Access, and Treatment (TREAT): linking telemedicine with diabetes self-management education to improve care in rural communities. *Diabetes Educ* 2014;40(6):797–805. doi: 10.1177/0145721714551993. Epub 2014 Sep 24

DIABETES TECHNOLOGY

Marconi Abreu, M.D.

CONTINUOUS GLUCOSE MONITORS

The world of glucose monitoring has evolved in the last 5 years. Real-time continuous glucose monitors (CGMs) are cheaper, smaller, more accurate, easier to insert, and require minimal or no calibration, and they can communicate with cellphones and wearable devices. They are a cost-effective approach to monitoring patients with a complex insulin regimen, those requiring frequent glycemic checks, and those at higher risk for hypoglycemia. Some are also approved as replacement for of traditional glucose meters in guiding insulin dosing decisions. The expectation over the next 5–10 years is that CGM technology will continue to get smaller and less expensive and will ultimately replace capillary blood glucose finger-stick checking in most patients with type 2 diabetes.

CGMs measure interstitial glucose, which correlates well with plasma glucose, although in most cases they incur a 5- to 10-min delay compared with real-time blood glucose measurements.[1] They have three components: a sensor (filament inserted on the skin, which measures the interstitial glucose), a transmitter (usually sits on top of the sensor and uses NFC or low-energy Bluetooth technology to transmit the information to the receiver), and the receiver (device used to read the blood glucose); an exception is the Eversense implantable CGM device where the sensor is implanted under the skin and can provide readings for 90–180 days (depending on country of approval). A smartphone, a smart watch, an insulin pump, or a separate device can be used as the receiver. CGM accuracy is represented by the mean absolute relative difference (MARD).[2] The MARD describes the average of the difference between glucose level measured by the CGM and the plasma glucose level assessed by standardized laboratory methods. It is expressed as a percentage number, and the lower the number, the "less inaccurate" the CGM device is. The Food and Drug Administration established that a CGM MARD <10% is required for that CGM data to be used as a replacement of capillary glucose to dose insulin.[3] The glucose reading from the CGM can lag behind 15–20 min from plasma glucose levels, and at times when blood glucose is moving rapidly, either up or down, the readings might be quite different than measured by capillary glucose. This difference is not due to a CGM defect or inaccuracy but rather represents a known limitation of the technology. CGM is also typically more inaccurate the day of sensor insertion. The reason is that the sensor filament requires some time to "soak" and react with interstitial fluid in order to improve its accuracy. Patients using CGM readings to make decisions on insulin dosing should consider using capillary glucose readings instead on the day of new sensor insertion.

There are currently four companies providing CGM systems in the U.S.: Abbot (Freestyle Libre), Dexcom (G5 & G6), Medtronic (Guardian), and Senseonics (Eversense). The Freestyle Libre is the only flash CGM.[4] It does not provide real-time glucose information or alerts for low or high glucose. Scanning takes about 1 sec (flash) and can be done using a cellphone or a separate reading device. Uploaded information includes the current interstitial glucose reading, an arrow indicating the glucose trend (rate of change), and the last 8 h of glucose information. The Freestyle Libre is a relatively low-cost (approximately $120 per month as per GoodRx information in Dec 2019), user-friendly, disposable system with a near-painless insertion kit that is currently approved for use only in the back of the arm. Its current version has a MARD of 9.4%, has a warm-up period of only 1 h, and can be continuously be used for 14 days. It comes factory calibrated and does not require additional finger-stick checks. One limitation of the Libre system is that it can be inaccurate in the lower glucose range, with readings typically reported lower in the CGM than by capillary blood glucose testing. It also does not provide alerts. Libre 2 is the updated version of the Libre, expected to enter the U.S. market in 2020. While still requiring flash scanning, it is expected to have a MARD of 9.2%, alarms for low and high blood glucose levels, along with better accuracy in the low glucose range.

All other available CGMs are categorized as real-time CGMs, as glucose readings are displayed continuously on the receiver in real time. They provide alerts for interstitial glucose levels that are high, low, or predicted to become low. The Dexcom G6 is factory precalibrated (can allow optional calibrations), has a MARD of 9.0%, can be inserted with just one hand, and is approved for use in the abdominal area.[5] Once the sensor is inserted, the patient attaches a transmitter on top of the sensor, which transfers the data to the receiver (separate device or a smartphone with the Dexcom app). Patients can set alarms for high or low glucose readings, which can alert the patient ≤30 min before a glucose level falls <80 mg/dl, making this device particularly useful for patients on complex insulin therapy with a high risk for hypoglycemia or those with hypoglycemia unawareness. When using a cellphone as a receiver, data are uploaded in real time to the cloud and can be shared in real time with others (e.g., caregivers, providers). Patients can use this feature as a back-up system by having a family member check on them if they fail to respond to a critical glucose level (i.e., hypoglycemia) for a prolonged period of time. The next generation Dexcom G7 should be available in 2020. It will be smaller than the current system, have a flat surface, be disposable, and have a lower cost.

The Medtronic Guardian is a system similar to the Dexcom G6 but requires several calibrations (three or more daily) to achieve good accuracy.[6] It has a warm-up period of 2 h and a MARD of 10.5% with one to two calibrations and 9.64% with three to four calibrations. The next generation of Medtronic CGM is also expected for 2020 and should be more accurate and require zero or one calibration. The Eversense from Senseonics is the first and only long-term implantable CGM on the market.[7] Its sensor is inserted subcutaneously via a 20-min in-office procedure and can be worn for ≤90 days (approved for 180 days in Europe). Patients use a rechargeable transmitter over the skin on top of the area of sensor insertion. It has a MARD of 8.5% with two calibrations, making it the most accurate CGM available in the U.S. Glucose data are transmitted to a cellphone, reader, or wearable device.

CGMs download offers more comprehensive glucose data to both patients and providers. It allows patients to understand the impact of individual foods on their glucose in real-time and can drive behavior modification. Several studies have demonstrated improvement in A1C of approximately 0.5% by simply using a real-time or flash CGM device.[8] It also helps providers to easily identify patterns of hypo- and hyperglycemia, which can guide medication adjustments and enhance provider-to-patient education.

PATCH PUMPS

The V-GO is the only patch pump available in the U.S.[9] The device is applied on top of the skin and has a subcutaneous infusion catheter that can simplify basal bolus insulin therapy in patients with type 2 diabetes, possibly increasing compliance in those requiring more complex insulin regimens. It is currently available in three reservoir sizes, providing three fixed basal insulin doses (20, 30, or 40 units/day), delivered continuously over 24 h. All three reservoir sizes also allow ≤36 units of additional insulin to be delivered as prandial or correction boluses in 2-unit increments by the press of a button on the device. The V-GO is a mechanical device with no screens or electronics, thus appealing to those patients with an aversion to technology. It is approved for use in the abdomen and in the arm.

SMART INSULIN PENS

Several smart insulin pens/pen caps will be available in the U.S. market by 2020.[10] They will either use insulin cartridges or be adapted to the current disposable insulin pens. Smarts pens/pen caps connect to cellphone apps, which can track the insulin dose delivered. These apps can often integrate CGM or blood glucose meter data and allow patients to input their carbohydrate intake and exercise activity.

INSULIN PUMPS

There are currently three insulin pump companies that provide insulin delivery systems in the U.S.: Insulet, Medtronic, and Tandem.[9] Omnipod (from Insulet) is the only tubeless system. Insulin is delivered from a reservoir attached to the patient's skin and controlled remotely. The MiniMed 670G tubed pump is a CGM-augmented hybrid pump system which uses data from the Medtronic Guardian CGM to deliver basal insulin in a semi-automatic fashion. The Tandem T: Slim X2 system is another tubed pump which uses CGM-augmented technology to control the insulin delivery via the pump. It adjusts basal insulin and provides an automated correction bolus with the goal to keep glucose values between 112.5 mg/dl (6.2 mmol/L) and 160 mg/dL (8.9 mmol/L). When glucose values are predicted to drop <112.5 mg/dL (<6.2 mmol/L), the delivery of basal insulin delivery is reduced, and when they are predicted to be <70 mg/dL (<3.9 mmol/L), delivery is stopped. When glucose values are predicted to be >160 mg/dL (>8.9 mmol/L) in the next 30 min, basal insulin is increased, and if values are predicted to be >180 mg/dL (>10 mmol/L), the pump calculates a correction bolus with a target of 110 mg/dL (6.1 mmol/L) and delivers 60% of that value up to once an hour as needed.[11] The T: Slim X2 is the only pump that can add new features solely via a software update. A more detailed discussion on pump therapy is beyond the scope of this book.

REFERENCES

1. Schmelzeisen-Redeker G, Schoemaker M, Kirchsteiger H, Freckmann G, Heinemann L, Del Re L. Time delay of CGM sensors: relevance, causes,

and countermeasures. *J Diabetes Sci Technol* 2015;9(5):1006–1015. doi: 10.1177/1932296815590154. Epub 2015 Aug 6. PubMed PMID: 26243773; PubMed Central PMCID: PMCPMC4667340

2. Cappon G, Vettoretti M, Sparacino G, Facchinetti A. Continuous glucose monitoring sensors for diabetes management: a review of technologies and applications. *Diabetes Metab J* 2019;43(4):383–397. doi: 10.4093/dmj.2019.0121. Epub 2019 Aug 24. PubMed PMID: 31441246; PubMed Central PMCID: PMCPMC6712232

3. Kovatchev BP, Patek SB, Ortiz EA, Breton MD. Assessing sensor accuracy for non-adjunct use of continuous glucose monitoring. *Diabetes Technol Ther* 2015;17(3):177–186. doi: 10.1089/dia.2014.0272. PubMed PMID: 25436913

4. Blum A. Freestyle libre glucose monitoring system. *Clin Diabetes* 2018;36(2):203–204. doi: 10.2337/cd17-0130. Epub 2018 Apr 25.PubMed PMID: 29686463; PubMed Central PMCID: PMCPMC5898159

5. Forlenza GP, Kushner T, Messer LH, Wadwa P, Sankaranarayanan S. Factory-calibrated continuous glucose monitoring: how and why it works, and the dangers of reuse beyond approved duration of wear. *Diabetes Technol Ther* 2019;21(4):222–229. doi: 10.1089/dia.2018.0401. PubMed PMID: 30817171

6. Tubiana-Rufi N, Riveline JP, Dardari D. Real-time continuous glucose monitoring using Guardian®RT: from research to clinical practice. *Diabetes Metab* 2007;33(6):415–420. doi: https://doi.org/10.1016/j.diabet.2007.05.003

7. Deiss D, Szadkowska A, Gordon D, Mallipedhi A, Schutz-Fuhrmann I, Aguilera E, Ringsell C, De Block C, Irace C. Clinical practice recommendations on the routine use of Eversense, the first long-term implantable continuous glucose monitoring system. *Diabetes Technol Ther* 2019;21(5):254–264. doi: 10.1089/dia.2018.0397. PubMed PMID: 31021180

8. American Diabetes Association. 6. Glycemic targets: standards of medical care in diabetes 2020. *Diabetes Care* 2020;43(Suppl. 1):S66–S76. doi: 10.2337/dc20-S006. Epub 2019 Dec 22. PubMed PMID: 31862749

9. Ginsberg BH. Patch pumps for insulin. *J Diabetes Sci Technol* 2019;13(1):27–33. doi: 10.1177/1932296818786513. Epub 2018 Aug 3. PubMed PMID: 30070604; PubMed Central PMCID: PMCPMC6313281

10. Klonoff DC, Kerr D. Smart pens will improve insulin therapy. *J Diabetes Sci Technol* 2018;12(3):551–553. doi: 10.1177/1932296818759845. Epub 2018 Feb 8. PubMed PMID: 29411641; PubMed Central PMCID: PMCPMC6154228

11. Brown SA, Kovatchev BP, Raghinaru D, Lum JW, Buckingham BA, Kudva YC, et al. Six-month randomized, multicenter trial of closed-loop control in type 1 diabetes. *N Engl J Med* 2019;381(18):1707–1717. doi: 10.1056/NEJMoa1907863

Special Therapeutic Situations

Highlights

Diabetes in Pregnancy
  Preconception Care and Counseling
  Prepregnancy and Pregnancy Metabolic Metrics
  Gestational Diabetes Mellitus
  Diabetes Care in Pregnancy

Diabetes in Youth
  Differentiation of Type 1 and Type 2 Diabetes in Youth
  Screening for Type 2 Diabetes in Youth
  Treating Type 2 Diabetes in Youth
  When to Consider Specialty Consultation

Diabetes in Hospitalized and Critically Ill Patients
  Glucose Monitoring
  Glycemic Targets
  Choice of Therapy
  Hypoglycemia
  Enteral/Parenteral Feeds
  Glucocorticoid Therapy
  Considerations for the Surgical Patient
  Transition from Hospital to Home

Major Acute Complications
  Hyperosmolar Hyperglycemic State
  Hypoglycemia
  Diabetic Ketoacidosis
  Infection

Elderly and Diabetes
  Diabetes Trials in Older Patients
  Glycemic Goals
  Treatment Regimens

Highlights
Special Therapeutic Situations

DIABETES IN PREGNANCY

■ Glycemic control at the time of conception and throughout pregnancy is critical. Consensus on specific glycemic targets has not been achieved, but an A1C as near to normal as possible without significant hypoglycemia is recommended.

■ Insulin should be used in all pregnant patients with preexisting diabetes who fail dietary management.

■ Care for the pregnant diabetic woman should utilize a team with experience in the care of this high-risk group.

DIABETES IN YOUTH

■ Inactive youth with obesity and a strong family history of type 2 diabetes are at high risk for type 2 diabetes.

■ The presence of ketoacidosis does not rule out the presence of type 2 diabetes in children.

■ Metformin is the only approved oral medication for type 2 diabetes in children. Liraglutide is the only noninsulin injectable drug approved to treat type 2 diabetes in pediatric patients.

■ Insulin should be used in children who have metabolic decompensation or who do not achieve adequate control with diet, exercise, or metformin therapy.

■ Young people with type 2 diabetes have a high risk for cardiovascular disease and should be treated aggressively for hypertension, dyslipidemia, and nephropathy.

DIABETES IN HOSPITALIZED AND CRITICALLY ILL PATIENTS

■ Intravenous insulin is the treatment of choice in hospitalized patients with hyperglycemia.

■ Care of the critically ill patients with type 2 diabetes should be provided through a collaboration of nursing, nutrition, and pharmacy, as well as the medical staff and patient. Institutional protocols should be developed and staff trained to allow strict glycemic control.

- Goals of therapy in hospitalized patients should be as follows:
  - Critically ill patients: 140–180 mg/dl.
  - For noncritically ill patients on general medicine and surgical units, glycemic goals are less definite:
    - Preprandial: 140 mg/dL; targets <110 mg/dL are not recommended.
    - Peak postprandial and all random glucose levels: <180 mg/dl.

MAJOR ACUTE COMPLICATIONS

- The major acute complications of diabetes include hyperosmolar hyperglycemic syndrome (HHS) and diabetic ketoacidosis, often precipitated by infection and hypoglycemia.

- The four major clinical features of HHS are as follows:
  - Severe hyperglycemia.
  - Absence of or slight ketosis.
  - Plasma or serum hyperosmolality.
  - Profound dehydration.

- Hypoglycemia can be precipitated by the following:
  - Decreased food intake.
  - Intensive exercise.
  - Alcohol and/or other drugs in combination with exogenous insulin, sulfonylureas, and meglitinides.

- Hypoglycemia is classified as level 1 (glucose <70 mg/dl [<3.9 mmol/L] and ≥54 mg/dl [≥3 mmol/L]), level 2 (glucose <54 mg/dl [<3.0 mmol/L]), or level 3 (severe hypoglycemia). Severe hypoglycemia is diagnosed in the setting of altered mental and/or physical status when third-party assistance is required to overcome a hypoglycemic event.

- If the patient is conscious, hypoglycemia should be treated by oral ingestion of some form of sugar. In the unconscious state or for the patient unable to ingest oral carbohydrate, either glucagon (parenteral or intranasal) or 50% dextrose by intravenous route is the intervention of choice.

ELDERLY AND DIABETES

- Glycemic targets in the elderly should consider their medical, psychological, and functional status. A1C targets for this population range from 7.5% for healthier individuals to 8.5% for those with complex health issues or advanced cognitive impairment.

- Favor medications with a low risk for hypoglycemia; sulfonylureas, especially glyburide, are generally not recommended.

Special Therapeutic Situations

DIABETES IN PREGNANCY

Nancy Drobycki, RN, MSN, CDCES

Diabetes is the most common medical complication of pregnancy,[1] and the prevalence of gestational diabetes mellitus (GDM) is steadily increasing, giving diabetes care providers many opportunities to positively impact the healthcare and health outcomes of both mother and child. Diabetes management in pregnancy poses a significant challenge for both the person with diabetes and the diabetes care team. The purpose of this section is to discuss the role of the healthcare professional in providing preconception care and counseling, prepregnancy/pregnancy metabolic metrics, GDM, and general aspects of diabetes care in pregnancy, as well as post pregnancy. The importance of establishing a relationship-based diabetes care team that places the woman with diabetes at the center of her care will be emphasized.

Women with preexisting diabetes have a four- to fivefold increase in perinatal mortality and a four- to sixfold increase in stillbirth when compared with women without diabetes.[2] The desired end point of this partnership is the prevention of stillbirth and other potentially devastating sequelae of uncontrolled diabetes in pregnancy, with subsequent outcomes of a safe pregnancy and delivery of a healthy baby.

Research reveals better diabetes and pregnancy outcomes when care has been delivered by a multidisciplinary healthcare team, with a focus on improved glucose control.[3]

PRECONCEPTION CARE AND COUNSELING

At the start of the 20th century, a successful pregnancy in a woman with pre-existing diabetes was almost unheard of. The perinatal mortality rate was ≤65%, and the maternal mortality rate was ≤35%.[2] The discovery and use of insulin was beneficial in reducing the maternal mortality rate, but the perinatal mortality rate did not improve until the 1960s. Advancements in medical technology, laboratory screening, surveillance of metabolic metrics, and prenatal care are all credited with reduced mortality rates, but there are other significant factors impacting outcomes of women with diabetes in pregnancy, especially obesity.[2,3]

With the increase in obesity and change in screening guidelines for diagnosing diabetes in pregnancy, there is an expectant increase in the prevalence of both GDM and pregestational diabetes.[3,4] Although obesity contributes to the rising prevalence of diabetes in pregnancy, not all women with diabetes in pregnancy are overweight or obese. Insulin resistance during pregnancy is a physiologic phenomenon driven by the metabolic demands of the maternal-fetal unit, stress, and pregnancy-induced hormonal changes. These changes can occur in women of any size.[5]

Almost half of all pregnancies are unplanned, and women with chronic illnesses are much more likely to have an unintended pregnancy than women without a chronic illness.[4] One study of pregnant women with preexisting diabetes showed that 70% of women were not using contraception, and thus a major barrier to their receiving preconception care was conceiving sooner than anticipated.[4]

Due to the risks of hyperglycemia-associated complications, the American Diabetes Association recommends that all women with reproductive capability receive preconception counseling and care as a part of routine diabetes care.[3] Counseling should address the importance of glucose control at the time of conception (A1C <6.5% [48 mmol/mol] if safely possible), family planning, use of effective contraception, and assessment of the woman's readiness to conceive.[1,3]

Preconception visits should include laboratory assessments, prescriptions, medication review with needed changes, and referrals (see Table 4.1). The risks associated with unplanned pregnancies should be explained to all women with diabetes who are of childbearing potential.

Table 4.1–Recommended Preconception Visit Assessment Items

Preconception education	**Comprehensive diabetes self-management education** ■ Overweight/obese ■ Meal planning to help achieve glycemic targets prior to conception ■ Correction of dietary nutritional deficiencies ■ Caffeine consumption ■ Safe food handling and preparation **Lifestyle recommendations for:** ■ Moderate exercise ■ Adequate sleep ■ Avoidance of hyperthermia (hot tubs/hot baths) **Comprehensive nutrition assessment with recommendations for:** **Counseling on diabetes in pregnancy per current standards to include:** ■ Insulin resistance of pregnancy and postpartum ■ Glycemic targets in preconception period ■ Avoidance of glycemic variability: severe hyperglycemia/diabetic ketoacidosis and severe hypoglycemia ■ Progression of retinopathy ■ Polycystic ovary syndrome—if indicated ■ Fertility in individuals with diabetes ■ Genetics of diabetes

(continued)

Table 4.1 *(continued)*

	Maternal and fetal risks including: ■ Miscarriage/fetal demise ■ Macrosomia ■ Congenital malformations ■ Preterm labor and delivery ■ Hypertensive disorders of pregnancy
Medical assessment and plan	**General evaluation of overall health** **Evaluation of diabetes-related complications and comorbidities, with a management plan to include:** ■ Nephropathy ■ Retinopathy ■ Neuropathy (sensorimotor and autonomic) ■ Macrovascular disease ■ Thyroid dysfunction ■ Dyslipidemia ■ Hypertension ■ Severe hypoglycemia/hypoglycemia unawareness ■ Nonalcoholic fatty liver disease ■ Barriers to receiving healthcare **Evaluation of obstetric/gynecologic history including:** ■ Cesarean section ■ Congenital malformations/fetal demise ■ Current methods of contraception with a plan to prevent pregnancy until glycemic targets are achieved ■ Hypertensive disorders of pregnancy ■ Postpartum hemorrhage ■ Preterm delivery ■ Previous macrosomia ■ Rh incompatibility ■ Thrombotic events
Laboratory assessments	■ Complete blood count ■ Rubella titer ■ Syphilis ■ Human immunodeficiency virus ■ Hepatitis C ■ A1C ■ Thyroid-stimulating hormone ■ Serum creatinine ■ Urinary albumin-to-creatinine ratio ■ Blood typing ■ Papanicolau testing ■ Chlamydia trachomatis/Neisseria gonorrhea ■ Genetic carrier status (based on history): cystic fibrosis, sickle cell anemia, Thallesemia, Tay-Sachs disease, others (as indicated)
Diabetes medication assessment and glycemic management plan	■ Implementation of a medication/insulin management plan to achieve glycemic targets prior to conception ■ Implementation of appropriate self-monitoring of blood glucose or use of a continuous glucose monitoring system ■ Assessment for desire to implement continuous subcutaneous insulin infusion technology

(continued)

Table 4.1 *(continued)*

Prescription recommendations	■ Prenatal vitamin (with ≥400 µg folic acid) ■ Alternative antihypertensive medication (if needed) ■ Low-dose aspirin (60–150 mg/day) with the alternative of starting this by week 16 gestation (if no contraindication)
Medication review and elimination of potentially hazardous medications	■ Angiotensin-converting enzyme inhibitors ■ Angiotensin receptor blockers ■ Diuretics ■ Atenolol (but other β-blockers may be used as needed) ■ Statins ■ Over-the-counter medications and supplements ■ Other medications deemed teratogenic
Referrals for ancillary health-care services	■ Smoking cessation (if needed) ■ Diabetes self-management education services ■ Medical nutritional therapy ■ Comprehensive eye exam, with ongoing monitoring in the presence of retinopathy

Source: American Diabetes Association.[3]

PREPREGNANCY AND PREGNANCY METABOLIC METRICS

Approximately 50% of women are overweight or obese at the time of conception.[6] Experts recommend that healthcare professionals assess for excessive weight gain in early pregnancy and intervene immediately to help prevent the complications of excessive maternal weight gain (with its coexisting insulin resistance), which increases the risk of preeclampsia, fetal macrosomia, cesarean delivery, and deterioration of metabolic metrics.[7]

Additional consequences of excessive weight gain on the offspring include an increased prevalence of childhood obesity, with its accompanying early onset of metabolic disorders, including cardiovascular disease and type 2 diabetes.[3]

Women should be educated on the appropriate weight gain recommendations in pregnancy. The Institute of Medicine has no specific weight gain recommendations for pregnant women with diabetes; therefore, these guidelines apply to all pregnant women[3,8] (Table 4.2).

Even though weight gain recommendations are the same for women with or without diabetes, the characteristics and treatment regimens for preexisting diabetes in pregnancy and GDM are slightly different. These are outlined in Table 4.3.

Diabetic ketoacidosis (DKA) occurs in 1%–3% of pregnant women with preexisting type 1 diabetes with a fetal mortality rate of between 9% and 36% and a maternal risk of death of >1%.[9] DKA is more common in the second and third trimesters as insulin demands increase. For this reason, consistent basal-bolus insulin administration should be emphasized to prevent the onset of DKA. Glucose and ketones cross the placenta; maternal dehydration and acidosis may lead to fetal hypoxia.

The Hyperglycemia and Adverse Pregnancy Outcome (HAPO) study as well as other observational studies have demonstrated the link between increas-

Table 4.2–Institute of Medicine Weight Gain in Pregnancy Guidelines

Pregestational Body Mass Index (BMI)	Total Weight Gain Range (lb)	Mean Rate of Weight Gain in Second and Third Trimesters (Range in lb/week)
Underweight <18.5	28–40	1 (1–1.3)
Normal weight 18.5–24.9	25–35	1 (0.8–1)
Overweight 25.0–29.9	15–25	0.6 (0.5–0.7)
Obese ≥30	10–20	0.5 (0.4–0.6)

Source: American College of Obstetricians and Gynecologists.[8]

Table 4.3–Comparison of Preexisting Diabetes in Pregnancy and Gestational Diabetes

	Preexisting Type 1 Diabetes	Preexisting Type 2 Diabetes	Gestational Diabetes Mellitus
Characteristics	■ Autoimmune β-cell dysfunction ■ Insulin sensitivity followed by progressive insulin resistance	■ Nonimmune β-cell dysfunction ■ May have insulin sensitivity in first trimester ■ Insulin resistance	■ Onset of glucose intolerance in second and third trimesters ■ Not preexisting overt diabetes ■ Progressive insulin resistance
Insulin needs	■ Variable ■ Insulin sensitive in first 16 weeks ■ Weeks 17–35: 60%–200% rise in insulin need	■ Improved glucose levels in first 16 weeks ■ Insulin doses may double by mid-second trimester and triple by term of pregnancy	■ Progressive insulin resistance throughout the second and third trimesters (with a leveling off with placental aging)
Treatment regimen	■ Monitoring ■ Medical nutritional therapy (MNT) ■ Regular physical activity ■ Stress management ■ Insulin	■ Monitoring ■ MNT ■ Regular physical activity ■ Stress management ■ Insulin	■ Monitoring ■ MNT ■ Regular physical activity ■ Stress management ■ Insulin (if needed)
Glucose targets	■ Fasting: <95 mg/dL (5.3 mmol/L) ■ 1-h postprandial: <140 mg/dL (7.8 mmol/L) ■ 2-h postprandial: <120 mg/dL (6.7 mmol/L)	■ Fasting: <95 mg/dL (5.3 mmol/L) ■ 1-h postprandial: <140 mg/dL (7.8 mmol/L) ■ 2-h postprandial: <120 mg/dL (6.7 mmol/L)	■ Fasting: <95 mg/dL (5.3 mmol/L) ■ 1-h postprandial: <140 mg/dL (7.8 mmol/L) ■ 2-h postprandial: <120 mg/dL (6.7 mmol/L)

(continued)

Table 4.3 *(continued)*

	Preexisting Type 1 Diabetes	Preexisting Type 2 Diabetes	Gestational Diabetes Mellitus
A1C target	■ 6%–6.5% (42–48 mmol/mol) (if achievable without significant hypoglycemia)	■ 6%–6.5% (42–48 mmol/mol) (if achievable without significant hypoglycemia)	■ A1C considered as a secondary measure of glucose control
Urine ketone testing	■ Any time glucose is >200 mg/dL (11.1 mmol/L) ■ When newly diagnosed ■ Every 4 h if ill, until ketones clear	■ At start of MNT (1–2 weeks) ■ If rapid weight loss occurs ■ Any time glucose is >200 mg/dL (11.1 mmol/L)	■ If persistent weight loss occurs ■ If concerns about adequate calorie/ carbohydrate consumption

Source: American Diabetes Association[3] and American College of Obstetricians and Gynecologists.[8]

ing A1C values in pregnancy and poor outcomes.[3] It is important to note that A1C values are lower in a normal pregnancy due to faster red blood cell turnover. In addition, since the A1C represents the estimated average glucose, it may not provide critical information about postprandial glucose control. Therefore, self-monitoring of blood glucose (SMBG) is the recommended first-line measure of glycemic control in pregnancy.[3]

Early in gestation, an A1C value <6%–6.5% (<42 mmol/mol– 48 mmol/mol) is associated with the lowest rate of adverse fetal outcomes, while in the second and third trimesters values <6% (<42 mmol/mol) reduce the risk of macrosomia, preterm delivery, and preeclampsia.[3] An A1C value <6% (<42 mmol/mol) in pregnancy may be ideal, if it can be achieved without frequent hypoglycemia. On the other hand, in the setting of frequent hypoglycemia, the A1C target may need to be loosened to <7% (<53 mmol/mol) due to the association of hypoglycemia in pregnancy with low birth weight and other deleterious outcomes.[3]

GESTATIONAL DIABETES MELLITUS

GDM is defined as diabetes that is diagnosed in the second or third trimester of pregnancy and is not clearly either preexisting type 1 or type 2 diabetes.[3] Approximately 9%–18% of all pregnancies are impacted by GDM, depending on the population and method of diagnosis.[10]

GDM screening guidelines[3,11] are as follows:

■ Screen for undiagnosed diabetes or prediabetes at the first prenatal visit in those with risk factors, using standard diagnostic criteria.
■ Screen for GDM at 24–28 weeks' gestation in pregnant women without a prior diagnosis of diabetes using a "one-step" 75 g oral glucose tolerance test (OGTT) with plasma glucose measurement fasting, 1 h and 2 h (Table 4.4). Alternatively, screen for GDM using a "two-step" approach with a 50-g nonfasting screen, followed by a 100 g OGTT for those who screen positive (Table 4.5).[12]

Table 4.4–One-Step Strategy: 75 g Glucose Load with Overnight Fast of 8 h or More

Glucose Measure	Glucose Concentration Threshold
Fasting plasma glucose	>92 mg/dL (≥5.1 mmol/L)
1-h plasma glucose	>180 mg/dL (>10.0 mmol/L)
2-h plasma glucose	>153 mg/dL (>8.5 mmol/L)

Source: American Diabetes Association[11] and Feldman.[13]

- Following delivery in women with GDM, screen for persistent diabetes 4–12 weeks postpartum using a 75 g OGTT and clinically appropriate, nonpregnancy diagnostic criteria.
- Women with a history of GDM should have lifelong screening for the development of diabetes or prediabetes every 1–3 years if the 75 g OGTT is normal.
- Women with a history of GDM found to have prediabetes should receive intensive lifestyle interventions and/or metformin to prevent diabetes.

The two-step strategy for diagnosing GDM is listed in Table 4.5. The American College of Obstetricians and Gynecologists supports this method, stating that in their studies the one-step approach did not decrease the incidence of

Table 4.5–Two-Step Strategy

Glucose Measure	Glucose Concentration Threshold
Step 1: Perform a 50 g glucose load test (nonfasting) with plasma glucose measurement 1 h post glucose load, at 24–28 weeks' gestation in women not previously diagnosed with diabetes.	If the plasma glucose measured after the load is ≥130 mg/dL, 135 mg/dL, or 140 mg/dL (7.2 mmol/L, 7.5 mmol/L, or 7.8 mmol/L, respectively), proceed to a 100 g oral glucose tolerance test (OGTT)
Step 2: Perform a 100 g OGTT (fasting), with plasma glucose measurements fasting, and 1 h, 2 h, and 3 h post–glucose load.	The diagnosis of GDM is made when at least two of the four readings meet or exceed the following: **(Carpenter-Coustan criteria)** Fasting: 95 mg/dL (5.3 mmol/L) 1 h: 180 mg/dL (10 mmol/L) 2 h: 155 mg/dL (8.6 mmol/L) 3 h: 140 mg/dL (7.8 mmol/L) **American College of Obstetricians and Gynecologists notes that 1 elevated value can be used for diagnosis.**

Source: American Diabetes Association[11] and Feldman.[13]

macrosomia or large-for-gestational-age infants but did increase the rate of primary cesarean deliveries.[13] The Carpenter/Coustan criteria are more sensitive and may diagnose more women with GDM.

Clinical experts in all groups strongly agree that reaching a consensus on the optimal diagnostic criteria for GDM is paramount. Long-term studies are ongoing and should enable the eventual establishment of uniform criteria.

Although obesity contributes to the rising prevalence of GDM,[14] not all women with GDM are overweight.[5] Insulin resistance during pregnancy is a physiologic phenomenon driven by the metabolic demands of the maternal-fetal unit, stress, and pregnancy-induced hormonal changes.

The recurrence of GDM in a subsequent pregnancy is not uncommon; women with a history of GDM have a 40%–60% probability of developing a metabolic disorder in a future pregnancy.[15] In addition, women with a history of GDM have a risk for developing type 2 diabetes of around 50%–70% over the ensuing 15–25 years.[3] As such, women with GDM should be screened at 4–12 weeks following delivery with a 75 g OGTT using nonpregnancy criteria and then every 1–3 years thereafter using any recommended glycemic evaluation (A1C, fasting plasma glucose, or 75 g OGTT).[3] Despite these guidelines, evidence indicates that less than half of women with GDM receive appropriate postpartum screening for type 2 diabetes in most populations.[16] Barriers to screening may be related to the person (e.g., lack of awareness regarding risk status), provider (e.g., uncertainty regarding recommended screening intervals), system (e.g., lack of communication between obstetric and postpartum providers), or access to the healthcare system. It has been noted that many women feel abandoned by the healthcare system after a pregnancy with GDM in that they do not receive the needed ongoing healthcare and support to maintain a healthy lifestyle and reduce the risks of diabetes and cardiovascular disease. Referral to diabetes education has the potential to play a vitally important role in addressing these barriers and may also serve as a bridge between the prenatal and postnatal care teams.[17,18]

The American Diabetes Association further recommends that women with a history of GDM found to have prediabetes should receive lifestyle interventions or metformin to prevent diabetes. The combination of metformin and lifestyle intervention has been shown to prevent or delay progression to overt diabetes.[18]

DIABETES CARE IN PREGNANCY

Diabetes care in pregnancy involves monitoring, healthy eating, being active, managing medication, and healthy coping.

Monitoring

Experts recommend that women with preexisting diabetes and GDM perform SMBG fasting and 2 h after the start of meals.[3] The American Diabetes Association and the American College of Obstetrics and Gynecology recommend the following SMBG targets: fasting <95 mg/dL (5.3 mmol/L) and 1-h postprandial <140 mg/dL (7.8 mmol/L) or 2-h postprandial <120 mg/dL (6.7 mmol/L).[3,19] Additional preprandial SMBG readings are often required for appropriate meal coverage and correction insulin dosing. Providers should take into account prescribing additional blood glucose testing supplies to enable more frequent SMBG requirements.

In addition to learning proper SMBG technique, the woman with diabetes should be instructed on ways to use SMBG as a problem-solving tool to enable effective self-management of her meal plan, physical activity routine, and assessment of potential insulin need. Use of continuous glucose monitoring systems in pregnancy is still being studied.

With pregnancy being a ketogenic state, women with type 1 diabetes and some women with type 2 diabetes are at risk for developing DKA at a lower blood glucose level than in the nonpregnant state.[3] Ketone test strips should be available for testing at home. Otherwise, routine urine ketone testing is not generally recommended unless there is persistent weight loss or a concern that the woman is not consuming enough calories or carbohydrate.

Healthy Eating

It is clear that nutrition-based interventions are effective for glucose management; yet experts cannot agree on the definition of the ideal meal plan for diabetes in pregnancy. The goal is to establish good nutrition, appropriate weight gain, and glycemic control.[3] A referral to a registered dietitian who is familiar with nutritional management in pregnancy with diabetes and GDM is recommended to enable the establishment of an individualized meal plan with insulin-to-carbohydrate ratio and to ascertain gestational weight gain goals. In addition to focusing on macronutrients, meal-planning instruction should also emphasize food safety tips to help prevent foodborne illnesses such as Listeriosis and Salmonella as well as avoiding fish that are high in methylmercury.

General dietary guidelines for all pregnant women indicate the dietary reference intakes for carbohydrate are a minimum of 175 g per day, for protein are a minimum of 71 g per day, and for fiber are a minimum of 28 g per day.[3] Because pregnancy presents a challenge with carbohydrate tolerance, an individualized distribution pattern of three smaller meals, plus two to three snacks throughout the day, may temper the glucose excursions associated with consuming large amounts of carbohydrate at one time in diet-treated patients. The amount and quality of the carbohydrate (high versus low glycemic index and load) consumed will impact glucose control, especially postprandial glucose levels.[3]

Being Active

Being physically active is known to be beneficial in establishing and maintaining glycemic control and maintaining a healthy gestational weight. The American College of Obstetricians and Gynecologists endorses that women who were previously active (either on a recreational or professional level) remain physically active with modifications as medically indicated.[20] Healthy women who were previously inactive should strive for 150 min of moderate intensity aerobic activity per week unless there are obstetrical or medical conditions that pose contraindications to being physically active.[3] Even activity intervals of 10 min duration can be effective.[1] Experts state that pregnancy is not the time to initiate a strenuous activity routine; however, most women are able to tolerate walking. A 15- to 20-min walk can potentially lower blood glucose by 20–40 mg/dL. Women with diabetes in pregnancy should be encouraged to be as physically active as possible and encouraged to find enjoyable ways to incorporate physical activity into their daily routine.

Medication Management

Many pharmacological agents used to treat type 2 diabetes outside of pregnancy cross the placenta and may be contraindicated for use in pregnancy. In addition, they may be insufficient in overcoming the progressive insulin resistance of pregnancy. Human insulin has not been shown to cross the placenta; it remains the first-line agent for glucose management in pregnancy.[3]

For pregnant women with preexisting diabetes, insulin management may present a formidable challenge. A recent Cochrane systematic review revealed there is no specific insulin regimen that is superior to another for the treatment of diabetes in pregnancy. Multiple daily injections and continuous subcutaneous insulin infusion have been deemed equally effective insulin delivery methods in pregnancy.[3]

In the woman with preexisting diabetes, the first trimester is characterized by an initial increase in insulin demand, followed by a period of heightened insulin sensitivity from weeks 9–16 of gestation. Hypoglycemia is more likely to occur during this time. From around 16 weeks' gestation through delivery, there is progressive insulin resistance that mandates insulin titration upwards of about 5% each week. By the end of the third trimester, there is generally a doubling of the total daily dose of insulin required to maintain glucose readings in the target range, accompanied by a leveling off as the placenta ages.[3,21] It is recommended that less than 50% of the total daily dose should be given as basal, and more than 50% should be given as prandial insulin.[3]

Upon delivery of the placenta, there is heightened insulin sensitivity, and the total daily dose of insulin may be as much as 34% lower than prepregnancy requirements. Breastfeeding combined with unpredictable sleeping and eating schedules may contribute to postpartum hypoglycemia. Women should be made aware of this in order to be adequately prepared to prevent and manage hypoglycemia.[3]

Insulin is also the first-line pharmacological agent for glucose management in women with GDM not controlled by lifestyle modification. While metformin and glyburide have been used to treat glucose excursions in pregnancy, they have been shown to cross the placenta.[3] In addition, two studies demonstrated that glyburide and metformin failed to provide adequate glucose control in 23% and 25%–28% (respectively) of women with GDM. Consequently, insulin was required for adequate glucose management in these women. A meta-analysis of randomized controlled trials showed that glyburide was associated with increased risk of neonatal hypoglycemia, high maternal weight gain, high neonatal birthweight, and macrosomia.[22] The long-term effects of both medications on the offspring remain unknown.

Women with preexisting diabetes in pregnancy are at increased risk for developing preeclampsia. The U.S. Preventative Services Task Force recommends the use of low-dose aspirin (81 mg/day) as a preventative after week 12 of gestation.[3]

Healthy Coping

Diabetes in pregnancy and a diagnosis of GDM can be very stressful for most women. They may suddenly perceive pregnancy as a disease state, experience anxiety and frustration over the urgent need to make immediate lifestyle changes, and/or fear suffering maternal and fetal complications of uncontrolled diabetes.[3] Care providers have the opportunity to address concerns, answer questions, and provide emotional support for women dealing with the psychological impact of diabetes in pregnancy. Referral to a mental health specialist who is familiar with diabetes management for evaluation and treatment may be helpful in certain situations.[17]

REFERENCES

1. Reader DM TA. *Pregnancy with Diabetes.* 4th ed. Cornell S HC, Ed. Chicago, American Association of Diabetes Educators, 2017

2. Starikov R, Dudley D, Reddy UM. Stillbirth in the pregnancy complicated by diabetes. *Curr Diabetes Rep* 2015;15(3):11. doi: 10.1007/s11892-015-0580-y

3. American Diabetes Association. 14. Management of diabetes in pregnancy: standards of medical care in diabetes 2020. *Diabetes Care* 2020;43 (Suppl. 1):S183–S192. doi: 10.2337/dc20-S014. Epub 2019 Dec 22. PubMed PMID: 31862757

4. Boggess KA, Berggren EK. Preconception care has the potential for a high return on investment. *Am J Obstet Gynecol* 2015;212(1):1–3. doi: 10.1016/j.ajog.2014.10.030

5. Kim SY, England L, Wilson HG, Bish C, Satten GA, Dietz P. Percentage of gestational diabetes mellitus attributable to overweight and obesity. *Am J Public Health* 2010;100(6):1047-52. doi: 10.2105/ajph.2009.172890. Epub 2010 Apr 17. PubMed PMID: 20395581; PubMed Central PMCID: PMCPMC2866592

6. Stang J. Preconception and internatal nutrition recommendations for women with diabetes. *On the Cutting Edge* 2016;37(4):10–14

7. Whitaker KM, Wilcox S, Liu J, Blair SN, Pate RR. Patient and provider perceptions of weight gain, physical activity, and nutrition counseling during pregnancy: a qualitative study. *Womens Health Issues* 2016;26(1):116–122. doi: 10.1016/j.whi.2015.10.007. Epub 2015 Dec 2. PubMed PMID: 26621605; PubMed Central PMCID: PMCPMC4690786

8. American College of Obstetricians and Gynecologists. Weight gain during pregnancy. Committee Opinion No. 548. *Obstet Gynecol* 2013;121: 210–212

9. Sibai BM, Viteri OA. Diabetic ketoacidosis in pregnancy. *Obstet Gynecol* 2014;123(1):167–178. doi: 10.1097/aog.0000000000000060. Epub 2014 Jan 28. PubMed PMID: 24463678

10. Metzger BE, Buchanan TA, Coustan DR, de Leiva A, Dunger DB, Hadden DR, et al. Summary and recommendations of the fifth international workshop-conference on gestational diabetes mellitus. *Diabetes Care* 2007;30(Suppl. 2):S251–S260. doi: 10.2337/dc07-s225

11. American Diabetes Association. 2. Classification and diagnosis of diabetes: standards of medical care in diabetes 2020. *Diabetes Care* 2020;43 (Suppl 1):S14–S31. doi: 10.2337/dc20-S002. Epub 2019 Dec 22. PubMed PMID: 31862745

12. O'Sullivan JB, Mahan CM. Criteria for the oral glucose tolerance test in pregnancy. *Diabetes* 1964;13:278–285. Epub 1964 May 1. PubMed PMID: 14166677

13. Feldman RK, Tieu RS, Yasumura L. Gestational Diabetes Screening: The International Association of the Diabetes and Pregnancy study groups compared with Carpenter-Coustan Screening. *Obstet Gynecol* 2016;127(1):10–17. doi: 10.1097/AOG.0000000000001132. Epub 2015 Dec 10. PubMed PMID: 26646142

14. Koivusalo SB, Rono K, Klemetti MM, Roine RP, Lindstrom J, Erkkola M, et al. Gestational diabetes mellitus can be prevented by lifestyle intervention: the Finnish Gestational Diabetes Prevention Study (Radiel): a randomized controlled trial. *Diabetes Care* 2016;39(1):24–30. doi: 10.2337/dc15-0511. Epub 2015 Aug 1. PubMed PMID: 26223239

15. Getahun D, Fassett MJ, Jacobsen SJ. Gestational diabetes: risk of recurrence in subsequent pregnancies. *Am J Obstet Gynecol* 2010;203(5):467.e1–e6. doi: 10.1016/j.ajog.2010.05.032. Epub 2010 Jul 16. PubMed PMID: 20630491

16. Smirnakis KV, Chasan-Taber L, Wolf M, Markenson G, Ecker JL, Thadhani R. Postpartum diabetes screening in women with a history of gestational diabetes. *Obstet Gynecol* 2005;106(6):1297–1303. doi: 10.1097/01. Aog.0000189081.46925.90. PubMed PMID: 00006250-200512000-00014

17. American Diabetes Association. 5. Facilitating behavior change and well-being to improve health outcomes: standards of medical care in diabetes 2020. *Diabetes Care* 2020;43(Suppl. 1):S48–S65. doi: 10.2337/dc20-S005. Epub 2019 Dec 22. PubMed PMID: 31862748

18. American Diabetes Association. 3. Prevention or delay of type 2 diabetes: standards of medical care in diabetes 2020. *Diabetes Care* 2020;43 (Suppl. 1):S32–S36. doi: 10.2337/dc20-S003. Epub 2019 Dec 22. PubMed PMID: 31862746

19. ACOG Practice Bulletin No. 190: gestational diabetes mellitus. *Obstet Gynecol* 2018;131(2):e49–e64. doi: 10.1097/aog.0000000000002501. Epub 2018 Jan 26. PubMed PMID: 29370047

20. ACOG Committee Opinion No. 650: physical activity and exercise during pregnancy and the postpartum period. *Obstet Gynecol* 2015;126(6):e135–e142. doi: 10.1097/aog.0000000000001214. Epub 2015 Nov 26. PubMed PMID: 26595585

21. Yeh T, Yeung M, Mendelsohn Curanaj FA. Inpatient glycemic management of the pregnant patient. *Curr Diabetes Rep* 2018;18(10):73. doi: 10.1007/s11892-018-1045-x

22. Jiang YF, Chen XY, Ding T, Wang XF, Zhu ZN, Su SW. Comparative efficacy and safety of OADs in management of GDM: network meta-analysis of randomized controlled trials. *J Clin Endocrin Metab* 2015;100(5): 2071–2080. doi: 10.1210/jc.2014-4403. Epub 2015 Mar 25. PubMed PMID: 25803270

DIABETES IN YOUTH

Olga Gupta, MD
Abha Choudhary, MD

The prevalence of type 2 diabetes in youth has increased dramatically over the past several decades, especially among racial and ethnic minority groups.[1] Current information on epidemiology, pathophysiology, and treatment approaches in youth with type 2 diabetes comes from the SEARCH (Search for Diabetes in Youth), RISE (Restoring Insulin Secretion), and TODAY (Treatment Options for Type 2 Diabetes in Adolescents and Youth) studies.[1-4] The pathophysiology of type 2 diabetes in young individuals is multifactorial, with obesity, genetics/epigenetics, minority race/ethnicity, low socioeconomic status, and physiologic insulin resistance of puberty identified as contributing risk factors in the setting of multiple stressors and other social determinants of health that are often difficult to address in a clinic setting.[5,6] Evidence suggests that type 2 diabetes in youth is different not only from type 1 diabetes but also from type 2 diabetes in adults. Youth appear to have greater insulin resistance and hyperresponsive insulin secretion than their adult counterparts.[2,3,5] These physiologic differences cause a faster rate of deterioration of β-cell function and accelerated development of diabetes complications, suggesting that type 2 diabetes has a more aggressive course in youth than adults.

DIFFERENTIATION OF TYPE 1 AND TYPE 2 DIABETES IN YOUTH

Distinguishing between type 1 and type 2 diabetes can be challenging since defining characteristics are not unique to either condition. With the increasing prevalence of childhood obesity, children with type 1 diabetes can be affected by overweight and obesity.[7] Likewise, pancreatic autoantibodies may be detected in patients with clinical features suggestive of type 2 diabetes.[8] The diabetes type may be uncertain during the first few weeks of treatment, and many youth with type 2 diabetes may present with ketoacidosis and hyperglycemia requiring insulin therapy, similar to youth with type 1 diabetes.[9] However, treatment regimens, dietary recommendations, and long-term management differ between type 1 and type 2 diabetes, so it is important to provide families with an accurate diagnosis at a subsequent clinical encounter. Current guidelines recommend checking a panel of pancreatic autoantibodies (GAD, insulin, tyrosine phosphatases IA-2 and IA-2b, ZnT8) in all youth in whom the diagnosis of type 2 diabetes is being considered to exclude the diagnosis of type 1 diabetes.[5] In addition, genetic testing for monogenic diabetes should be considered since 4.5%–8.0% of youth with clinical features suggestive of type 2 diabetes were subsequently diagnosed with monogenic diabetes.[10]

SCREENING FOR TYPE 2 DIABETES IN YOUTH

The American Diabetes Association has criteria for risk-based screening for type 2 diabetes in the pediatric population (Table 4.6). They recommend testing after the onset of puberty or after 10 years of age (whichever occurs earlier) in

Table 4.6–Risk-Based Screening for Type 2 Diabetes in Asymptomatic Children and Adolescents in a Clinical Setting

Testing should be considered in youth* who are overweight (BMI ≥ 85 percentile) or obese (BMI ≥ 95 percentile) and who have one or more additional risk factors based on the strength of their association with diabetes:

- Maternal history of diabetes or gestational diabetes during the child's gestation
- Family history of type 2 diabetes in first- or second-degree relative
- Race/ethnicity (e.g., Native American, African American, Latino, Asian American, and Pacific Islander)
- Signs of insulin resistance or conditions associated with insulin resistance (e.g., acanthosis nigricans, hypertension, dyslipidemia, polycystic ovary syndrome, or small-for-gestational-age birthweight)

*After the onset of puberty or ≥10 years of age, whichever occurs earlier. If tests are normal, repeat testing at a minimum of 3-year intervals, or more frequently if BMI is increasing.

Source: American Diabetes Association, 2020.[12]

youth with overweight (BMI ≥85th percentile) or obesity (BMI ≥95th percentile) and who have one or more additional risk factors for diabetes.[5] The laboratory glycemia-based criteria for diagnosis of type 2 diabetes are the same for youth as adults (please refer to Chapter 1). However, these diagnostic definitions are based on population studies that did not include pediatric participants, so it is unclear if these cutoffs are appropriate for all age groups.[5]

It is not recommended that clinicians screen for organic causes of obesity unless there is clinical evidence for diseases such as hypothyroidism. Obesity-related comorbidities may need to be addressed, including nonalcoholic fatty liver disease, polycystic ovary syndrome, orthopedic complications, and psychosocial stressors.

TREATING TYPE 2 DIABETES IN YOUTH

Goals of treatment in children and adolescents with type 2 diabetes treated with oral agents alone is <7% (<53 mmol/mol).[11] A1C targets for youth with type 2 diabetes on insulin should be individualized, taking into consideration long-term health benefits as well as low rates of adverse effects such as hypoglycemia.[11] Given the early onset of type 2 diabetes and longer potential duration of the disease, aggressive therapies are required to mitigate subsequent risk for macrovascular and microvascular complications. Culturally appropriate lifestyle intervention directed toward long-term weight management is an essential part of the therapeutic plan. Especially important is education of the patient and family, with the goal of increasing intake of nutrient-dense, high-quality foods and decreasing consumption of calorie-dense and nutrient-poor foods, particularly sugar-added beverages.[11] In addition, a family-based progressive increase in physical activity and reduction of sedentary activities should be emphasized. It is important for providers to recognize that many youth with type 2 diabetes experience psychosocial stressors, which may negatively impact adherence and response to therapy.

Personalized diabetes management with special attention to mental/behavioral health and eating disorders (particularly binge eating disorder) is a key component of optimizing care.

Unfortunately, weight loss and lifestyle interventions for obesity in youth have had disappointing results, and there is a lack of safe, effective, and tolerable pharmacologic agents for weight loss in this population. Metabolic surgery yields weight loss that is superior to nonsurgical management and may be considered for the treatment of adolescents with type 2 diabetes who are obese (BMI >35 kg/m²) and who have uncontrolled glycemia and/or serious comorbidities despite lifestyle and pharmacologic intervention or adolescents with BMI >40 kg/m² with or without a comborbidity.[11] Long-term studies show that adolescents experience similar degrees of weight loss and diabetes remission as their adult counterparts for at least 3 years after surgery.[13] However, the benefits of surgery must be weighed against the risks of surgical perioperative complications, and longer-term potential micronutrient deficiencies and reduced bone mineral density.[14] Metabolic surgery should be performed only by a surgeon with experience in the pediatric population working with an interdisciplinary team, including a pediatric endocrinologist, a nutritionist, and a behavioral health specialist.[11]

While more than 10 different classes of antidiabetes medications are available to treat type 2 diabetes in adults, current pharmacologic treatment options for youth-onset type 2 diabetes were limited to two drugs—insulin and metformin—until the recent U.S. Food and Drug Administration (FDA) approval of liraglutide in June 2019.[15] In the ELLIPSE (Evaluation of Liraglutide in Pediatrics with Diabetes) study, pediatric patients with uncontrolled type 2 diabetes ≥10 years and BMI >85th percentile received liraglutide (≤1.8 mg a day) for 52 weeks and experienced a lower A1C level (difference with placebo at 52 weeks was –1.3% [14.2 mmol/mol]) but higher rates of hypoglycemia and gastrointestinal side effects.[15] Use of medications not approved by the FDA for youth with type 2 diabetes is not recommended outside of research trials. In metabolically stable patients (A1C <8.5% [<69 mmol/mol]) with normal renal function and no acidosis, metformin is the initial pharmacologic agent. Approximately half of the participants in the TODAY study achieved glycemic control (A1C ≤8% [≤64 mmol/mol]) for 6 months using metformin monotherapy,[16] which is a lower-than-predicted success rate compared to the positive experience that adult patients have with metformin. Patients with significant hyperglycemia (blood glucose ≥250 mg/dL [≥13.9 mmol/L] and A1C ≥8.5% [≥69 mmol/mol]) without acidosis at diagnosis who are symptomatic (polyuria, polydipsia, nocturia, and/or weight loss) should be treated initially with basal insulin 0.5 units/kg/day with escalation every 2–3 days based on self-monitoring of blood glucose. Metformin is initiated and titrated up to 2,000 mg per day as tolerated. If glycemic targets are no longer met with metformin (with or without basal insulin), liraglutide therapy should be considered in children ≥10 years if they have no past medical history of medullary thyroid carcinoma or multiple endocrine neoplasia type 2. Patients treated with basal insulin ≤1.5 units/kg/day who do not meet the A1C target should be moved to multiple daily injections with basal and premeal bolus insulins. Once glucose control is established in patients initially treated with insulin and metformin, it may be possible to transition the patient to oral medications by tapering insulin over 2–6 weeks by decreasing the insulin dose 10%–30% every few days.[11]

Diabetes-related complications, including nephropathy, retinopathy, and neuropathy, may be present at the time of diagnosis of type 2 diabetes in youth. To aid in evaluation, the clinician should obtain blood pressure measurement, random albumin-to-creatinine ratio, dilated eye examination, and comprehensive foot examination (inspection; assessment of foot pulses; pinprick; and 10-g monofilament sensation tests, testing of vibration sensation using 128-Hz tuning fork, and ankle reflexes) at the time of diagnosis.[11] Lipid testing should be performed when glycemic and metabolic control have been achieved. As in adults, dyslipidemia and hypertension should be treated aggressively. Goals for therapy are outlined in Table 4.7.

WHEN TO CONSIDER SPECIALTY CONSULTATION

With increasing rates of type 2 diabetes in youth and a short supply of pediatric endocrinologists, primary care physicians may start seeing more of these patients in their clinics. The management of diabetes outside of a tertiary care clinic may pose a challenge for primary healthcare. It is important to recognize that all youth with type 2 diabetes and their families should receive assessment by appropriately trained educators for evaluation of education requirements, diabetes self-management education, glucose management training, medical nutrition therapy, identification and prevention of complications, and activity/exercise guidance that is culturally competent and specific to youth.[11] An interdisciplinary diabetes team

Table 4.7–Recommendations for Prevention and Management of High Blood Pressure and Dyslipidemia in Youth

High Blood Pressure
- Please refer to the American Academy of Pediatrics' clinical practice guidelines for the diagnosis, evaluation, and treatment of high blood pressure in children and adolescents.[17]
- If blood pressure is >95th percentile for age, sex, and height, increased emphasis should be placed on lifestyle management to promote weight loss.
- If blood pressure remains above the 95th percentile for age, sex, and height after 6 months, or ≥140/90 mmHg in adolescents ≥13 years, antihypertensive therapy with angiotensin-converting enzyme inhibitors or angiotensin receptor blockers should be initiated.

Dyslipidemia
A lipid profile should be obtained after glycemic control has been achieved and annually thereafter.
Optimal goals are as follows:

- LDL cholesterol <100 mg/dl (<2.0 mmol/L)
- HDL cholesterol >35 mg/dl (>0.905 mmol/L)
- Triglycerides <150 mg/dl (<1.7 mmol/L)

If the LDL cholesterol level is >100 mg/dl (>2.6 mmol/L), an exercise and diet plan should be prescribed. If LDL cholesterol remains >130 mg/dl after 6 months of dietary intervention, consider statin therapy with a goal of LDL <100 mg/dl.

including a physician, diabetes care and education specialist, registered dietitian, and psychologist or social worker is essential to target the complex social and environmental challenges impacting youth with type 2 diabetes and their families.[11] Referral to a diabetes specialist should be considered when these educational resources are not readily available, especially when the A1C warrants insulin therapy (A1C ≥8.5% [69 mmol/mol]).

REFERENCES

1. Dabelea D, Mayer-Davis EJ, Saydah S, Imperatore G, Linder B, Divers J, et al. Prevalence of type 1 and type 2 diabetes among children and adolescents from 2001 to 2009. *JAMA* 2014;311(17):1778–1786. doi: 10.1001/jama.2014.3201. PubMed PMID: 24794371; PubMed Central PMCID: PMCPMC4368900

2. The RISE Consortium. Metabolic contrasts between youth and adults with impaired glucose tolerance or recently diagnosed type 2 diabetes: I. observations using the hyperglycemic clamp. *Diabetes Care* 2018;41(8):1696–1706. doi: 10.2337/dc18-0244. Epub 2018 Jun 25. PubMed PMID: 29941497; PubMed Central PMCID: PMCPMC6054493

3. The RISE Consortium. Metabolic contrasts between youth and adults with impaired glucose tolerance or recently diagnosed type 2 diabetes: II. observations using the oral glucose tolerance test. *Diabetes Care* 2018;41(8):1707–1716. doi: 10.2337/dc18-0243. Epub 2018 Jun 25. PubMed PMID: 29941498; PubMed Central PMCID: PMCPMC6054494

4. Group TS, Zeitler P, Epstein L, Grey M, Hirst K, Kaufman F, et al. Treatment options for type 2 diabetes in adolescents and youth: a study of the comparative efficacy of metformin alone or in combination with rosiglitazone or lifestyle intervention in adolescents with type 2 diabetes. *Pediatr Diabetes* 2007;8(2):74–87. doi: 10.1111/j.1399-5448.2007.00237.x. PubMed PMID: 17448130; PubMed Central PMCID: PMCPMC2752327

5. Arslanian S, Bacha F, Grey M, Marcus MD, White NH, Zeitler P. Evaluation and management of youth-onset type 2 diabetes: a position statement by the American Diabetes Association. *Diabetes Care* 2018;41(12):2648–2668. doi: 10.2337/dci18-0052. PubMed PMID: 30425094

6. Nadeau KJ, Anderson BJ, Berg EG, Chiang JL, Chou H, Copeland KC, et al. Youth-onset type 2 diabetes consensus report: current status, challenges, and priorities. *Diabetes Care* 2016;39(9):1635–1642. doi: 10.2337/dc16-1066. Epub 2016 Aug 2. PubMed PMID: 27486237; PubMed Central PMCID: PMCPMC5314694

7. Corbin KD, Driscoll KA, Pratley RE, Smith SR, Maahs DM, Mayer-Davis EJ, et al. Obesity in type 1 diabetes: pathophysiology, clinical impact, and mechanisms. *Endocr Rev* 2018;39(5):629–663. doi: 10.1210/er.2017-00191. PubMed PMID: 30060120

8. Klingensmith GJ, Pyle L, Arslanian S, Copeland KC, Cuttler L, Kaufman F, et al. The presence of GAD and IA-2 antibodies in youth with a type 2 diabetes phenotype: results from the TODAY study. *Diabetes Care* 2010;33(9):1970–1975. doi: 10.2337/dc10-0373. Epub 2010 Jun 2. PubMed PMID: 20519658; PubMed Central PMCID: PMCPMC2928346

9. Pinhas-Hamiel O, Dolan LM, Zeitler PS. Diabetic ketoacidosis among obese African-American adolescents with NIDDM. *Diabetes Care* 1997;20(4): 484–486. PubMed PMID: 9096965

10. Kleinberger JW, Copeland KC, Gandica RG, Haymond MW, Levitsky LL, Linder B, et al. Monogenic diabetes in overweight and obese youth diagnosed with type 2 diabetes: the TODAY clinical trial. *Genet Med* 2018;20(6):583–590. doi: 10.1038/gim.2017.150. Epub 2017 Oct 12. PubMed PMID: 29758564; PubMed Central PMCID: PMCPMC5955780

11. American Diabetes Association. 13. Children and adolescents: standards of medical care in diabetes 2020. *Diabetes Care* 2020;43(Suppl. 1):S163–S182. doi: 10.2337/dc20-S013. PubMed PMID: 31862756

12. American Diabetes Association. 2. Classification and diagnosis of diabetes: standards of medical care in diabetes 2020. *Diabetes Care* 2020;43 (Suppl. 1):S14–S31. doi: 10.2337/dc20-S002. PubMed PMID: 31862745

13. Inge TH, Courcoulas AP, Jenkins TM, Michalsky MP, Helmrath MA, Brandt ML, et al. Weight loss and health status 3 years after bariatric surgery in adolescents. *N Engl J Med* 2016;374(2):113–123. doi: 10.1056/ NEJMoa1506699. Epub 2015 Nov 6. PubMed PMID: 26544725; PubMed Central PMCID: PMCPMC4810437

14. Stefater MA, Inge TH. Bariatric surgery for adolescents with type 2 diabetes: an emerging therapeutic strategy. *Curr Diab Rep* 2017;17(8):62. doi: 10.1007/ s11892-017-0887-y. PubMed PMID: 28681327; PubMed Central PMCID: PMCPMC5841547

15. Tamborlane WV, Barrientos-Perez M, Fainberg U, Frimer-Larsen H, Hafez M, Hale PM, et al. Liraglutide in children and adolescents with type 2 diabetes. *New Engl J Med* 2019;381(7):637–646. doi: 10.1056/NEJMoa1903822. Epub 2019 Apr 30. PubMed PMID: 31034184

16. Group TS, Zeitler P, Hirst K, Pyle L, Linder B, Copeland K, et al. A clinical trial to maintain glycemic control in youth with type 2 diabetes. *N Engl J Med* 2012;366(24):2247–2256. doi: 10.1056/NEJMoa1109333. Epub 2012 Apr 29. PubMed PMID: 22540912; PubMed Central PMCID: PMCPMC3478667

17. Flynn JT, Kaelber DC, Baker-Smith CM, Blowey D, Carroll AE, Daniels SR, et al. Clinical practice guideline for screening and management of high blood pressure in children and adolescents. *Pediatrics* 2017;140(3):ii. doi: 10.1542/ peds.2017-1904. Epub 2017 Aug 21. PubMed PMID: 28827377

DIABETES IN HOSPITALIZED AND CRITICALLY ILL PATIENTS

Sasan Mirfakhraee, MD
Anitha Litty, DNP, FNP-C, CDCES

Hyperglycemia in hospitalized patients is common and is associated with increased mortality and poor clinic outcomes.[1] However, overly aggressive management of type 2 diabetes in the inpatient setting increases the risk of hypoglycemia, which has been shown to increase mortality and the length of stay.[2] While some early randomized trials in the intensive care population showed that tight glycemic control could improve mortality and reduce complications,[3,4] subsequent data[5] have shown a lack of benefit with intensive glycemic control and high risk for severe hypoglycemia.[5,6] Inpatient glycemic goals should therefore aim to reduce the rates of both hyperglycemia and hypoglycemia.[7]

GLUCOSE MONITORING

Hospitalized patients with a history of diabetes or those on hypoglycemic agents should have their glucose monitored routinely. Glucose monitoring should be performed before meals and at bedtime for those who are eating and every 4–6 h for those who are not eating or on enteral or parenteral nutrition. More frequent glucose monitoring (e.g., every 30 min to every 2 h) is required in patients who are receiving intravenous insulin therapy.[7] The majority of glucose measurements in the hospital are performed using a fingertip capillary blood sample with point-of-care glucose monitors. However, the accuracy of point-of-care glucose monitoring is not established in the intensive care unit (ICU) setting, as capillary glucose values can be altered due to issues with perfusion, edema, anemia/erythrocytosis, and various medications.[7] Therefore, when there is doubt as to the accuracy of the glucose result, the value must be confirmed through a serum sample sent urgently to the clinical laboratory.

GLYCEMIC TARGETS

While glycemic recommendations for the critically ill patient population are based upon randomized clinical trial results, those for non–critically ill, hospitalized patients are based on clinical experience and judgment, as prospective randomized clinical trial data are lacking. Guidelines for the management of hyperglycemia in the hospital advocate glycemic targets depending on patient location (e.g., ward vs. ICU) and prognosis (see Table 4.8). In the non-ICU population, a premeal glucose of <140 mg/dL (<7.8 mmol/L) and random glucose of <180 mg/dL (<10.0 mmol/L) is recommended by both the American Association of Clinical Endocrinologists/American College of Endocrinology and the Endocrine Society.[7–9] In the ICU setting, a target glucose range of 140–180 mg/dL (7.8–10.0 mmol/L) is recommended by the American Diabetes Association and the American Association of Clinical Endocrinologists/American College of Endocrinology.[8] The accuracy of capillary blood glucose monitoring in theICU is not established, especially in patients with hypovolemia or hypotension; in these patients glucose measurements should be performed with IV samples and a STAT analyzer. More stringent (e.g., 110–140 mg/dL [6.1–7.8 mmol/L]) or less strict targets (e.g., >180 mg/dL [>10.0 mmol/L]) may be appropriate for select patients, depending on medical comorbidities and prognosis. Achieving such levels of glycemic control in the hectic inpatient environment provides a formidable challenge to patients, healthcare/healthcare providers, and healthcare systems and requires the collaboration of nursing, nutrition, and pharmacy, in addition to the medical staff and patient.[7] To optimize glycemic control in the inpatient setting, standardized recommendations (i.e., written or computerized protocols, structured order sets) allow for precise insulin delivery based on glucose variability.[7]

An important caveat is that these glycemic targets are appropriate only if they can be safely achieved. Hypoglycemia should be avoided in the inpatient setting, and the treatment regimen should be modified if glucose levels fall <70 mg/dL (<3.9 mmol/L), with prompt implementation of the hypoglycemia treatment protocol (see Hypoglycemia section below).[7]

CHOICE OF THERAPY

In the ICU setting, intravenous infusion of insulin is a safe and effective means of correcting and maintaining glucose levels at goal. Through continuous intravenous insulin infusion, insulin delivery can be promptly modified via standardized protocol to maintain glycemic control despite fluctuating clinical variables, such as diet, concurrent medications, stress, and the severity of illness. While there may be subtle differences in the protocols of varying institutions,

Table 4.8–Glycemic Targets Based on Various Guidelines

Organization	Recommendation
American Diabetes Association (2020)[7]	■ Insulin therapy should be initiated for treatment of persistent hyperglycemia starting at a threshold 180 mg/dL. ■ Once insulin therapy is started, a target glucose range of 140–180 mg/dL (7.8–10.0 mmol/L) is recommended for the majority of critically ill patients and non–critically ill patients. ■ More stringent goals, such as 110–140 mg/dL (6.1–7.8 mmol/L), may be appropriate for selected patients if this can be achieved without significant hypoglycemia.
American Association of Clinical Endocrinologists/ American College of Endocrinology (2015)[8]	■ For most hospitalized individuals with hyperglycemia in the ICU, a glucose range of 140–180 mg/dL (7.8–10.0 mmol/L) is recommended, provided this target can be safely achieved. ■ For general medicine and surgery patients in non-ICU settings, a premeal glucose target <140 mg/dL (<7.8 mmol/L) and a random blood glucose <180 mg/dL (<10.0 mmol/L) are recommended.
Endocrine Society (2012)[9]	■ For the majority of hospitalized patients with non-critical illness, a premeal glucose target <140 mg/dL (<7.8 mmol/L) and a random blood glucose <180 mg/dL (<10.0 mmol/L) are recommended. ■ For patients with a terminal illness and/or with limited life expectancy or at high risk for hypoglycemia, a higher target range (glucose <200 mg/dL [<11.1 mmol/L]) may be reasonable.

insulin infusion protocols share by design the ability to quickly and safely correct patients' blood glucose to a predefined range.

When transitioning a patient from insulin infusion to subcutaneous (SQ) insulin therapy, a dose of SQ long-acting insulin should be given ≥2–4 h before the infusion is discontinued to ensure overlap between intravenous insulin and SQ insulin therapy; some have advocated for an overlap ≤12 h.[10] A variety of protocols exist to facilitate the transition from intravenous to SQ insulin therapy.[11,12] In general, the total daily dose of insulin by intravenous infusion should be reduced by 20%–40%, and this new total should be divided evenly as basal and bolus insulin. For example, for a patient receiving 60 units per day through insulin infusion, first reduce by 20% to achieve a new daily total of 48 units. Next, divide this evenly into 24 units of basal insulin daily and 8 units of rapid-acting insulin with meals.

For patients not in the critical care setting, SQ insulin therapy is the preferred strategy for achieving glycemic targets. Basal/bolus insulin therapy allows for long-acting insulin to maintain basal (i.e., fasting) glycemic control, with the addition of rapid-acting, prandial insulin to control postprandial glycemic excursions and rapid-acting, supplemental insulin to correct glucose levels that are above goal. The use of "sliding scale" insulin—short-acting insulin given on a scheduled basis to correct elevated glucose levels, without associated prandial insulin coverage—should be discouraged, as this reactive approach is associated with more glycemic variation than basal/bolus insulin therapy.[13] Additionally, premixed insulin therapy (e.g., insulin 70:30) has been shown to result in similar glycemic outcomes to basal/bolus insulin therapy but with a significantly increased incidence of hypoglycemia[14]; it should therefore be avoided in the inpatient setting.

Currently, there is no high-quality evidence to support the use of non-insulin therapy for glucose lowering in the hospital setting. Smaller studies have supported the safety and efficacy of incretin therapy for hospitalized patients with type 2 diabetes.[15-17] While metformin has traditionally been held in the hospital setting owing to a theoretical increased risk of lactic acidosis, the actual risk is likely quite low,[18] and some experts recommend continuing metformin therapy for stable patients with an acceptable estimated glomerular filtration rate. However, the evidence supporting the use of metformin in the inpatient setting is weak and inconsistent. Sulfonylurea therapy is generally avoided due to an elevated risk of hypoglycemia when meals are held or delayed in the inpatient setting.[19] There are insufficient data supporting the use of sodium–glucose cotransporter 2 (SGLT2) inhibitor therapy in the inpatient setting, and concerns for hospital use include SGLT2 inhibitor–associated diabetic ketoacidosis, increased risk of infection, and worsening renal function.[20] Further studies are ongoing to establish the efficacy and safety of non-insulin therapy in the hospital setting.

HYPOGLYCEMIA

Hypoglycemia in the inpatient setting is common[21] and is associated with factors such as older age, decreased caloric intake, compromised renal/hepatic function, critical illness, and deviation from hospital protocol.[22,23] Furthermore, hypoglycemia among hospitalized patients on insulin has been associated with an increased risk of mortality and increased hospital length of stay.[24] A standardized, nurse-initiated hypoglycemia treatment protocol should be available to immediately correct a blood glucose level <70 mg/dL and to prompt an adjustment to a patient's overall treatment regimen.[7]

ENTERAL/PARENTERAL FEEDS

Hospitalized patients who are at high nutritional risk, are unable to sustain volitional intake, and are expected to remain in the hospital ≥3 days are candidates for specialized nutrition therapy.[25] Generally, enteral nutrition is preferred to parenteral nutrition due to reduced cost, reduced risk of infectious complications, and lower incidence of hyperglycemia.[26] As opposed to parenteral nutrition, enteral feedings play an integral part in maintaining the gastrointestinal mucosal function, barrier function, immunologic function, and gastric motility.[27] Enteral feeds can be given continuously or run over a preset length of time (e.g., overnight) to provide adequate macro- and micronutrient supplementation.

In patients who develop hyperglycemia while on enteral feeds, it is important to note the specific formulation being used, as the carbohydrate content differs (see Table 4.9). For continuous tube feeds, the nutritional component can be covered with regular insulin (given every 6 h) or rapid-acting insulin analogs (given every 4 h) based on a 1:10 carbohydrate ratio (if BMI >30) or 1:15 carbohydrate ratio (if BMI ≤30). For example, if a patient with a BMI of 32 is given TwoCal tube feeds continuously at 50 cc/h every 4 h, the patient would receive 200 cc of formula containing 43.8 g carbohydrate. Using a 1:10 carbohydrate ratio, the patient would receive 4 units of rapid-acting insulin subcutaneously every 4 h to cover the carbohydrate content.

For bolus tube feeds, the calculated insulin dose can be given subcutaneously prior to each feed based on the carbohydrate ratios listed above. The basal insulin

Table 4.9–Carbohydrate Content per Liter of Enteral Formula

Formula	Carb Content (per L)
Ensure Plus	211 g
Glucerna 1.2	115 g
Glucerna 1.5	133 g
Jevity 1.2	169 g
Jevity 1.5	216 g
Nepro	160 g
Osmolite	136 g
Osmolite 1.2	158 g
Peptamen AF	112 g
Peptamen 1.5	188 g
Pivot 1.5	172 g
Promote	130 g
TwoCal	219 g

coverage can be given as split-dosed NPH or once-daily long-acting insulin while the patient is receiving tube feeds.[28] If a patient's enteral feeds are unexpectedly stopped or interrupted, dextrose 10% solution should be given intravenously (generally at the same rate that the enteral feeds had been running) until the risk of hypoglycemia from SQ insulin coverage has abated.

For a patient receiving parenteral nutrition, regular insulin can be added to the total parenteral nutrition solution by the pharmacy so that the patient receives insulin concurrently with the parenteral feed. Insulin at concentrations below 1U/cc adheres to plastic tubing and can reduce insulin delivery until the plastic is saturated[29]; some centers pretreat the tubing with albumin to mitigate this risk. A carbohydrate ratio of 1 unit of regular insulin: 10 g of dextrose in the parenteral feed is recommended as a starting dose, with daily adjustments on an as-needed basis.[28] If parenteral feeds are interrupted, the risk of hypoglycemia is reduced, since parenteral insulin delivery is also halted.

GLUCOCORTICOID THERAPY

The effects of glucocorticoids on blood glucose are well established.[30] The magnitude and duration of glycemic effect depends on the type and dose of glucocorticoid used. For glucocorticoids with a long half-life (e.g., dexamethasone), a once-daily dose of glargine or detemir attenuates the rise in the postprandial blood glucose. For shorter-acting glucocorticoids (e.g., prednisone), an intermediate-acting insulin such as NPH is preferred. Table 4.10 lists the estimated starting dose

Table 4.10–Estimated Insulin Dose Needed to Treat Glucocorticoid-Induced Hyperglycemia, Based on Glucocorticoid Type and Dose

Intermediate-Acting Steroids (Half-Life: 12–16 h)	
Prednisone/Methylprednisolone Dose (mg/day)	NPH Insulin Dose (unit/kg/day)
≥40	0.4
30	0.3
20	0.2
10	0.1

Long-Acting Steroid (Half-life: 20–36 h)	
Dexamethasone Dose (mg/day)	Insulin Glargine/Detemir Dose (unit/kg/day)
≥8	0.4
6	0.3
4	0.2
2	0.1

of insulin based on glucocorticoid dose and type.[31] If a different glucocorticoid is used, it should be converted to one of the glucocorticoids in the table based on equivalent glucocorticoid dosing as follows: hydrocortisone 20 mg, prednisolone 4 mg, prednisone 5 mg, dexamethasone 0.75 mg.

The dose of insulin given to cover a given glucocorticoid would be in addition to the "baseline (and basal)" insulin dose used to manage a patient's hyperglycemia. For example, a 100 kg patient who takes glargine 25 units at bedtime—who is then started on prednisone 30 mg each morning—should be given NPH insulin 30 units along with the glucocorticoid dose in addition to his or her usual dose of glargine 25 units at bedtime. The clinician must be mindful to reduce the insulin dose as the glucocorticoid dose is tapered to prevent hypoglycemia.

CONSIDERATIONS FOR THE SURGICAL PATIENT

The target range for blood glucose in the perioperative period should be 80–180 mg/dL (4.4–10 mmol/L).[7] Unless the surgical condition is an emergency, the patient should be allowed sufficient time to achieve acceptable control of hyperglycemia before surgery. The objectives of perioperative management are to prevent hypoglycemia—which can lead to seizure and death—and to prevent excessive hyperglycemia (180–200 mg/dl [10.0–11.1 mmol/L] or higher), which can complicate postoperative care by increasing the risk of major infections, thrombosis, dehydration, excessive protein loss, and electrolyte imbalance. Sub-optimal glycemic control in the perioperative setting has been associated with an increased rate of complications and reduced long-term survival after surgery.[32-34] Clinicians may refer to the following guidelines that detail the perioperative management of diabetes.[35,36]

TRANSITION FROM HOSPITAL TO HOME

Discharge planning should start early in the course of the hospitalization to allow for adequate teaching and to help familiarize a patient with the routine that he or she will continue in the outpatient setting. An inpatient regimen that effectively manages a patient's blood glucose may not result in adequate glycemic control in the outpatient setting. Inpatient factors such as scheduled, consistent carbohydrate meals and regularly administered medications may not represent the real-world scenario that a patient may experience outside of the closely monitored hospital environment. For this reason, it is critical that hypoglycemia/hyperglycemia precautions be given and that timely, outpatient follow-up be made with a patient's diabetes provider for reevaluation of a given diabetes regimen. A significant number of patients will no longer require insulin therapy following discharge. A hospital discharge algorithm (see Table 4.11) can be used to determine a patient's discharge diabetes regimen based on admission A1C.[37]

Table 4.11–Example of a Hospital Discharge Algorithm Based on A1C

A1C	Diabetes Discharge Plan
<7% (<53.0 mmol/mol)	Continue preadmission regimen
7%–9% (53.0–74.9 mmol/mol)	Preadmission regimen + glargine at 50% of hospital daily dose
>9.0% (>74.9 mmol/mol)	On oral antidiabetes agents + glargine or basal bolus regimen at 80% of inpatient dose

REFERENCES

1. Umpierrez GE, Isaacs SD, Bazargan N, You X, Thaler LM, Kitabchi AE. Hyperglycemia: an independent marker of in-hospital mortality in patients with undiagnosed diabetes. *J Clin Endocrinol Metab* 2002;87(3):978–982. doi: 10.1210/jcem.87.3.8341. Epub 2002 Mar 13. PubMed PMID: 11889147

2. Turchin A, Matheny ME, Shubina M, Scanlon JV, Greenwood B, Pendergrass ML. Hypoglycemia and clinical outcomes in patients with diabetes hospitalized in the general ward. *Diabetes Care* 2009;32(7):1153–1157. doi: 10.2337/dc08-2127. Epub 2009 Jul 1. PubMed PMID: 19564471; PubMed Central PMCID: PMCPMC2699723

3. Van den Berghe G, Wouters P, Weekers F, Verwaest C, Bruyninckx F, Schetz M, et al. Intensive insulin therapy in critically ill patients. *N Engl J Med* 2001;345(19):1359–1367. doi: 10.1056/NEJMoa011300. Epub 2002 Jan 17. PubMed PMID: 11794168

4. Van den Berghe G, Wilmer A, Hermans G, Meersseman W, Wouters PJ, Milants I, et al. Intensive insulin therapy in the medical ICU. *N Engl J Med* 2006;354(5):449–461. doi: 10.1056/NEJMoa052521. Epub 2006 Feb 3. PubMed PMID: 16452557

5. Investigators N-SS, Finfer S, Chittock DR, Su SY, Blair D, Foster D, et al. Intensive versus conventional glucose control in critically ill patients. *N Engl J Med* 2009;360(13):1283–1297. doi: 10.1056/NEJMoa0810625. Epub 2009 Mar 26. PubMed PMID: 19318384

6. Kansagara D, Fu R, Freeman M, Wolf F, Helfand M. Intensive insulin therapy in hospitalized patients: a systematic review. *Ann Intern Med* 2011;154(4):268–282. doi: 10.7326/0003-4819-154-4-201102150-00008. Epub 2011 Feb 16. PubMed PMID: 21320942

7. American Diabetes Association. 15. Diabetes care in the hospital: standards of medical care in diabetes 2020. *Diabetes Care* 2020;43(Suppl. 1):S193–S202. doi: 10.2337/dc20-S015. Epub 2019 Dec 22. PubMed PMID: 31862758

8. Handelsman Y, Bloomgarden ZT, Grunberger G, Umpierrez G, Zimmerman RS, Bailey TS, et al. American Association of Clinical Endocrinologists

and American College of Endocrinology—clinical practice guidelines for developing a diabetes mellitus comprehensive care plan—2015. *Endocr Pract* 2015;21(Suppl. 1):1–87. doi: 10.4158/EP15672.GL. Epub 2015 Apr 15. PubMed PMID: 25869408; PubMed Central PMCID: PMCPMC4959114

9. Umpierrez GE, Hellman R, Korytkowski MT, Kosiborod M, Maynard GA, Montori VM, et al. Management of hyperglycemia in hospitalized patients in non-critical care setting: an endocrine society clinical practice guideline. *J Clin Endocrinol Metab* 2012;97(1):16–38. doi: 10.1210/jc.2011-2098. Epub 2012 Jan 10. PubMed PMID: 22223765

10. Hsia E, Seggelke S, Gibbs J, Hawkins RM, Cohlmia E, Rasouli N, et al. Subcutaneous administration of glargine to diabetic patients receiving insulin infusion prevents rebound hyperglycemia. *J Clin Endocrinol Metab* 2012;97(9):3132–3137. doi: 10.1210/jc.2012-1244. Epub 2012 June 12. PubMed PMID: 22685233

11. Bode BW, Braithwaite SS, Steed RD, Davidson PC. Intravenous insulin infusion therapy: indications, methods, and transition to subcutaneous insulin therapy. *Endocr Pract* 2004;10(Suppl. 2):71–80. doi: 10.4158/EP.10.S2.71. Epub 2004 Jul 15. PubMed PMID: 15251644

12. Wilson M, Weinreb J, Hoo GW. Intensive insulin therapy in critical care: a review of 12 protocols. *Diabetes Care* 2007;30(4):1005–1011. doi: 10.2337/dc06-1964. Epub 2007 Jan 11. PubMed PMID: 17213376

13. Baldwin D, Villanueva G, McNutt R, Bhatnagar S. Eliminating inpatient sliding-scale insulin: a reeducation project with medical house staff. *Diabetes Care* 2005;28(5):1008–1011. doi: 10.2337/diacare.28.5.1008. Epub 2005 Apr 28. PubMed PMID: 15855558

14. Bellido V, Suarez L, Rodriguez MG, Sanchez C, Dieguez M, Riestra M, et al. Comparison of basal-bolus and premixed insulin regimens in hospitalized patients with type 2 diabetes. *Diabetes Care* 2015;38(12):2211–2216. doi: 10.2337/dc15-0160. Epub 2015 Oct 16. PubMed PMID: 26459273; PubMed Central PMCID: PMCPMC4657612

15. Umpierrez GE, Gianchandani R, Smiley D, Jacobs S, Wesorick DH, Newton C, et al. Safety and efficacy of sitagliptin therapy for the inpatient management of general medicine and surgery patients with type 2 diabetes: a pilot, randomized, controlled study. *Diabetes Care* 2013;36(11):3430–3435. doi: 10.2337/dc13-0277. Epub 2013 Jul 24. PubMed PMID: 23877988; PubMed Central PMCID: PMCPMC3816910

16. Macdonald JJ, Neupane S, Gianchandani RY. The potential role of incretin therapy in the hospital setting. *Clin Diabetes Endocrinol* 2015;1:4. doi: 10.1186/s40842-015-0005-5. Epub 2015 Jul 1. PubMed PMID: 28702223; PubMed Central PMCID: PMCPMC5469200

17. Perez-Belmonte LM, Osuna-Sanchez J, Millan-Gomez M, Lopez-Carmona MD, Gomez-Doblas JJ, Cobos-Palacios L, et al. Glycaemic efficacy and safety of linagliptin for the management of non-cardiac surgery patients with

type 2 diabetes in a real-world setting: Lina-Surg study. *Ann Med* 2019; 51(3-4):252–261. doi: 10.1080/07853890.2019.1613672. Epub 2019 May 1. PubMed PMID: 31037970

18. Salpeter SR, Greyber E, Pasternak GA, Salpeter EE. Risk of fatal and nonfatal lactic acidosis with metformin use in type 2 diabetes mellitus. *Cochrane Database Syst Rev* 2010(4):CD002967. doi: 10.1002/14651858.CD002967. pub4. Epub 2010 Apr 16. PubMed PMID: 20393934

19. Deusenberry CM, Coley KC, Korytkowski MT, Donihi AC. Hypoglycemia in hospitalized patients treated with sulfonylureas. *Pharmacotherapy* 2012;32(7):613–617. doi: 10.1002/j.1875-9114.2011.01088.x. Epub 2012 May 10. PubMed PMID: 22570146

20. Levine JA, Karam SL, Aleppo G. SGLT2-I In the hospital setting: diabetic ketoacidosis and other benefits and concerns. *Curr Diab Rep* 2017;17(7):54. doi: 10.1007/s11892-017-0874-3. Epub 2017 Jun 10. PubMed PMID: 28597228

21. Wexler DJ, Meigs JB, Cagliero E, Nathan DM, Grant RW. Prevalence of hyper- and hypoglycemia among inpatients with diabetes: a national survey of 44 U.S. hospitals. *Diabetes Care* 2007;30(2):367–369. doi: 10.2337/dc06-1715. Epub 2007 Jan 30. PubMed PMID: 17259511

22. Fischer KF, Lees JA, Newman JH. Hypoglycemia in hospitalized patients. Causes and outcomes. *N Engl J Med* 1986;315(20):1245–1250. doi: 10.1056/NEJM198611133152002. Epub 1986 Nov 13. PubMed PMID: 3534567

23. Smith WD, Winterstein AG, Johns T, Rosenberg E, Sauer BC. Causes of hyperglycemia and hypoglycemia in adult inpatients. *Am J Health Syst Pharm* 2005;62(7):714–719. doi: 10.1093/ajhp/62.7.714. Epub 2005 Mar 26. PubMed PMID: 15790798

24. Brodovicz KG, Mehta V, Zhang Q, Zhao C, Davies MJ, Chen J, et al. Association between hypoglycemia and inpatient mortality and length of hospital stay in hospitalized, insulin-treated patients. *Curr Med Res Opin* 2013;29(2):101–107. doi: 10.1185/03007995.2012.754744. Epub 2012 Dec 4. PubMed PMID: 23198978

25. McClave SA, DiBaise JK, Mullin GE, Martindale RG. ACG clinical guideline: nutrition therapy in the adult hospitalized patient. *Am J Gastroenterol* 2016;111(3):315–334; quiz 35. doi: 10.1038/ajg.2016.28. Epub 2016 Mar 10. PubMed PMID: 26952578

26. Petrov MS, Zagainov VE. Influence of enteral versus parenteral nutrition on blood glucose control in acute pancreatitis: a systematic review. *Clin Nutr* 2007;26(5):514–523. doi: 10.1016/j.clnu.2007.04.009. Epub 2007 Jun 15. PubMed PMID: 17559987

27. Schorghuber M, Fruhwald S. Effects of enteral nutrition on gastrointestinal function in patients who are critically ill. *Lancet Gastroenterol Hepatol* 2018;3(4):281–287. doi: 10.1016/S2468-1253(18)30036-0. Epub 2018 Mar 14. PubMed PMID: 29533200

28. Gosmanov AR, Umpierrez GE. Management of hyperglycemia during enteral and parenteral nutrition therapy. *Curr Diab Rep* 2013;13(1):155–162. doi: 10.1007/s11892-012-0335-y. Epub 2012 Oct 16. PubMed PMID: 23065369; PubMed Central PMCID: PMCPMC3746491

29. Weisenfeld S, Podolsky S, Goldsmith L, Ziff L. Adsorption of insulin to infusion bottles and tubing. *Diabetes* 1968;17(12):766–771. Epub 1968 Dec 1. doi: 10.2337/diab.17.12.766. PubMed PMID: 5726255

30. Hwang JL, Weiss RE. Steroid-induced diabetes: a clinical and molecular approach to understanding and treatment. *Diabetes Metab Res Rev* 2014;30(2):96–102. doi: 10.1002/dmrr.2486. Epub 2013 Oct 15. PubMed PMID: 24123849; PubMed Central PMCID: PMCPMC4112077

31. Perez A, Jansen-Chaparro S, Saigi I, Bernal-Lopez MR, Minambres I, Gomez-Huelgas R. Glucocorticoid-induced hyperglycemia. *J Diabetes* 2014;6(1):9–20. doi: 10.1111/1753-0407.12090. Epub 2013 Oct 10. PubMed PMID: 24103089

32. Gandhi GY, Nuttall GA, Abel MD, Mullany CJ, Schaff HV, Williams BA, et al. Intraoperative hyperglycemia and perioperative outcomes in cardiac surgery patients. *Mayo Clin Proc* 2005;80(7):862–866. doi: 10.4065/80.7.862. Epub 2005 Jul 13. PubMed PMID: 16007890

33. Dronge AS, Perkal MF, Kancir S, Concato J, Aslan M, Rosenthal RA. Long-term glycemic control and postoperative infectious complications. *Arch Surg* 2006;141(4):375–380; discussion 80. doi: 10.1001/archsurg.141.4.375. Epub 2006 Apr 19. PubMed PMID: 16618895

34. Golden SH, Peart-Vigilance C, Kao WH, Brancati FL. Perioperative glycemic control and the risk of infectious complications in a cohort of adults with diabetes. *Diabetes Care* 1999;22(9):1408–1414. doi: 10.2337/diacare.22.9.1408. Epub 1999 Sep 10. PubMed PMID: 10480501

35. Jacober SJ, Sowers JR. An update on perioperative management of diabetes. *Arch Intern Med* 1999;159(20):2405–2411. doi:10.1001/archinte.159.20.2405. Epub 2000 Feb 9. PubMed PMID: 10665888

36. Smiley DD, Umpierrez GE. Perioperative glucose control in the diabetic or nondiabetic patient. *South Med J* 2006;99(6):580–589; quiz 90–91. doi: 10.1097/01.smj.0000209366.91803.99. Epub 2006 Jun 28. PubMed PMID: 16800413

37. Umpierrez GE, Reyes D, Smiley D, Hermayer K, Khan A, Olson DE, et al. Hospital discharge algorithm based on admission HbA1c for the management of patients with type 2 diabetes. *Diabetes Care* 2014;37(11):2934–2939. doi: 10.2337/dc14-0479. Epub 2014 Aug 30. PubMed PMID: 25168125; PubMed Central PMCID: PMCPMC4207201

MAJOR ACUTE COMPLICATIONS

Luigi Meneghini, MD, MBA

In this section, the acute metabolic complications of type 2 diabetes, specifically the hyperosmolar hyperglycemic state (HHS) and hypoglycemia and their management, are reviewed. Patients with type 2 diabetes are often treated with numerous medications, including hypoglycemic, antihypertensive, and hypolipidemic drugs, to treat their diabetes and common coexistent disorders. The adverse effects of these medications and their interactions are also reviewed, including the issue of diabetic ketoacidosis (DKA) induced by sodium-glucose cotransporter 2 (SGLT2) inhibitors.

Major acute complications of diabetes include metabolic problems, often precipitated by infection. The two metabolic problems of most concern in patients with type 2 diabetes are hyperosmolar hyperglycemic nonketotic syndrome and hypoglycemia, although patients with type 2 diabetes can present with ketoacidosis exacerbated by severe stressors.

HYPEROSMOLAR HYPERGLYCEMIC STATE

HHS is characterized by severe hyperglycemia, volume depletion, and resultant hyperosmolarity without evidence of ketoacidosis.[1] Most cases are encountered in older patients with type 2 diabetes, often in association with compromised renal function. The mortality from HHS can be as high as 20% and is affected by the patient's age, associated comorbidities, and degree of volume depletion. The pathogenesis of HHS involves a combination of insulin deficiency and increased counterregulatory hormones leading to decreased glucose utilization and increased gluconeogenesis and glycogenolysis. The resultant hyperglycemia leads to an osmotic diuresis, loss of fluid and electrolytes, and dehydration, which when combined with decreased fluid intake will lead to hyperosmolarity and impaired renal function.[1]

Precipitating Causes

There is almost always a precipitating factor (Table 4.12), the most common being infection, usually pneumonia and urinary tract infections,[2] although up to 20% of cases present as a new diagnosis of diabetes.[1] Other precipitating events include the use of drugs as well as stressful events such as stroke, myocardial infarction, or trauma, all of which are associated with the release of counterregulatory hormones. Abnormal thirst sensation (as can be seen in the elderly) or limited access to water (e.g., bedridden patients) also facilitate development of this syndrome.

Clinical Presentation

There are four major clinical features of HHS:[3–5]

1. Severe hyperglycemia (blood glucose >600 mg/dl [>33.3 mmol/l] and generally between 1,000 and 2,000 mg/dl [55.5–111.1 mmol/l]).
2. Absence of or slight ketosis.
3. Plasma or serum hyperosmolality (>350 mOsm/kg).
4. Profound dehydration.

Table 4.12–Factors Associated with HHS

Therapeutic Agents	Therapeutic Procedures	Chronic Diseases	Acute Situations
Glucocorticoids	Peritoneal dialysis	Renal disease	Infection
Diuretics	Hemodialysis	Heart disease	Diabetic gangrene
Diphenylhydantoin	Hyperosmolar	Hypertension	Urinary tract
α-Aderenergic-	Alimentation	Dementia	infections
blocking agents	Surgical stress	Old stroke	Septicemia
Diazoxide		Alcoholism	Extensive burns
L-Asparaginase		Psychiatric loss	Gastrointestinal
Immunosuppres-		of thirst	hemorrhage
sive agents			Cerebrovascular
			accident
			Myocardial infarction
			Pancreatitis

Source: Garcia de los Rio M: Nonketotic hyperosmolar coma. In World Book of Diabetes Practice 1982. Krall LP, Alberti KGMM, Eds. Amsterdam, Netherlands, Excerpta Medica, 1982, p. 96–99. Podolsky S: Hyperosmolar nonketotic coma. In Diabetes Mellitus. Vol. V. Rifkin H, Raskin P, Eds. Bowie, MD, Brady, 1981.

Typically, the patient develops excessive thirst, altered sensorium (coma or confusion), and physical signs of severe dehydration.

Treatment

The precipitating event should be determined and corrected as soon as possible, and lifesaving measures should be used immediately. Dehydration, hyperglycemia, electrolyte abnormalities, and the hyperosmolar condition should be corrected with the use of appropriate fluids, insulin, and potassium. Aggressive hydration should begin with isotonic saline, which on its own will result in a substantial reduction in hyperglycemia.

HYPOGLYCEMIA

While hypoglycemia is more frequent in patients with type 1 diabetes, it is increasingly recognized in patients with longer-standing type 2 diabetes, especially when treated with agents such as sulfonylureas (or glinides) and insulin.[6] More relevant to morbidity, mortality, and the cost of care is the incidence and rate of severe hypoglycemia (level 3 hypoglycemia based on American Diabetes Association criteria), which is characterized by an altered mental or physical state requiring third-party assistance.[7]

Precipitating Causes

Hypoglycemia results when there is an imbalance between needs and the appropriate dosage of drug therapy (i.e., sulfonylureas, meglitinides, insulin, or a combination of these drugs); it remains a major limiting factor to glycemic management, especially in long-standing, insulin-deficient type 2 diabetes.

It is important when evaluating potential management options for hyperglycemia to assess a patient's risk of treatment-associated hypoglycemia. Factors that are associated with an increased risk include the type of treatment (e.g., use of sulfonylureas and/or insulin), impaired renal or hepatic function, longer diabetes duration, older age or frailty, cognitive impairment, physical or intellectual disability, and diabetic autonomic neuropathy. Other factors include alcohol use and polypharmacy. Perhaps the strongest predictor of risk for severe hypoglycemia (an event requiring third-party assistance) is impaired counterregulatory response and hypoglycemia unawareness.[8-10] Hypoglycemia unawareness is characterized by an inadequate counterregulatory hormone response (glucagon, epinephrine), which is exacerbated by frequent episodes of hypoglycemia.[11] In addition, older patients experiencing episodes of severe hypoglycemia also have an increased risk of dementia; likewise, for patients with decreased cognitive function, the risk of severe hypoglycemia increases.[12,13]

Clinical Presentation

Hypoglycemia should be suspected in a patient who presents with symptoms indicative of altered mental and/or neurological function (changes in sensorium and behavior, coma, or seizure), as well as adrenergic responses (tachycardia, palpitations, increased sweating, and hunger). The diagnosis is confirmed with a plasma glucose level <70 mg/dl (<3.9 mmol/l). Hypoglycemia is currently classified as level 1 (glucose <70 mg/dl [<3.9 mmol/L] and ≥54 mg/dl [3 mmol/L]), level 2 (glucose <54 mg/dl [<3.0 mmol/L]), or level 3 (severe hypoglycemia, which is an event characterized by mental status changes and requiring third-party assistance for treatment).[7] Hypoglycemia can result in injury to patients or others around them, especially when in the setting of motor vehicle accidents or falls. Repeated episodes of level 2 hypoglycemia, or one or more events of level 3 hypoglycemia, warrant immediate intervention and timely adjustment of the treatment plan, behavioral intervention, and potentially the use of continuous monitoring glucose technologies.[7]

Treatment

The objective of treatment is to restore the plasma glucose level to normal. When the patient is conscious and cooperative, ingestion of some form of fast-acting carbohydrate by mouth (e.g., fruit juice, sugar cubes, glucose tablets, or a solution equivalent to 15–20 g carbohydrate) is usually followed by relief of symptoms, usually within 10–15 min from ingestion. A good sequence to remember is the rule of 15: Ingest 15 g carbohydrate, repeat blood glucose check in 15 min, and repeat if still hypoglycemic. For individuals in whom there is ongoing insulin activity (e.g., within a couple of hours of a prandial insulin injection), additional foods that contain carbohydrate may need to be ingested to prevent a recurrence of the hypoglycemia. In treating a hypoglycemic episode, pure glucose (available in tablets or gel form) is preferred, although any form of carbohydrate-containing glucose is appropriate, as long as it limits the amount of fat or protein, which can respectively slow glucose absorption and stimulate insulin response.[7] Once glucose levels have returned to normal, it might be prudent for the patient to eat a meal or snack to prevent recurrence of the event. In the unconscious or uncooperative patient, parenteral or intranasal glucagon or intravenous glucose (50 ml 50% dextrose or glucose followed by 5% or 10% dextrose drip) can be safely administered by nonmedical individuals who have been appropriately trained. In the setting of hypoglycemia secondary to sulfonylureas, hypoglycemia may be prolonged, and patients should be observed for at least 12–24 h.

Prevention of future episodes of hypoglycemia requires the appropriate monitoring technologies (e.g., self-monitoring of blood glucose, continuous glucose monitoring) and an awareness of situations that can precipitate hypoglycemia, such as fasting or skipped meals, increased physical activity, and alcohol consumption. While continuous glucose monitoring has been shown to reduce the time spent in hypoglycemia (54–70 mg/dl [3.0–3.9 mmol/L]) in individuals with type 1 diabetes, the impact in type 2 diabetes appears to be limited to modest improvement in A1C levels.[14]

Patients with hypoglycemia unawareness may concomitantly experience fear of hypoglycemia, especially if there is an underlying general anxiety disorder,[15] and this may affect a person's ability or willingness to correct hyperglycemia to appropriate target levels. Interventions exist for patients with fear of hypoglycemia and hypoglycemia unawareness, with structured training that can improve glycemic control, reduce the risk of severe hypoglycemia, and in some cases restore hypoglycemia awareness.[16,17]

DIABETIC KETOACIDOSIS

DKA has been described in patients with metabolic features of type 2 diabetes and no evidence of autoimmunity. This type of presentation has been labeled as atypical diabetes, type 1B diabetes, diabetes 1.5, and ketosis-prone type 2 diabetes.[18] Most adults with DKA present with acute symptoms of polyuria, polydipsia, and weight loss in the setting of new-onset diabetes.[19] Treatment of DKA follows usual protocols, and resolution of the acute metabolic decompensation is often followed by recovery of β-cell function; in many cases, the insulin resistance from the gluco- and lipo-toxic environment common in the presentation of DKA resolves over the ensuing several weeks with appropriate treatment of hyperglycemia, namely with insulin. Many of these patients can maintain excellent glycemic control with dietary management, although the use of sulfonylureas and metformin has been shown to prolong the duration of normoglycemia.[19,20]

SGLT2 inhibitors, which are used for the treatment of diabetes and are particularly effective in patients with atherosclerotic cardiovascular disease, with chronic kidney disease, and who are at risk for heart failure, are also associated with an increased risk of DKA.[21–23] The incidence of DKA was 1.0–1.6/1,000 person years in trials using SGLT2 inhibitors with one-third of patients presenting with plasma glucose levels <200 mg/dl (<11.1 mmol/L). Events of ketoacidosis can be precipitated by illness, reduction or discontinuation of insulin in insulin-deficient patients, surgery, dehydration, or the development of latent autoimmune diabetes in a patient previously diagnosed with type 2 diabetes.[24] Patients who are prescribed SGLT2 inhibitors and who might be at risk of developing ketoacidosis should be made aware of symptoms of DKA, cautioned to suspend the SGLT2 inhibitor during illness, and instructed to get in touch with their provider if they develop suspicious symptomatology.

INFECTION

Individuals with diabetes are more likely to experience infections, likely attributed to compromised immune function worsened by hyperglycemia, microvascular complications, age, and related comorbidities.[25] Common infections seen in patients with diabetes are listed in Table 4.13. The rapid diagnosis and treatment of infection in a patient with diabetes is absolutely necessary because infection is a leading cause of metabolic abnormalities that can result in severe hyperglycemia and precipitate HHS or DKA.

Table 4.13–Major Infections Associated with Diabetes

Respiratory infections
   Streptococcus pneumonia
   Influenza
   H1N1
   Tuberculosis

Urinary tract infections
   Asymptomatic bacteriuria
   Fungal cystitis
   Emphysematous cystitis
   Perinephric abscess

Gastrointestinal and liver infections
   H. pylori infection
   Oral and esophageal candidiasis
   Emphysematous cholecystitis
   Hepatitis C
   Hepatitis B
   Enteroviruses

Skin and soft tissue infections
   Foot infection
   Necrotizing fasciitis
   Fournier's gangrene

Head and neck infections
   Invasive external otitis
   Rhinocerebral mucormycosis

Other infections
   Human immunodeficiency virus

Source: Casqueiro.[26]

REFERENCES

1. Pasquel FJ, Umpierrez GE. Hyperosmolar hyperglycemic state: a historic review of the clinical presentation, diagnosis, and treatment. *Diabetes Care* 2014;37(11):3124–3131. doi: 10.2337/dc14-0984

2. Wachtel TJ. The diabetic hyperosmolar state. *Clin Geriatr Med* 1990;6(4): 797–806. Epub 1990 Nov 1. PubMed PMID: 2224747

3. Arieff AI, Carroll HJ. Nonketotic hyperosmolar coma with hyperglycemia: clinical features, pathophysiology, renal function, acid-base balance, plasma-cerebrospinal fluid equilibria and the effects of therapy in 37 cases. *Medicine (Baltimore)* 1972;51(2):73–94. doi: 10.1097/00005792-197203000-00001. Epub 1972 Mar 1. PubMed PMID: 5013637

4. Gerich JE, Martin MM, Recant L. Clinical and metabolic characteristics of hyperosmolar nonketotic coma. *Diabetes* 1971;20(4):228–238. doi: 10.2337/diab.20.4.228. Epub 1971 Apr 1. PubMed PMID: 4994561

5. Kitabchi AE, Umpierrez GE, Miles JM, Fisher JN. Hyperglycemic crises in adult patients with diabetes. *Diabetes Care* 2009;32(7):1335–1343. doi: 10.2337/dc09-9032. Epub 2009 Jul 1. PubMed PMID: 19564476; PubMed Central PMCID: PMCPMC2699725

6. Khunti K, Alsifri S, Aronson R, Cigrovski Berkovic M, Enters-Weijnen C, Forsen T, et al. Rates and predictors of hypoglycaemia in 27,585 people from 24 countries with insulin-treated type 1 and type 2 diabetes: the global HAT study. *Diabetes Obes Metab* 2016;18(9):907–15. doi: 10.1111/dom.12689. Epub 2016 May 11. PubMed PMID: 27161418; PubMed Central PMCID: PMCPMC5031206

7. American Diabetes Association. 6. Glycemic targets: standards of medical care in diabetes 2020. *Diabetes Care* 2020;43(Suppl. 1):S66–S76. doi: 10.2337/dc20-S006. Epub 2019 Dec 22. PubMed PMID: 31862749

8. American Diabetes Association. 4. Comprehensive medical evaluation and assessment of comorbidities: standards of medical care in diabetes 2020. *Diabetes Care* 2020;43(Suppl. 1):S37–S47. doi: 10.2337/dc20-S004. Epub 2019 Dec 22. PubMed PMID: 31862747

9. Shorr RI, Ray WA, Daugherty JR, Griffin MR. Incidence and risk factors for serious hypoglycemia in older persons using insulin or sulfonylureas. *Arch Intern Med* 1997;157(15):1681–1686. Epub 1997 Aug 11. PubMed PMID: 9250229

10. Lipska KJ, Ross JS, Wang Y, Inzucchi SE, Minges K, Karter AJ, et al. National trends in US hospital admissions for hyperglycemia and hypoglycemia among Medicare beneficiaries, 1999 to 2011. *JAMA Intern Med* 2014;174(7):1116–1124. doi: 10.1001/jamainternmed.2014.1824. Epub 2014 May 20. PubMed PMID: 24838229; PubMed Central PMCID: PMCPMC4152370

11. Cryer PE. Diverse causes of hypoglycemia-associated autonomic failure in diabetes. *N Engl J Med* 2004;350(22):2272–2229. doi: 10.1056/NEJMra031354. Epub 2004 May 28. PubMed PMID: 15163777

12. Punthakee Z, Miller ME, Launer LJ, Williamson JD, Lazar RM, Cukierman-Yaffee T, et al. Poor cognitive function and risk of severe hypoglycemia in type 2 diabetes: post hoc epidemiologic analysis of the ACCORD trial. *Diabetes Care* 2012;35(4):787–793. doi: 10.2337/dc11-1855. Epub 2012 Mar 1. PubMed PMID: 22374637; PubMed Central PMCID: PMCPMC3308284

13. Whitmer RA, Karter AJ, Yaffe K, Quesenberry CP, Jr., Selby JV. Hypoglycemic episodes and risk of dementia in older patients with type 2 diabetes mellitus. *JAMA* 2009;301(15):1565–1572. doi: 10.1001/jama.2009,460. Epub 2009 Apr 16. PubMed PMID: 19366776; PubMed Central PMCID: PMCPMC2782622

14. Dicembrini I, Mannucci E, Monami M, Pala L. Impact of technology on glycaemic control in type 2 diabetes: A meta-analysis of randomized trials on continuous glucose monitoring and continuous subcutaneous insulin infusion. *Diabetes Obes Metab* 2019;21(12):2619–2625. doi: 10.1111/dom.13845. Epub 2019 Aug 2. PubMed PMID: 31368658

15. Wild D, von Maltzahn R, Brohan E, Christensen T, Clauson P, Gonder-Frederick L. A critical review of the literature on fear of hypoglycemia in diabetes: implications for diabetes management and patient education. *Patient Educ Couns* 2007;68(1):10–15. doi: 10.1016/j.pec.2007.05.003. Epub 2007 Jun 22. PubMed PMID: 17582726

16. Cox DJ, Gonder-Frederick L, Polonsky W, Schlundt D, Kovatchev B, Clarke W. Blood glucose awareness training (BGAT-2): long-term benefits. *Diabetes Care* 2001;24(4):637–642. doi: 10.2337/diacare.24.4.637. Epub 2001 Apr 24. PubMed PMID: 11315822

17. Cox DJ, Kovatchev B, Koev D, Koeva L, Dachev S, Tcharaktchiev D, et al. Hypoglycemia anticipation, awareness and treatment training (HAATT) reduces occurrence of severe hypoglycemia among adults with type 1 diabetes mellitus. *Int J Behav Med* 2004;11(4):212–218. doi: 10.1207/s15327558ijbm1104_4. Epub 2005 Jan 20. PubMed PMID: 15657021

18. American Diabetes Association. 2. Classification and diagnosis of diabetes: standards of medical care in diabetes 2020. *Diabetes Care* 2020;43(Suppl. 1):S14–S31. doi: 10.2337/dc20-S002. Epub 2019 Dec 22. PubMed PMID: 31862745

19. Umpierrez GE, Smiley D, Kitabchi AE. Narrative review: ketosis-prone type 2 diabetes mellitus. *Ann Intern Med* 2006;144(5):350–357. doi: 10.7326/0003-4819-144-5-200603070-00011. Epub 2006 Mar 8. PubMed PMID: 16520476

20. McFarlane SI, Chaiken RL, Hirsch S, Harrington P, Lebovitz HE, Banerji MA. Near-normoglycaemic remission in African-Americans with type 2 diabetes mellitus is associated with recovery of beta cell function.

Diabet Med 2001;18(1):10–16. doi: 10.1046/j.1464-5491.2001.00395.x. Epub 2001 Feb 13. PubMed PMID: 11168335

21. Tang H, Li D, Wang T, Zhai S, Song Y. Effect of sodium-glucose cotransporter 2 inhibitors on diabetic ketoacidosis among patients with type 2 diabetes: a meta-analysis of randomized controlled trials. *Diabetes Care* 2016;39(8):e123–e124. doi: 10.2337/dc16-0885. Epub 2016 Jun 18. PubMed PMID: 27311492

22. Peters AL, Buschur EO, Buse JB, Cohan P, Diner JC, Hirsch IB. Euglycemic diabetic ketoacidosis: a potential complication of treatment with sodium-glucose cotransporter 2 inhibition. *Diabetes Care* 2015;38(9):1687–1693. doi: 10.2337/dc15-0843. Epub 2015 Jun 17. PubMed PMID: 26078479; PubMed Central PMCID: PMCPMC4542270

23. Bonora BM, Avogaro A, Fadini GP. Sodium-glucose co-transporter-2 inhibitors and diabetic ketoacidosis: An updated review of the literature. *Diabetes Obes Metab* 2018;20(1):25–33. doi: 10.1111/dom.13012. Epub 2017 May 19. PubMed PMID: 28517913

24. Burke KR, Schumacher CA, Harpe SE. SGLT2 inhibitors: a systematic review of diabetic ketoacidosis and related risk factors in the primary literature. *Pharmacotherapy* 2017;37(2):187–194. doi: 10.1002/phar.1881. Epub 2017 Jan 16

25. Magliano DJ, Harding JL, Cohen K, Huxley RR, Davis WA, Shaw JE. Excess risk of dying from infectious causes in those with type 1 and type 2 diabetes. *Diabetes Care* 2015;38(7):1274–1280. doi: 10.2337/dc14-2820. Epub 2015 Jun 14. PubMed PMID: 26070592

26. Casqueiro J, Casqueiro J, Alves C. Infections in patients with diabetes mellitus: a review of pathogenesis. *Indian J Endocrinol Metab* 2012;16 (Suppl. 1):S27–S36. doi: 10.4103/2230-8210.94253. Epub 2012 Jun 16. PubMed PMID: 22701840; PubMed Central PMCID: PMCPMC3354930

ELDERLY AND DIABETES

Sasan Mirfakhraee, MD
Nisha Jacob, DNP, FNP-C, CDCES, MBA

The prevalence of diabetes in elderly adults is high, with one-third of the elderly population having diabetes and three-quarters with either prediabetes or diabetes.[1] With the population continuing to age, it is projected that the number of diabetes diagnoses will more than quadruple from 2005 to 2050.[2] As the duration of diabetes and advancing age have been shown to independently predict diabetes morbidity and mortality,[3] it is imperative that clinicians familiarize themselves with the unique sets of challenges presented by older adults with diabetes.

DIABETES TRIALS IN OLDER PATIENTS

Randomized trials of subjects with type 2 diabetes have frequently excluded older adults, which limits their translation into clinical practice. Dedicated trials of older adults with type 2 diabetes have failed to show a benefit with intensive glycemic control in terms of reducing adverse cardiovascular outcomes. In the ADVANCE,[4] VADT,[5] and ACCORD[6] studies, despite a significant difference in achieved A1C between the intensive versus standard glycemic control groups, no difference was seen in the reduction of major macrovascular outcomes (Table 4.14). Despite the lack of reduction in macrovascular events with intensive glycemic control in these trials, clinicians should be mindful that A1C reduction clearly reduces the risk of microvascular complications,[7] and thus glycemic targets should not be abandoned in older adults with diabetes.

GLYCEMIC GOALS

Older adults with diabetes are at risk for multiple coexisting medical conditions, which may impact their glucose-managing abilities and diminish their quality of life. These include cognitive dysfunction, functional impairment, depression, polypharmacy, hearing/vision loss, urinary incontinence, injurious falls, and persistent pain.[8] The 2020 *Standards of Medical Care in Diabetes* recommends that the medical, psychological, and functional status of older adults with diabetes be considered in determining glycemic targets and therapeutic approaches.[9] In older adults with diabetes who are otherwise healthy with intact cognition and acceptable functional status, an A1C goal of 7.5% is reasonable; for those with multiple comorbidities or mild–moderate cognitive impairment, glycemic targets should be relaxed to an A1C 8%, and for those with very complex health with moderate to severe cognitive impairment, the A1C should approach 8.5% in order to prevent hypoglycemia.[9] The 2020 Endocrine Society Guidelines for the Treatment of Diabetes in Older Adults provide blood glucose targets depending on overall health category (defined as comorbid conditions, cognitive impairment, and/or affected instrumental activities of daily living) and the use of medications associated with hypoglycemia.[9] To assess for unrecognized cognitive impairment, older adults with diabetes should have periodic cognitive evaluations; if cognitive impairment is present, the medication regimen should be simplified to reduce the

Table 4.14–Trial Characteristics in the VADT, ADVANCE, and ACCORD Studies

Participant Characteristics	VADT	ADVANCE	ACCORD
n	1,791	11,140	10,251
Mean age (years)	60	66	62
Duration of DM (years)	11.5	8	10
Sex (male/female, %)	97/3	58/42	39/61
History of CVD (%)	40	32	35
A1C target	1.5% A1C reduction in intensive-therapy arm	≤6.5% vs. standard control per "local guidelines"	<6% vs. 7%–7.9%
Achieved median A1C (%) (standard vs. intensive therapy)	8.4/6.9	7/6.3	7.5/6.4
Primary outcome	Nonfatal MI, nonfatal CVA, CV death, heart failure hospitalization, revascularization	Combined macro-vascular (nonfatal MI, nonfatal CVA, CV death) and major microvascular events	Nonfatal MI, nonfatal stroke, CVD death
HR for primary outcome	0.88 (0.74–1.05)	0.9 (0.82–0.98)*	0.90 (0.78–1.04)

CV, cardiovascular; CVA, cerebrovascular accident; CVD, cardiovascular disease; DM, diabetes mellitus; HR, hazard ratio; MI, myocardial infarction.

*The slight reduction in hazard ratio in the ADVANCE trial was based on a reduction in nephropathy.

risk for hypoglycemia.[9] The avoidance of hypoglycemia is especially important in older adults, as the increased risk of mortality is likely influenced by a greater risk of cardiovascular death. The association of severe hypoglycemia and cardiovascular death was seen in the ADVANCE trial as well as in a large-scale retrospective observational study.[10] Additionally, control of hyperglycemia needs to be sufficient to prevent acute complications such as dehydration, poor wound healing, and hyperglycemic hyperosmolar coma.

TREATMENT REGIMENS

Similar to the recommendation for adult patients with diabetes, lifestyle changes are recommended as the initial intervention for older adults with diabetes. For those who are unable to achieve glycemic targets with lifestyle modifications, metformin should be the starting oral agent given the low cost, convenience, and efficacy, provided that there are no contraindications.[9] Metformin can cause gastrointestinal side effects and suppress appetite in some older adults.[9]

Extended-release metformin (i.e., metformin XR) has fewer gastrointestinal side effects than immediate-release metformin and is the preferred formulation given comparable cost.[11] Per the package insert, metformin should not be used in patients with an estimated glomerular filtration rate <30 mL/min/1.73 m². Also, metformin may lower vitamin B12 levels, so it is recommended to monitor B_{12} levels regularly in older patients on long-term metformin therapy.[12]

Given the increased convenience of oral versus injectable therapy, a variety of oral medications are generally used for the treatment of adults with type 2 diabetes when metformin is not sufficiently effective or is contraindicated. Sulfonylureas, while inexpensive and convenient to administer, are generally not recommended in older adults with diabetes given the increased risk of hypoglycemia, particularly with glyburide.[13] Dipeptidyl peptidase-4 (DPP-4) inhibitors are generally well tolerated and safe in older patients, including those with advanced chronic kidney disease; however, the high cost and increased rate of heart failure hospitalization with saxagliptin[14] could be of concern. Sodium–glucose cotransporter 2 (SGLT2) inhibitors have a modest effect on A1C reduction and are not associated with hypoglycemia; additionally, empagliflozin and canagliflozin have been shown to reduce atherosclerotic major adverse cardiovascular events, and all SGLT2 inhibitors reduce heart failure hospitalization and the progression of renal disease.[15–17] There is an increased risk of genital infection with SGLT2 inhibitor therapy; volume depletion has also been described in patients ≥75 years.[18]

Injectable therapy for type 2 diabetes consists of glucagon-like peptide 1 receptor (GLP-1) agonists and/or insulin. GLP-1 agonists stimulate glucose-dependent insulin release, reduce weight and appetite, and lower glucagon levels but are associated with nausea in a dose-dependent fashion.[19] Once-weekly GLP-1 agonists, such as semaglutide and dulaglutide, combine potent A1C reduction with added convenience over once-daily GLP-1 agonists (e.g., liraglutide). Additionally, the cardiovascular benefit seen with liraglutide,[20] semaglutide,[21] and dulaglutide[22] (mean age 64–66 years in the LEADER, SUSTAIN-6, and REWIND trials) further increases their appeal in older adults with type 2 diabetes at high risk for cardiovascular disease. However, GLP-1 receptor agonists may not be preferred in older adults who are experiencing unexplained weight loss.

In patients with type 2 diabetes who fail to reach glycemic goals despite the use of medications with low risk for hypoglycemia (e.g., metformin, DPP4 inhibitors, SGLT-2 inhibitors, GLP-1 agonists), insulin is generally added, provided that the patient or caregiver has the intellectual and physical ability to administer insulin. Basal insulin monotherapy is a typical starting strategy, as once-daily dosing increases patient convenience and acceptance, and appropriate patients can be taught to self-titrate their insulin dose based on predefined glycemic targets.[23] The use of longer-acting basal insulin analogs (compared with intermediate-acting insulin such as NPH) has been associated with a reduced risk for overnight hypoglycemia.[24] In patients with suboptimal glycemic control despite basal insulin monotherapy, prandial insulin can be carefully added (either with the largest meal of the day or with each meal). Since this adds to the complexity of the diabetes regimen, a twice-daily premixed insulin regimen may be a simpler method for getting some patients to goal,[25] but patients should be counseled to eat regular meals and a small bedtime snack to prevent low blood glucose. Another option consists of combination basal insulin plus GLP-1 agonist therapy in a single device, which provides a once-daily option to control basal and postprandial blood glucose.[26] For patients with type 1 diabetes, insulin monotherapy is recommended with avoidance of hypoglycemia as a priority.

Some elderly patients with multiple comorbidities may need their glycemic goals and treatment regimen to be de-intensified. For patients on oral agents, this can be achieved by lowering the doses of medications or discontinuing others. For patients on complex insulin schedules, especially ones that challenge their self-management abilities, simplification of the insulin regimen can decrease hypoglycemia risk and reduce disease-related distress without a loss in blood glucose control.[9,27] A useful algorithm for insulin de-escalation can be found in the 2020 *Standards of Medical Care in Diabetes.*[9]

REFERENCES

1. Corriere M, Rooparinesingh N, Kalyani RR. Epidemiology of diabetes and diabetes complications in the elderly: an emerging public health burden. *Curr Diab Rep* 2013;13(6):805–813. doi: 10.1007/s11892-013-0425-5. Epub 2013 Sep 11. PubMed PMID: 24018732; PubMed Central PMCID: PMCPMC3856245

2. Narayan KM, Boyle JP, Geiss LS, Saaddine JB, Thompson TJ. Impact of recent increase in incidence on future diabetes burden: U.S., 2005–2050. *Diabetes Care* 2006;29(9):2114–2116. doi: 10.2337/dc06-1136. Epub 2006 Aug 29. PubMed PMID: 16936162

3. Huang ES, Laiteerapong N, Liu JY, John PM, Moffet HH, Karter AJ. Rates of complications and mortality in older patients with diabetes mellitus: the diabetes and aging study. *JAMA Intern Med* 2014;174(2):251–258. doi: 10.1001/jamainternmed.2013.12956. Epub 2013 Dec 11. PubMed PMID: 24322595; PubMed Central PMCID: PMCPMC3950338

4. The ADVANCE Collaborative Group, Patel A, MacMahon S, Chalmers J, Neal B, Billot L, et al. Intensive blood glucose control and vascular outcomes in patients with type 2 diabetes. *N Engl J Med* 2008;358(24):2560–2572. doi: 10.1056/NEJMoa0802987. Epub 2008 Jun 10. PubMed PMID: 18539916

5. Duckworth W, Abraira C, Moritz T, Reda D, Emanuele N, Reaven PD, et al. Glucose control and vascular complications in veterans with type 2 diabetes. *N Engl J Med* 2009;360(2):129–139. doi: 10.1056/NEJMoa0808431. Epub 2008 Dec 19. PubMed PMID: 19092145

6. The Action to Control Cardiovascular Risk in Diabetes Study Group, Gerstein HC, Miller ME, Byington RP, Goff DC, Jr., Bigger JT, et al. Effects of intensive glucose lowering in type 2 diabetes. *N Engl J Med* 2008;358(24):2545–2559. doi: 10.1056/NEJMoa0802743. Epub 2008 Jun 10. PubMed PMID: 18539917; PubMed Central PMCID: PMCPMC4551392

7. Zoungas S, Arima H, Gerstein HC, Holman RR, Woodward M, Reaven P, et al. Effects of intensive glucose control on microvascular outcomes in patients with type 2 diabetes: a meta-analysis of individual participant data

from randomised controlled trials. *Lancet Diabetes Endocrinol* 2017;5(6):431–437. doi: 10.1016/S2213-8587(17)30104-3. Epub 2017 Apr 4. PubMed PMID: 28365411

8. Kirkman MS, Briscoe VJ, Clark N, Florez H, Haas LB, Halter JB, et al. Diabetes in older adults. *Diabetes Care* 2012;35(12):2650–2664. doi: 10.2337/dc12-1801. Epub 2012 Oct 27. PubMed PMID: 23100048; PubMed Central PMCID: PMCPMC3507610

9. American Diabetes Association. 12. Older adults: standards of medical care in diabetes 2020. *Diabetes Care* 2020;43(Suppl. 1):S152–S162. doi: 10.2337/dc20-S012. Epub 2019 Dec 22. PubMed PMID: 31862755

10. Johnston SS, Conner C, Aagren M, Smith DM, Bouchard J, Brett J. Evidence linking hypoglycemic events to an increased risk of acute cardiovascular events in patients with type 2 diabetes. *Diabetes Care* 2011;34(5):1164–1170. doi: 10.2337/dc10-1915. Epub 2011 Mar 23. PubMed PMID: 21421802; PubMed Central PMCID: PMCPMC3114512

11. Blonde L, Dailey GE, Jabbour SA, Reasner CA, Mills DJ. Gastrointestinal tolerability of extended-release metformin tablets compared to immediate-release metformin tablets: results of a retrospective cohort study. *Curr Med Res Opin* 2004;20(4):565–572. doi: 10.1185/030079904125003278. Epub 2004 May 4. PubMed PMID: 15119994

12. Reinstatler L, Qi YP, Williamson RS, Garn JV, Oakley GP, Jr. Association of biochemical B(1)(2) deficiency with metformin therapy and vitamin B(1)(2) supplements: the National Health and Nutrition Examination Survey, 1999–2006. *Diabetes Care* 2012;35(2):327–33. doi: 10.2337/dc11-1582. Epub 2011 Dec 20. PubMed PMID: 22179958; PubMed Central PMCID: PMCPMC3263877

13. Douros A, Yin H, Yu OHY, Filion KB, Azoulay L, Suissa S. Pharmacologic differences of sulfonylureas and the risk of adverse cardiovascular and hypoglycemic events. *Diabetes Care* 2017;40(11):1506–1513. doi: 10.2337/dc17-0595. Epub 2017 Sep 3. PubMed PMID: 28864502

14. Scirica BM, Bhatt DL, Braunwald E, Steg PG, Davidson J, Hirshberg B, et al. Saxagliptin and cardiovascular outcomes in patients with type 2 diabetes mellitus. *New Engl J Med* 2013;369(14):1317–1326. doi: 10.1056/NEJMoa1307684. Epub 2013 Sep 3. PubMed PMID: 23992601

15. Zinman B, Wanner C, Lachin JM, Fitchett D, Bluhmki E, Hantel S, et al. Empagliflozin, cardiovascular outcomes, and mortality in type 2 diabetes. *N Engl J Med* 2015;373(22):2117–2128. doi: 10.1056/NEJMoa1504720. Epub 2015 Sep 18. PubMed PMID: 26378978

16. Wiviott SD, Raz I, Bonaca MP, Mosenzon O, Kato ET, Cahn A, et al. Dapagliflozin and cardiovascular outcomes in type 2 diabetes. *N Engl J Med* 2019;380(4):347–357. doi: 10.1056/NEJMoa1812389. Epub 2018 Nov 13. PubMed PMID: 30415602

17. Neal B, Perkovic V, Mahaffey KW, de Zeeuw D, Fulcher G, Erondu N, et al. Canagliflozin and cardiovascular and renal events in type 2 diabetes. *N Engl J Med* 2017;377(7):644–657. doi: 10.1056/NEJMoa1611925. Epub 2017 Jun 13. PubMed PMID: 28605608

18. Kohler S, Zeller C, Iliev H, Kaspers S. Safety and tolerability of empagliflozin in patients with type 2 diabetes: pooled analysis of phase I-III clinical trials. *Adv Ther* 2017;34(7):1707–1726. doi: 10.1007/s12325-017-0573-0. Epub 2017 Jun 21 PubMed PMID: 28631216; PubMed Central PMCID: PMCPMC5504200

19. Bettge K, Kahle M, Abd El Aziz MS, Meier JJ, Nauck MA. Occurrence of nausea, vomiting and diarrhoea reported as adverse events in clinical trials studying glucagon-like peptide-1 receptor agonists: a systematic analysis of published clinical trials. *Diabetes Obes Metab* 2017;19(3):336–347. doi: 10.1111/dom.12824. Epub 2016 Nov 20. PubMed PMID: 27860132

20. Buse JB, the LSC. Liraglutide and cardiovascular outcomes in type 2 diabetes. *N Engl J Med* 2016;375(18):1798–1799. doi: 10.1056/NEJMc1611289. Epub 2016 Nov 3. PubMed PMID: 27806225

21. Marso SP, Bain SC, Consoli A, Eliaschewitz FG, Jodar E, Leiter LA, et al. Semaglutide and cardiovascular outcomes in patients with type 2 diabetes. *N Engl J Med* 2016;375(19):1834–1844. doi: 10.1056/NEJMoa1607141. Epub 2016 Sep 17. PubMed PMID: 27633186

22. Gerstein HC, Colhoun HM, Dagenais GR, Diaz R, Lakshmanan M, Pais P, et al. Dulaglutide and cardiovascular outcomes in type 2 diabetes (REWIND): a double-blind, randomised placebo-controlled trial. *Lancet* 2019;394(10193):121–130. doi: 10.1016/S0140-6736(19)31149-3. Epub 2019 Jun 14. PubMed PMID: 31189511

23. Riddle MC, Rosenstock J, Gerich J, Insulin Glargine Study I. The treat-to-target trial: randomized addition of glargine or human NPH insulin to oral therapy of type 2 diabetic patients. *Diabetes Care* 2003;26(11):3080–3086. PubMed PMID: 14578243

24. Yki-Jarvinen H, Dressler A, Ziemen M, Group HOEsS. Less nocturnal hypoglycemia and better post-dinner glucose control with bedtime insulin glargine compared with bedtime NPH insulin during insulin combination therapy in type 2 diabetes. HOE 901/3002 Study Group. *Diabetes Care* 2000;23(8):1130–1136. doi: 10.2337/diacare.23.8.1130. Epub 2000 Aug 11. PubMed PMID: 10937510

25. Raskin P, Allen E, Hollander P, Lewin A, Gabbay RA, Hu P, et al. Initiating insulin therapy in type 2 diabetes: a comparison of biphasic and basal insulin analogs. *Diabetes Care* 2005;28(2):260–265. doi: 10.2337/diacare.28.2.260. Epub 2005 Jan 29. PubMed PMID: 15677776

26. Rosenstock J, Diamant M, Aroda VR, Silvestre L, Souhami E, Zhou T, et al. Efficacy and safety of LixiLan, a titratable fixed-ratio combination of lix-isenatide and insulin glargine, versus insulin glargine in type 2 diabetes inad-

equately controlled on metformin monotherapy: the LixiLan proof-of-concept randomized trial. *Diabetes Care* 2016;39(9):1579–1586. doi: 10.2337/dc16-0046. Epub 2016 Jun 11. PubMed PMID: 27284114; PubMed Central PMCID: PMCPMC5001145

27. Munshi MN, Slyne C, Segal AR, Saul N, Lyons C, Weinger K. Simplification of insulin regimen in older adults and risk of hypoglycemia. *JAMA Intern Med* 2016;176(7):1023–105. doi: 10.1001/jamainternmed.2016.2288. Epub 2016 Jun 9. PubMed PMID: 27273335

Detection and Treatment of Chronic Complications

Highlights

Highlights
Detection and Treatment of Chronic Complications

ECONOMIC AND DISEASE BURDEN OF DIABETES

■ Diabetes was the seventh leading cause of death in the U.S. in 2015, according to death certificate data.

MACROVASCULAR COMPLICATIONS

■ One of the major complications of diabetes is macrovascular events, also known as atherosclerotic cardiovascular disease (ASCVD). They consist of coronary artery disease (CAD), cerebrovascular disease (CVD), and peripheral arterial disease (PVD).

■ Macrovascular complications are the leading cause of death in the U.S. and the major cause of morbidity and mortality in diabetes.

■ Adults with diabetes have a higher rate of ASCVD-related deaths, two to four times higher than adults without diabetes. Patients with type 2 diabetes have a three to sixfold increase in rate of myocardial infarction or stroke.

■ Diabetes caused significant financial burden at both the individual patient and health-system levels. People diagnosed with diabetes, on average, have medical expenditures ~2.3 times higher than those without diabetes.

■ Strategies to reduce macrovascular complications include pharmacological management of hypertension, hyperlipidemia, and hyperglycemia, as well as addressing modifiable risk factors such as smoking cessation and lifestyle modifications.

MICROVASCULAR COMPLICATIONS

DIABETIC RETINOPATHY

■ The risk of developing diabetic retinopathy is closely related to the duration of diabetes, the degree of antecedent hyperglycemia, and blood pressure control.

■ Worldwide, approximately 93 million individuals have diabetic retinopathy, with 28 million at risk for vision loss.

■ Approximately 12,000–24,000 new cases of diabetic retinopathy are diagnosed yearly in the U.S.

DIABETIC NEPHROPATHY

■ Diabetic nephropathy occurs in 20%–40% of individuals with diabetes, is the leading cause of end-stage renal disease, and accounts for over one-third of all new cases of kidney failure.

■ Native Americans, Hispanic individuals, Asians, and African Americans have a higher risk of developing diabetic kidney disease compared with non-Hispanic Caucasians.

DIABETIC FOOT PROBLEMS

■ Foot ulcers develop in 9.1–26.1 million people with diabetes annually worldwide.

■ 15%–25% of patients with diabetes will develop a foot ulcer during their lifetime.

■ Approximately 20% of moderate to severe diabetic foot infections lead to amputations.

DIABETIC NEUROPATHY

■ Lifetime prevalence of diabetic polyneuropathy is approximately 50%. Diabetic polyneuropathy is the most common complication of diabetes.

■ Diabetic neuropathies include the polyneuropathies of the upper and lower extremities, autonomic nervous system, lumbosacral plexus neuropathies, truncal radiculopathy, upper limb mononeuropathies, and cranial neuropathies.

■ Neuropathy and peripheral vascular disease are strongly associated with the development of diabetic foot ulcers.

■ The autonomic neuropathies include cardiovascular autonomic neuropathy (manifested mainly as impaired heart rate variability, resting tachycardia, and postural hypotension), gastroparesis, diabetic diarrhea/constipation, urologic dysfunction, impaired cardiovascular reflexes and orthostatic hypotension, impaired glucose counterregulation, and sexual dysfunction.

■ The presence of cardiovascular autonomic neuropathy is an important independent predictor of increased mortality risk in patients with diabetes.

■ Therapy is principally directed toward early diagnosis, prevention of foot complications, and improving symptoms.

Detection and Treatment of Chronic Complications

Many clinicians consider type 2 diabetes a mild form of diabetes compared with type 1 diabetes because, characteristically, patients with type 2 diabetes have less labile glucose profiles and can often be managed satisfactorily with nutrition and exercise therapy, plus noninsulin therapies. Consequently, the risk of chronic complications of type 2 diabetes was often overlooked, and the complications have traditionally not been treated aggressively.

However, people with type 2 diabetes have the same devastating litany of diabetes-specific long-term microvascular and neurological complications as patients with type 1 diabetes (Table 5.1). Several earlier clinical trials, such as the U.K. Prospective Diabetes Study (UKPDS)[1] and Kumamoto Study,[2] showed that improved glycemic control in individuals with type 2 diabetes reduced their rate of diabetic microvascular complications. The Action in Diabetes and Vascular Disease—Preterax and Diamicron Modified Release Controlled Evaluation (ADVANCE)[3] and Action to Control Cardiovascular Risk in Diabetes (ACCORD) trials[4] reported beneficial effects of intensive glucose control on some microvascular end points (as discussed below). In addition, type 2 diabetes generally affects an older population, who are already at risk for cardiovascular diseases (CVDs). This combination of characteristics magnifies the risk of premature cardiac, cerebral, and peripheral vascular disease two- to sevenfold compared with people without diabetes.[5]

These complications—loss of vision, renal failure requiring dialysis or transplantation, amputation, heart attack, stroke, and premature mortality—cause immense burden to patients and belie the notion that type 2 diabetes is mild. Because of the "silent" onset of type 2 diabetes in many, ≤50% of individuals already have complications at diagnosis.[6] Patients with diabetes who do not have any prior history of myocardial infarction (MI) have as high a risk of MI as nondiabetic patients with previous history of MI; therefore, diabetes is regarded as the CVD equivalent.[7]

ECONOMIC AND DISEASE BURDEN OF DIABETES

Kyaw Soe, MD

Diabetes was the seventh leading cause of death in the U.S. in 2015 according to death certificate data.[8] Atherosclerotic cardiovascular disease (ASCVD), which consists of coronary artery disease (CAD), cerebrovascular disease, and

Table 5.1–Chronic Complications Associated with Type 2 Diabetes

Vascular diseases

- Macrovascular
  - Accelerated coronary atherosclerosis
  - Accelerated cerebrovascular atherosclerosis
  - Accelerated peripheral vascular disease
- Microvascular
  - Retinopathy
  - Nephropathy
  - Neuropathy

Diabetic peripheral neuropathies syndromes and outcomes

- Generalized sensorimotor polyneuropathies
  - Symmetrical polyneuropathy, bilateral (lower > upper limbs)
    - ☐ Pain
    - ☐ Foot deformity
    - ☐ Ulceration
  - Mononeuropathy
    - ☐ Lumbosacral
    - ☐ Thoracic
    - ☐ Cervical
    - ☐ Radiculoplexus
    - ☐ Mononeuropathy multiplex
  - Diabetic amyotrophy
  - Neuropathic cachexia

- Autonomic neuropathy
- Hypoglyecmia unawareness
- Cardiovascular autonomic neuropathy
- Diabetic gastroparesis and enteropathy
- Neurogenic bladder
- Sexual dysfunction

Mixed vascular and neuropathic diseases

- Leg ulcers
- Foot ulcers

peripheral arterial disease, is the leading cause of death in the U.S. Patients with diabetes have a two- to fourfold increased risk of cardiovascular (CV) mortality compared with patients without diabetes; hence, ASCVD is the major cause of morbidity and mortality of diabetes.[9] The total estimated cost of diabetes in 2017 is $327 billion, including $237 billion in direct medical costs and $90 billion in reduced productivity. The cost for ASCVD-related spending in diabetes is estimated to be $37.3 billion per year. After adjusting for inflation, economic costs of diabetes increased by 26% from 2012 to 2017 due to the increased prevalence of diabetes and the increased expenditure per person with diabetes. People diagnosed with diabetes, on average, have medical expenditures ~2.3 times higher than what expenditures would be in the absence of diabetes.[10] Type 2 diabetes is the single most common cause of new cases of end-stage renal disease and chronic kidney disease annually.[11] It is also the leading cause of new cases of blindness among adults age 20–74 years and the leading cause of nontraumatic amputations.[12] Despite this huge burden of diabetes, recent reports have shown a significant reduction in all-cause mortality and CV mortality in people with diabetes within the last two decades.[13,14] Similarly, the U.S. National Health Interview Survey from 1988 to 2015 showed a greater decline in all-cause mortality and vascular disease–related mortality among people with diabetes than in people without diabetes.[15]

RATIONALE FOR OPTIMIZING GLYCEMIC CONTROL IN TYPE 2 DIABETES

Kyaw Soe, MD

A strong association between hyperglycemia and microvascular disease risk has emerged from epidemiologic studies; intervention studies were eventually conducted to assess whether improved glucose control delays the development and progression of retinopathy, nephropathy, and neuropathy in patients with diabetes. In type 2 diabetes, evidence supporting the role of treating hyperglycemia in the reduction of diabetic microvascular complications initially emerged in the Kumamoto Study[2] and was confirmed in the larger UKPDS.[1] The UKPDS evaluated the effects of intensive blood glucose control (to achieve a fasting plasma glucose goal <108 mg/dl [<6 mmol/l]) with sulfonylurea, metformin, or insulin, versus less intensive treatment with nutrition therapy and conventional treatment (to maintain a fasting plasma glucose goal of <270 mg/dl [<15 mmol/l] without symptoms of hyperglycemia) on the risk of microvascular and macrovascular complications in patients with newly diagnosed type 2 diabetes. Over 10 years, A1C averaged 7.0% (53 mmol/mol) in the intensive group compared with 7.9% (63 mmol/mol) in the conventionally treated group—an 11% reduction. Compared with less intensive therapy, intensive therapy reduced the risk by 12% for any diabetes-related end points. Most of this benefit was due to a 25% relative risk reduction in microvascular complications, including the need for retinal photocoagulation.[1] Moreover, achieving and maintaining A1C goals for a prolonged period appeared to reduce the risk of subsequently developing complications in the long term, even if the glucose control became deteriorated.[16] The term *metabolic memory*, or *legacy effect*, has been invoked to describe this benefit. These data strongly support the beneficial results of effective antihyperglycemic therapy on the prevention of microvascular disease, regardless of the pathophysiology of the hyperglycemia.

The UKPDS showed that improved glycemic control resulted in nonstatistically significant reduction in the incidence of macrovascular complications in patients with newly diagnosed type 2 diabetes.[17] There was a 16% risk reduction of MI and sudden death, but diabetes-related mortality and all-cause mortality did not differ between the intensive and conventionally treated groups. However, a significant persistent benefit for MI and all-cause mortality was reported after intensive glycemic control and metformin therapy in this cohort during 10 years of posttrial follow-up of the UKPDS participants.[16]

Further evidence by other large multicenter clinical trials, such as ACCORD, ADVANCE, and VADT, showed that an intensive glucose control did not improve CV outcome in patients with type 2 diabetes. The ACCORD trial was designed to test whether intensive intervention to control hyperglycemia to a near-normal range (A1C <6%) in patients with type 2 diabetes can reduce CV risks.[18] It also included randomized comparisons of two targets for blood pressure control and two regimens for plasma lipid control and randomized 10,251 participants with either history of a CV event or significant CV risk. Due to an unexpected higher all-cause mortality with the intensive treatment strategy (1.4% vs. 1.1% per patient-year [257 vs. 203 total deaths during follow-up], a hazard ratio [HR] of 1.22 [95% CI 1.02 to 1.44], $P = 0.04$), this arm was discontinued early, after median follow-up of 3.4 years rather than the planned 5.6 years.[19] These trends for increased all-cause and CV mortality in ACCORD persisted during the 9-year follow-up period.[20]

Several predefined microvascular end points, including the main UKPDS end points, were also analyzed in ACCORD. Intensive glycemia treatment in ACCORD had no significant effect on the two prespecified composite microvascular outcomes; (i) advanced renal and eye complications, or (ii) the above two plus evidence of peripheral neuropathy. Intensive treatment did reduce the development of urinary albumin-to-creatinine ratio (UACR) ≥ 300 mg/g, loss of three lines of visual acuity, and peripheral neuropathy. However, in a subgroup of 2,856 participants evaluated with seven-field stereoscopic fundus photographs, intensive glycemia treatment significantly reduced the progression of diabetic retinopathy by three or more steps on the Early Treatment Diabetic Retinopathy Study Severity Scale or the development of diabetic retinopathy, necessitating laser photocoagulation or vitrectomy after 4 years.[21] These benefits must be weighed against the overall risks of increase in mortality, lack of any effect on CV events, increased weight gain, and higher risk of severe hypoglycemia in the intensively treated patients.

The Memory in Diabetes (MIND) substudy of ACCORD found no benefit nor adverse effect of the intensive glycemia treatment on cognitive outcomes or brain magnetic resonance imaging at the time of study and at 80 months follow-up.[22] Analysis of the ACCORD data did not identify a clear explanation for the higher mortality in the intensive treatment arm, and hypoglycemia cannot be directly attributed to adverse outcomes.[4]

Two other large trials related to intensive glycemic control, ADVANCE and VADT, showed no significant reduction in CV outcomes with intensive glycemic control. The ADVANCE study randomized 11,140 participants to a strategy of intensive glycemic control (with primary therapy being the sulfonylurea gliclazide and additional medications as needed to achieve a target A1C ≤6.5% [≤48 mmol/mol]) or to the standard therapy. The primary outcome of ADVANCE was a combination of microvascular events (nephropathy and retinopathy) and major adverse CV events (MI, stroke, and CV death). Intensive glycemic control significantly reduced the primary end points (HR 0.90 [95% CI 0.82–0.98], $P = 0.01$), although this was due to a significant reduction in the microvascular outcome (HR 0.86 [95% CI 0.77–0.97], $P = 0.01$), primarily development of UACR ≥300 mg/g, with no significant reduction in the macrovascular outcome (HR 0.94 [95% CI 0.84–1.06], $P = 0.32$).[3]

VADT randomized 1,791 U.S. military veterans with a mean age of 60.4 years, a mean duration of diabetes of 11.5 years, and 40% of patients with established CVDs and uncontrolled diabetes (median entry A1C 9.4% [79 mmol/mol]) to a strategy of intensive glycemic control (goal A1C <6.0% [<42 mmol/mol]) or standard glycemic control, with a planned A1C separation of at least 1.5%.[23]

Median A1C levels of 6.9% (52 mmol/mol) and 8.5% (69 mmol/mol) were achieved in the intensive and standard arms, respectively, within the first year of the study. Other CVD risk factors were treated aggressively and equally in both groups, with the trial achieving excellent blood pressure control, high levels of aspirin and statin usage, and a high degree of smoking cessation.[23]

The primary outcome of VADT was a composite of CVD events (MI, stroke, CV death, revascularization, hospitalization for heart failure, and amputation due to ischemia). During a median 5.6-year follow-up period, the cumulative incidence of the primary outcome was not significantly lower in the intensive therapy arm (HR 0.88 [95% CI 0.74–1.05], *P* = 0.12). There were nonstatistically significant more CV deaths in the intensive therapy arm than in the standard therapy arm (38 vs. 29, sudden deaths 11 vs. 4). No significant benefit on microvascular outcomes was also noted in the intensive therapy arm.

A meta-analysis that included a total of 27,049 participants with type 2 diabetes and 2,370 major vascular events, mainly combining the ACCORD, ADVANCE, UKPDS, and VADT trials, reported that targeting intensive glucose lowering over a 4.4-year period modestly reduced major macrovascular events and increased major hypoglycemia, while not affecting overall mortality.[23a]

POST-TRIAL FOLLOW-UP STUDIES

A 6-year posttrial follow-up study of the ADVANCE trial has shown no evidence of CV benefit or harm, but the end-stage renal disease rate was lower in the intensive treatment group.[24]

VADT subjects were subsequently observed over 10–15 years of follow-up periods using the central data bases and surveys. The difference in A1C values between the two groups (intensive therapy versus standard therapy) declined from 1.5% at the completion of the trial to 0.2%–0.3% by 3 years after the trial ended. Over a period of 15 years of follow-up (active trial period plus post-trial observation), there was no difference in the risks of major CV events or death between the intensive-therapy group and the standard-therapy group (for primary outcome, HR 0.9 [95% CI 0.78–1.06]; *P* = 0.23; for death, HR 1.02 [95% CI 0.88–1.18]).[25] ACCORD and ADVANCE follow-up studies also showed similar findings of no evidence of legacy effect or a mortality benefit with intensive glycemic control.[20,24]

It is noteworthy to pay attention to the difference in the study design, characteristics of the studied population, glycemic targets, and prespecified outcomes across these large clinical trials before coming to any conclusion. In the view of current evidence, it can be concluded that the good glycemic control reflected by a A1C goal <7% (<53 mmol/mol) is associated with important benefits, mainly from a microvascular standpoint; it may have longer-term benefits for CVD risk in patients with newly diagnosed type 2 diabetes and should be advocated in relatively young patients with no significant CVD risk and comorbid conditions. However, more stringent goals (i.e., a normal A1C <6% [42 mmol/mol]) are not currently recommended in patients with diabetes who have high CV risks, given increased risk for harm. Therefore, glycemic targets should always be individualized, taking into consideration the patient's age, risk of hypoglycemia, underlying comorbid disease burden, and prognosis.

MACROVASCULAR COMPLICATIONS

Kyaw Soe, MD

DIABETES AS A CV RISK FACTOR

In the patient with diabetes, ASCVD or CVD involving the coronary, cerebrovascular, and peripheral vessels can occur at an earlier age and with greater frequency than it does in those without diabetes and is responsible for two-thirds of the mortality in adults with the disease. Patients with diabetes have a two to three times higher risk of CVDs than those without. CV mortality among patients with diabetes is two to four times higher than in adults without diabetes.[26]

Diabetes was also associated with a significantly higher long-term mortality in both men and women after an acute MI. CVD currently contributes to about one-quarter to one-half of all deaths in individuals with 10–19 years' duration of type 1 diabetes, whereas it accounts for more than half of all-cause mortality in those with duration of diabetes greater than 20 years.[27]

Therefore, diabetes itself is regarded as an independent risk factor for macrovascular disease. In addition, other risk factors such as hypertension, dyslipidemia (decreased HDL-C, increased triglycerides, and alterations in LDL-C particle size and number), hypercoagulability, and obesity commonly coexist among patients with diabetes and metabolic syndrome. According to 2017 Centers for Disease Control and Prevention data, 16% of patients with diabetes were active smokers; 87.5% were overweight or obese (BMI ≥25 kg/m²); 40.8% were physically inactive; 73.6% were hypertensive (blood pressure ≥140/90 mmHg or used prescription medications for hypertension); and 58% were adults (≥21 years) without any self-reported CVD who were eligible for statin therapy but were not taking any statin.[12] These data indicate that aggressive management of coexisting modifiable risk factors is much needed as an integral part of diabetes management.

The pattern of obesity is also important, with central fat distribution (waist circumference >40 inches [>101.6 cm] in men and >35 inches [>88.9 cm] in women) associated with dyslipidemia, hypertension, and higher prevalence of CVD, independent of obesity. Renal failure, CV autonomic neuropathy, UACR between 30–299 mg/g, blindness, and foot ulcers and amputations are additional markers of high CV risk.

SCREENING FOR CVD

Silent MI is very common among patients with diabetes, accounting for up to one-third of the all events resulting in higher risk of mortality.[28] Despite individuals with diabetes having exceedingly high CVD risks compared with individuals without diabetes, routine screening of CVD in asymptomatic patients with diabetes, using investigations such as echo or stress tests, remains controversial.[29,30] The DIAD study showed that indiscriminate screening for silent CAD is not likely to improve clinical outcomes.[31] Therefore, routine screening of CVD among asymptomatic patients is not recommended as there is no additional benefit if patients have already been on intensive medical therapy for CVD prevention.

Screening for CAD should include a careful history, physical examination, and resting electrocardiogram (ECG). Additional diagnostic testing for CAD should be considered in patients with either typical or atypical cardiac symptoms or an abnormal resting ECG. Exercise ECG testing with or without echocardiography may be used as the initial test. A pharmacologic stress test or nuclear stress imaging can be used for those who cannot exercise or those with underlying ECG abnormalities such as left bundle branch block or ST-T abnormalities. In patients with diabetes who have very high pretest probability of an abnormal test, a cardiac catheterization may be appropriate.

The coronary artery calcium score (CACS), a quantitative assessment of the calcium deposit within the coronary arteries (as a marker of atherosclerosis), is a promising screening test. However, currently there are no randomized prospective trials that showed improvement during clinical outcomes by using CACS screening. The American Heart Association (AHA) and American Diabetes Association's joint statement states that CACS is reasonable for CV risk assessment in asymptomatic adults with diabetes ≥40 years of age,[32] although probably this becomes most valuable when trying to decide on statin therapy in patients with intermediate risk.

CV RISK ASSESSMENT IN PATIENTS WITH DIABETES

The American College of Cardiology/American Heart Association ASCVD risk calculator (Risk Estimator Plus) and Framingham risk calculator are generally useful tools to estimate 10-year ASCVD risk (http://tools.acc.org/ASCVD-Risk-Estimator-Plus). These calculators have diabetes as a CVD equivalent, but there is no further risk stratification among patients with diabetes. Therefore, it is important to note that not all patients with diabetes have the same CVD risk; additional risk enhancers such as glycemic control, the duration of diabetes, and the presence of diabetes-related complications, such as albuminuria, retinopathy, and peripheral arterial disease (Ankle-Brachial Index <0.9), should be taken into consideration. For prevention and management of both ASCVD and heart failure, CV risk factors should be systematically assessed at least annually in all patients with diabetes. These risk factors include obesity/overweight, hypertension, dyslipidemia, smoking, family history of premature coronary disease, chronic kidney disease, and the presence of albuminuria.

MODIFICATION OF VASCULAR RISK FACTORS

Lifestyle Modification

Lifestyle modifications, including weight reduction and regular exercise for overweight or obese patients with type 2 diabetes, are the most cost effective and safest modes of therapy and should be the cornerstone of all diabetes treatment regimens. In the Look-AHEAD Trial, which compared the effect of an intensive lifestyle intervention with a control regimen of diabetes support and education among overweight or obese patients with type 2 diabetes, the intensive lifestyle intervention group showed more weight loss (mean weight loss of 4.7% at 8 years) and maintenance of weight loss throughout the study. Approximately 50% of intensive lifestyle intervention participants lost and maintained ≥5% of their initial body weight at 8 years; 27% lost and maintained ≥10%. Those who lost weight in the intensive lifestyle intervention group were noted to require fewer medications less medication for blood pressure, cholesterol, and blood glucose control.[33]

However, intensive lifestyle intervention failed to reduce the CV outcome despite achieving greater weight loss, greater reductions in A1C, and greater initial improvements in fitness and all CV risk factors, except for LDL-C levels.[34]

Pharmacological Management of Associated Risk Factors

Since all patients with type 2 diabetes are at high ASCVD risk, all modifiable risk factors such as hypertension and hyperlipidemia should be treated aggressively. The STENO-2 Diabetes trial proved that aggressively controlling the multiple CVD risk factors simultaneously lowered both macrovascular and microvascular complications; a 53% reduction in death and MI at median followed-up at 7.8 years.[35] The CV benefit of multifactorial intervention was sustained even after the end of the active intervention period, when measured at a mean of 13.3 years (7.8 years of active intervention and an additional 5.5 years of follow-up).[36]

Antiplatelet Therapy

The 2020 American Diabetes Association recommendations for antiplatelet therapy are as follows:

- Aspirin therapy (75–162 mg/day) can be used as a secondary CVD prevention in patients with diabetes and a history of ASCVD.
- Aspirin therapy (75–162 mg/day) can be considered as a primary CVD prevention in patients who are at increased CV risk after a discussion with the patient regarding the benefit of CV prevention and the risk of bleeding.
- For patient with established ASCVD and documented aspirin allergy, clopidogrel (75 mg/day) should be used.
- Dural antiplatelet therapy (low-dose aspirin and P2Y12 inhibitor) can be used after acute coronary syndrome (ACS).
- Aspirin is not recommended for those at low ASCVD risk (e.g., men and women age <50 years with diabetes but no other ASCVK risk factors) as the risk of bleeding is likely to outweigh the benefit of the drug.[37]

Aspirin (65–162 mg/day) has a clear indication as secondary CVD prevention in high-risk patients with diabetes and a previous history of MI or stroke, but the role of aspirin in primary CV prevention among patients with diabetes without any ASCVD remains controversial due to an increased risk of bleeding.[38]

Most recently, the ASCEND (A Study of Cardiovascular Events iN Diabetes) trial showed that use of aspirin has some benefit in primary CV prevention but increased the risk of a major bleed.[39] ASCEND randomized 15,480 patients with diabetes but no evident CVD to either aspirin 100 mg daily or a placebo. During a mean follow-up of 7.4 years, there was a significant 12% reduction (8.5% vs. 9.6%; $P = 0.01$) in the primary efficacy end point (vascular death, MI, or stroke or transient ischemic attack) but an increase in major bleeding (mostly gastrointestinal bleeding and other extracranial bleeding) in the aspirin group (4.1% vs. 3.2%; $P = 0.003$). There were no significant differences by sex, weight, or duration of diabetes or other baseline factors, including the ASCVD risk score. In addition, there was no overall benefit of prophylactic aspirin use in patients with diabetes when receiving contemporary ASCVD preventive treatments, such as evidence-based antihypertension and cholesterol-lowering therapies.

Two other large, randomized trials of use of aspirin for primary prevention in patients without diabetes (ARRIVE trial)[40] and in the elderly (ASPREE trial),[41] which included only 11% of patients with diabetes, found no benefit of aspirin on the primary efficacy end point and an increased risk of bleeding.

According to a 2010 Position Statement of the American Diabetes Association, AHA, and American College of Cardiology Foundation (ACCF) on joint recommendations for primary prevention, low-dose (75–162 mg/day) aspirin use for primary prevention is reasonable for patients with diabetes with no previous history of vascular disease who are at increased CVD risk (10-year risk of CVD events >10%) and who are not at increased risk for bleeding. This generally includes most men >50 years and women >60 years who also have one or more of the major risk factors such as smoking, hypertension, dyslipidemia, family history of premature CVD, and albuminuria. However, aspirin is no longer recommended for those at low CVD risk (<50 years of age with diabetes and no major CVD risk factors; 10-year CVD risk <5%) as the minimal benefit is likely to be outweighed by the risks of significant bleeding.[42]

Aspirin dosing. Average daily dosages used in most clinical trials involving patients with diabetes ranged from 50 mg to 650 mg but were mostly in the range of 100–325 mg/day.[43] In the U.S., the most common low-dose aspirin tablet is 81 mg. The benefit of ASCVD risk reduction by low-dose aspirin is equivalent to that for high-dose aspirin but with a lower risk of bleeding.[44] Since there is little evidence to support any specific dose, it is safer to use the lowest possible dose, which may help to reduce side effects.

Other antiplatelet agents. For patients with ASCVD and a documented aspirin allergy, a P2Y12 inhibitor, such as clopidogrel (75 mg/day), should be used. Dual antiplatelet therapy (with low-dose aspirin and a P2Y12 inhibitor) is reasonable for ≥1 year after an ACS and may have benefits beyond this period. Evidence supports the use of either ticagrelor or clopidogrel if no percutaneous coronary intervention was performed and clopidogrel, ticagrelor, or prasugrel if a percutaneous coronary intervention was performed.[45] In patients with diabetes and prior MI (1–3 years before), adding ticagrelor to aspirin significantly reduces the risk of recurrent ischemic events, including CV death.[46]

Management of Hypertension and Blood Pressure Targets

Hypertension, defined as a sustained blood pressure ≥140/90 mmHg, is very common among patients with diabetes and is also a leading cause of mortality and morbidity related to diabetes. Treatment of hypertension in individuals with diabetes reduces the development and progression of CAD, stroke, and nephropathy.

The American Diabetes Association recommends that blood pressure should be measured at every routine clinical care visit, and patients with a blood pressure ≥140/90 mmHg should have a diagnosis of hypertension confirmed using multiple readings, including measurements on separate days. All hypertensive patients with diabetes should be educated to self-monitor blood pressure with a home blood pressure monitoring machine regularly to identify white-coat hypertension and to improve medication adherence. The blood pressure target for most people with diabetes and hypertension should be <140 mmHg systolic and <90 mmHg diastolic.[37] Lower blood pressure targets, such as <130/80 mmHg, may be appropriate for individuals at high risk of CVD if the blood pressure targets can be achieved without an undue treatment burden.[47]

Randomized controlled trials of intensive versus standard blood pressure control. Several major randomized clinical trials such as UKPDS,[48] Hypertension Optimal Treatment (HOT),[49] or Heart Outcomes Prevention Evaluation (HOPE)[50] demonstrated that improving blood pressure control was particularly beneficial in patients with diabetes in reducing major CV events.

The UKPDS explored the benefits of blood pressure control (blood pressure target <150/85mmHg vs. <180/105 mmHg) on microvascular and macrovascular end points in subjects with type 2 diabetes. It proved that a 10/5 mmHg systolic/diastolic blood pressure reduction lowered the incidence of microvascular complications by 37%, and major CV events, including death, by 32%. In this study, the greatest benefits were observed in subjects achieving both glycemic and hypertension control.[48]

Intensification of antihypertensive therapy to target blood pressures lower than <140/90 mmHg may be beneficial for selected patients with diabetes. The Hypertension Optimal Treatment (HOT) trial studied 18,000 patients with hypertension, among which 1,500 had diabetes. There was no overall CV benefit but a 51% reduction in major CV events in patients with diabetes that achieved a diastolic blood pressure ≤80 mmHg, compared with target group subjects ≤90 mmHg (p for trend = 0.005) (Table 5.2).[49]

The ACCORD blood pressure trial examined the CV benefit of intensive blood pressure control (systolic blood pressure [SBP] <120mmHg) versus standard blood pressure control (SBP <140mmHg) among people with type 2 diabetes with high CVD risk. The blood pressure achieved was 119/64 mmHg in the intensive group with an average of 3.4 medications per participant compared with 133/70 mmHg in the standard group with 2.1 medications. The ACCORD blood pressure showed no significant reduction in total atherosclerotic CV events (nonfatal MI, nonfatal stroke, and CV death) (in the intensive group, HR 0.88 [95% CI 0.73–1.06]; $P = 0.20$) but statistically significant reduction in stroke risk.[51] Therefore, it can be concluded that for patients with diabetes with high CV risk, aggressive control of SBP (<120 mmHg) does not confer any CV benefit compared with less aggressive SBP control (<140 mmHg), but it is reasonable to get aggressive blood pressure control (SBP <120 mmHg) for some patients who have no significant treatment burden and side effects of medications and have a higher risk of stroke (Table 5.2).

The ADVANCE blood pressure trial reported that treatment with an angiotensin converting enzyme inhibitor (Perindopril) and a thiazide-type diuretic (Indapamide) reduced the rate of death but not the composite macrovascular outcome.[3] However, the ADVANCE trial had no specified blood pressure targets, and the achieved mean SBP in the intensive group of ADVANCE (135 mmHg) was higher than the achieved mean SBP in the ACCORD blood pressure standard therapy group (<120 mmHg) (Table 5.2).

A post hoc analysis of blood pressure control in 6,400 patients with diabetes and CAD enrolled in the International Verapamil-Trandolapril (INVEST) trial demonstrated that "tight control" (SBP <130 mmHg) was not associated with improved CVD outcomes compared with "usual care" (SBP 130–140 mmHg).[52]

The SPRINT trial, which studied patients without diabetes with high CV risk, showed intensive SBP control (target SBP <120 mmHg) and lowered risk of primary composite outcomes (MI, ACS, stroke, heart failure, and CV death) by 25%.

Table 5.2–Randomized Controlled Trials of Intensive Versus Standard Hypertension Treatment Strategies

Clinical trial	Studied population	Intensive Rx	Standard Rx	Outcomes
ACCORD BP[51]	4,733 participants with type 2 diabetes age 40–79 years with prior evidence of CVD or multiple CV risk factors	SBP target: <120 mmHg Achieved (mean) SBP/DBP: 119.3/64.4 mmHg	SBP target: 130–140 mmHg Achieved (mean) SBP/DBP: 13.5/70.5 mmHg	No benefit in primary end point: composite of nonfatal MI, nonfatal stroke, and CVD death ■ Stroke risk reduced 41% with intensive control, not sustained through follow-up beyond the period of active treatment ■ Adverse events more common in intensive group, particularly elevated serum creatinine and electrolyte abnormalities
ADVANCE BP[3]	11,140 participants with type 2 diabetes age ≥55 years with prior evidence of CVD or multiple CV risk factors	Intervention: a single-pill, fixed-dose combination of perindopril and indapamide Achieved (mean) SBP/DBP: 136/73 mmHg	Control: placebo Achieved (mean) SBP/DBP: 141.6/75.2 mmHg	Intervention reduced risk of primary composite end point of major macrovascular and microvascular events (9%), death from any cause (14%), and death from CVD (18%) ■ 6-year observational follow-up found reduction in risk of death in intervention group attenuated but still significant
HOT[49]	18,790 participants, including 1,501 with diabetes	DBP target: ≤80 mmHg	DBP target: ≤90 mmHg	In the overall trial, there was no CV benefit with more intensive targets ■ In the subpopulation with diabetes, an intensive DBP target was associated with a significantly reduced risk (51%) of CVD event
SPRINT[53]	9,361 participants without diabetes	SBP target: <120 mmHg Achieved (mean): 121.4 mmHg	SBP target: <140 mmHg Achieved (mean): 136.2 mmHg	Intensive SBP target lowered risk of the primary composite outcome 25% (MI, ACS, stroke, heart failure, and death due to CVD) ■ Intensive target reduced risk of death 27% ■ Intensive therapy increased risks of electrolyte abnormalities and AKI

ACS, acute coronary syndrome; AKI, Acute Kidney Injury; CV, cardiovascular; CVD, cardiovascular disease; DBP, diastolic blood pressure; MI, myocardial infarction; Rx, prescription; SPB, systolic blood pressure.

Source: American Diabetes Association.[37]

The Intensive treatment arm had a higher incidence of electrolyte abnormalities and acute renal injury[53] (Table 5.2).

From the above-mentioned evidence, it can be concluded that among patients with diabetes and high CV risk, lowering SBP from the low 130s to <120 mmHg does not reduce coronary events or death further and that most of the CV benefit from lowering blood pressure is achieved by targeting a goal of SBP <140 mmHg.

According to the 2020 American Diabetes Association guideline for CVD and risk management, it is recommended to set the blood pressure target according to the individual CV risk profile and potential side effects of antihypertensive medications. A blood pressure target of <130/80 mmHg is reasonable for patients with diabetes and hypertension at higher CV risk (established ASCVD or 10-years ASCVD risk ≥15%) if the target blood pressure can be achieved safely. A less aggressive blood pressure target of <140/90 mmHg should be used for individuals with diabetes and hypertension who are at relatively lower risk of CV risk (i.e., 10-years ASCVD risk <15%).[37]

This approach is also consistent with the guideline from the American College of Cardiology/American Heart Association, which recommended a blood pressure target <130/80 mmHg for all patients, with or without diabetes.[54] Potential side effects of antihypertensive therapy, such as orthostatic hypotension, syncope, acute renal failure, and electrolyte abnormalities, should be taken into consideration, especially among frail elderly patients who have underlying multiple comorbid conditions and who are at high risk of adverse effects of polypharmacy.

Hypertension control for type 1 diabetes. There is no randomized trial regarding clinical outcome in type 1 diabetes with hypertension. The effects of antihypertension management can only be extrapolated from trials in type 2 diabetes like ACCORD blood pressure and nondiabetes like SPRINT.

Hypertension during pregnancy. There is limited high-quality evidence regarding antihypertensive therapy in pregnant women with diabetes. In CHIPS (Control of Hypertension in Pregnancy Study), which studied women with chronic hypertension, the targeting diastolic blood pressure of 85 mmHg during pregnancy was associated with a reduced risk of accelerated maternal hypertension but no difference in the risk of pregnancy loss and maternal complication and no demonstrable adverse outcome for infants compared with a higher diastolic blood pressure (target diastolic blood pressure = 100 mmHg). However, this study consisted of a small number of gestational diabetes (6.3% in tight control arm and 6.4% in less tight control arm). Women with gestational diabetes also showed similar outcomes compared with patients without diabetes.

In CHIPS, the mean SBP, 133.1 ± 0.5 mmHg, and the mean diastolic blood pressure 85.3 ± 0.3 mmHg, blood pressure were achieved in the more intensively treated group.[55] The American Diabetes Association 2020 edition of *Standards of Medical Care in Diabetes* supports controlling blood pressure to these levels, with a target of ≤135/85 mmHg.[37] A similar approach is supported by the International Society for the Study of Hypertension in Pregnancy, which specifically recommends use of antihypertensive therapy to maintain SBP between 110 mmHg and 140 mmHg and diastolic blood pressure between 80 mmHg and 85 mmHg.[56]

During pregnancy, antihypertensive treatment with ACE inhibitors (ACEi), angiotensin receptor blockers (ARBs), and spironolactone are contraindicated due to fetal complication. Antihypertensive medications such as methyldopa, labetalol, and long-acting nifedipine and hydralazine have been used and proven to be effective and safe for pregnant women.[57]

Lifestyle management for hypertension. Lifestyle management is an important part of hypertension management because it not only lowers blood pressure, but it also enhances the effectiveness of antihypertensive medications and promotes the other aspects of metabolic and vascular health. All patients with diabetes and hypertension should be counseled for lifestyle modification as a mandatory part of hypertension management. Although there are no well-controlled studies of diet and exercise in the treatment of hypertension in individuals with diabetes, the Dietary Approaches to Stop Hypertension (DASH) study in individuals without diabetes has shown antihypertensive effects of dietary modification (diet rich in fruit, vegetable and low fat diet) resulted in similar antihypertensive effect compared to pharmacological monotherapy[58]

Lifestyle therapy consists of body weight reduction through caloric restriction, restricting sodium intake (<2,300 mg/day), increasing consumption of fruits and vegetables (8–10 servings per day) and low-fat dairy products (two to three servings per day), avoiding excessive alcohol consumption (no more than two servings per day in men and no more than one serving per day in women), and increasing physical activity. Therefore, in individuals with diabetes and mild hypertension (systolic blood pressure of 120–160 mmHg or diastolic blood pressure of 80–100 mmHg), a short trial of lifestyle modification may be attempted initially. Pharmacological therapy should be instituted if these interventions fail.[47]

Pharmacotherapy of hypertension. Pharmacologic therapy is recommended, along with lifestyle therapy, for patients with confirmed office-based blood pressure readings of ≥140/90 mmHg.[59] For patients with higher confirmed blood pressure readings (≥160/100 mmHg), dual drug or single-pill combination drug therapy is warranted.[59] Refer to Fig. 1.1.[47]

ACEi and ARBs, thiazide-like diuretics, and dihydropyridine calcium-channel antagonists have all been shown to reduce CV events in diabetes. The selection of appropriate antihypertensive agent depends on the clinical characteristics of the individual patient, such as age, underlying comorbid conditions, and associated diabetic complications. In particular, elderly patients with diabetes should have their blood pressure lowered gradually, because they can experience significant hypotension on initiation of therapy. Commonly, multiple drug therapy may be needed to achieve blood pressure targets. However, combinations of ACEi and ARBs or either drug class in combination with direct renin inhibitors should not be used due to a lack of additional ASCVD benefit and an increased rate of an adverse event such as hyperkalemia, syncope, and acute renal injury.[59]

ACEi or ARBs are the first-line antihypertensive treatment in patients with diabetes and persistent albuminuria (UACR ≥30 mg/g) because of their renal protective effects. However, the potential side effects of ACEi and ARB, such as acute renal injury (AKI) and hyperkalemia, should be considered and monitored. Diuretics can also be associated with AKI, and both hypokalemia or hyperkalemia, depending on the mechanism of action. Since diabetic nephropathy is already associated with an increased risk of hyperkalemia due to hyporeninemic hypoaldosteronism, ACEi and ARBs may further exacerbate hyperkalemia in such patients. Therefore, for patients treated with ACEi, ARBS, and/or diuretics, the serum creatinine/estimated glomerular filtration rate (eGFR) and serum potassium levels should be monitored. ARBs may be substituted for ACEi if unacceptable side effects occur; these agents tend to cause less hyperkalemia and cough. While clear benefit exists for ACEi or ARB therapy among patients with diabetic kidney disease and hypertension, the benefits for patients with ASCVD in the absence of these conditions are less clear, especially when LDL-C is already at target.[60,61] ACEi and ARBs have not been found to afford superior cardio-protection when compared with other antihypertensive agents.[62]

Based on multiple studies, a **thiazide diuretic** such as indapamide (1.5 mg/day) or chlorthalidone (25 mg/day) should be used among the first two drugs for managing hypertension in patients with diabetes if the glomerular filtration rate (GFR) is >30 ml/min/1.73m.[2] The benefit of thiazide diuretics may be particularly relevant in African American patients. In patients with GFR <30 ml/min or evidence of volume overload, a more intensive diuresis by the addition of loop diuretics to reduce intravascular volume can be effective. Caution is necessary when initiating ACEi therapy in patients on diuretics because hypotension may occur.[63]

Patients with diabetes and prior MI, angina, or congestive heart failure (HFrEF) should be treated with a β-**blocker,** since these agents have been shown to reduce the risk of death in these specific populations.[59,64,65] β-Blockers should be used cautiously in patients at high risk of hypoglycemia as they can reduce or mask hypoglycemia symptoms by interfering with adrenergic responses. At risk patients should be counseled about identifying and treating asymptomatic hypoglycemia.

Calcium channel blockers (CCBs) are among the most effective blood pressure–lowering agents. As monotherapy in head-to-head studies, they have generally had more modest effects on CVD risk than the other classes listed above. However, the dihydropyridine CCBs clearly has a place in combination with ACEi and ARBs in treating hypertension and reducing CVD risk in diabetes. The Avoiding Cardiovascular Events through Combination Therapy in Patients Living with Systolic Hypertension (ACCOMPLISH) trial showed a decrease in morbidity and mortality in those receiving benazapril and amlodipine versus benazapril and hydrochlorothiazide, which suggests an additional benefit with combinations of ACEi and CCBs.[66]

Other antihypertensive agents such as a central sympatholytic agent (i.e., clonidine, alpha-methyldopa) may worsen orthostatic hypotension and sexual dysfunction, while β-blockers used as monotherapy have been associated with a higher risk of masking the hypoglycemia symptoms and the exacerbation of congestive heart failure, and it should not be used as first-line therapy in managing hypertension.

Mineralocorticoid receptor antagonist therapy should be considered for hypertensive patients who are not meeting blood pressure targets on three classes of antihypertensive medications (including a diuretic).[67] Mineralocorticoid receptor antagonists also reduce albuminuria and have additional CV benefits.[68,69] Adding a mineralocorticoid receptor antagonist to a regimen including an ACEi or ARB may increase the risk for hyperkalemia, emphasizing the importance of regular monitoring for serum creatinine and potassium in these patients. Long-term outcome studies are needed to better evaluate the role of mineralocorticoid receptor antagonists in blood pressure management. Please refer to the treatment flow diagram in Fig 5.1 for treatment of hypertension in patients with diabetes.[47]

Direct renin inhibitors (i.e., aliskiren) failed to show noninferiority compared with ACEi or ARB treatment in large clinical trials evaluating CV clinical end points. The addition of aliskiren to standard therapy with renin-angiotensin blockade in patients with type 2 diabetes who are at high risk for CV has no benefit and may even have harmful effects. There is an increased risk of hyperkalemia and

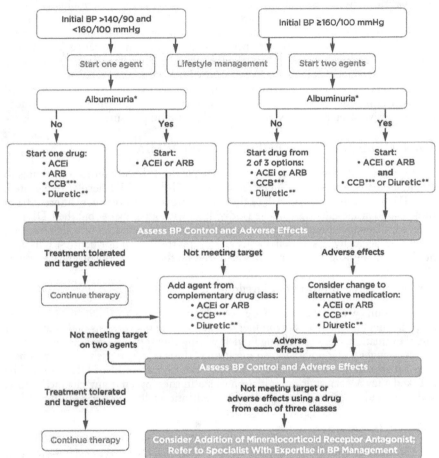

Figure 5.1 Recommendations for the treatment of confirmed hypertension in people with diabetes. BP, blood pressure. *An ACE inhibitor (ACEi) or angiotensin receptor blocker (ARB) is suggested to treat hypertension for patients with UACR 30–299 mg/g creatinine and strongly recommended for patients with UACR ≥300 mg/g creatinine. **Thiazide-like diuretic; long-acting agents shown to reduce cardiovascular events, such as chlorthalidone and indapamide, are preferred. ***Dihydropyridine calcium channel blocker (CCB). *Source*: Adapted from American Diabetes Association position statement de Boer et al, 2017.[47]

renal impairment with the use of aliskiren in addition to baseline ACEi and ARB therapy.[69,70]

Resistant hypertension is defined as blood pressure ≥140/90 mmHg despite a therapeutic strategy that includes appropriate lifestyle management plus a diuretic and two other antihypertensive drugs of different classes at adequate doses.[59] Prior to establishing a diagnosis of resistant hypertension, providers should exclude other factors such as white-coat hypertension, medication nonadherence (a common drive of poor blood pressure control), and secondary hypertension (e.g., primary hyperaldosteronism). Sleep apnea can contribute to uncontrolled hypertension and is associated with increased CV risk; hence, it should be screened and treated in all patients with diabetes who are obese and at risk for the condition. Treatment of obstructive sleep apnea has proven to reduce blood pressure.[71]

MANAGEMENT OF DIABETIC DYSLIPIDEMIA

In type 2 diabetes, an increased prevalence of lipid abnormalities contributes to accelerated atherosclerosis. Characteristically, TG-rich VLDL levels are elevated, and HDL-C levels are decreased. LDL-C levels are usually not much different from those found in age- and sex-matched individuals without diabetes, but the LDL particles may be smaller and denser, more oxidized, and glycated, all of which increase their atherogenicity. Associated obesity aggravates the lipid abnormalities. This lipid profile is the result of a combination of altered synthesis, catabolism, and clearance.

Screening and Monitoring of Dyslipidemia

For adults with diabetes who are not taking statins or any lipid-lowering therapy, a fasting lipid profile is recommended at the time of diagnosis of diabetes or at initial evaluation, prior to starting lipid-lowering therapy, and periodically thereafter. In younger patients with longer duration of disease (e.g., those with youth-onset type 1 diabetes), more frequent lipid profiles may be reasonable. LDL-C should be checked a few weeks after the initiation of statin therapy, after any change in dose, and on an individual basis to monitor for medication adherence and efficacy.[59]

Lifestyle Intervention

Lifestyle modification includes weight loss, increased physical activity, and nutritional intervention. Nutritional intervention should be individualized, and it should focus on the application of a Mediterranean diet[72] or the Dietary Approaches to Stop Hypertension (DASH) dietary pattern, reducing saturated and trans-fat intake and increasing plant stanols/sterols, n-3 fatty acids, and viscous fiber (e.g., oats, legumes, and citrus) intake.[73]

Pharmacotherapy of Hyperlipidemia

Treatment of elevated LDL-C is considered to have first priority over treatment of hypertriglyceridemia or low HDL-C. The Heart Protection Study demonstrated that in people with diabetes >40 years with total cholesterol >135 mg/dl (>3.5 mmol/l), LDL-C reductions of ~30% by taking simvastatin were associated with ~25% reduction in coronary events, independent of baseline LDL-C levels, prior vascular disease, or diabetes (type 1 or 2).[74] Similarly, in the CARDS trial, atorvastatin 10 mg daily had a significant reduction (~36%) in major CV events, including stroke, compared with a placebo among patients with type 2 diabetes.[75]

CV Benefit of Statin in Patients with Diabetes Statin has been the first-line treatment of hyperlipidemia in patients with diabetes due to its proven efficacy and excellent safety profile. Multiple clinical trials have demonstrated the beneficial effects of statin therapy on ASCVD outcomes in subjects with and without CVD.[76,77] Meta-analyses, including data from >18,000 patients with diabetes from 14 randomized trials of statin therapy (mean follow-up 4.3 years) demonstrate a 9% proportional reduction in all-cause mortality and a 13% reduction in vascular mortality for each 1 mmol/L (39 mg/dL) reduction in LDL cholesterol.[77] Hence, statin is recommended for both primary and secondary CV prevention in patients with diabetes.

For primary prevention, in addition to lifestyle modification, moderate-dose statin therapy is recommended for patients with diabetes between 40 and 75 years old without ASCVD. High-intensity statin therapy is reasonable to be used as a primary CV prevention in patients with additional ASCVD risk factors or age 50–70 years and for secondary CVD prevention for those with established ASCVD.[74] The evidence is strong for patients with diabetes age 40–75 years, an age-group well represented in statin trials showing benefit, but the strength of evidence is lower for patients age >75 years due to less representation of this age-group in CVD prevention trials.[74,79]

Indications for statin.[38] Recommendations for statin therapy and intensification with combination therapy in adults are based on patient age and ASCVD risk. Moderate- or high-intensity statin therapy is prescribed for patients with type 2 diabetes due to high CV risk when indicated and can be combined with either ezetimibe or PCSK9 (proprotein convertase subtilisin/kexin type 9) inhibitors for additional LDL-C lowering effect (see Table 5.3).

Table 5.3–High-Intensity and Moderate-Intensity Statin Therapy (Once-Daily Dosing)

High-intensity statin Rx (lower LDL-C by ≥50%)	Moderate-intensity statin Rx (lower LDL-C by 30%–49%)
Atorvastatin 40–80 mg	Atorvastatin 10–20 mg
Rosuvastatin 20–40 mg	Rosuvastatin 5–10 mg
	Simvastatin 20–40 mg
	Pravastatin 40–80 mg
	Lovastatin 40 mg
	Fluvastatin XL 80 mg
	Pitavastatin 1–4 mg

Source: American Diabetes Association.[37]

American Diabetes Association recommendations for primary prevention are as follows:[37]

■ For patients with diabetes age 40–75 years without ASCVD, use moderate-intensity statin therapy in addition to lifestyle therapy.

■ For patients with diabetes age 20–39 years with additional ASCVD risk factors, it may be reasonable to initiate statin therapy in addition to lifestyle therapy.

■ In patients with diabetes at higher risk, especially those with multiple ASCVD risk factors or age 50–70 years, it is reasonable to use high-intensity statin therapy.

■ In adults with diabetes and a 10-year ASCVD risk of 20% or higher, it may be reasonable to add ezetimibe to maximally tolerated statin therapy to reduce LDL cholesterol levels ≥50%.

American Diabetes Association recommendations for secondary prevention are as follows:

■ For patients of all ages with diabetes and ASCVD, high-intensity statin therapy should be added to lifestyle therapy.

■ For patients with diabetes and ASCVD considered very high risk using specific criteria, if LDL cholesterol is ≥70 mg/dL on a maximally tolerated statin dose, consider adding additional LDL-lowering therapy (e.g., ezetimibe or PCSK9 inhibitor). Ezetimibe may be preferred due to its lower cost.

■ For patients who do not tolerate the intended intensity, the maximally tolerated statin dose should be used.

■ In adults with diabetes age >75 years already on statin therapy, it is reasonable to continue statin treatment.

■ In adults with diabetes age >75 years, it may be reasonable to initiate statin therapy after discussion of potential benefits and risks.

■ Statin therapy is contraindicated in pregnancy.

Diabetes risk with statin use. There is a minimal risk of developing diabetes related to both the dose and potency of statins, although the benefits of therapy almost always outweigh the risk. Compared with pravastatin (the reference drug in all analyses), there is an increased risk of incident diabetes with atorvastatin (adjusted HR 1.22 [95% CI 1.15–1.29]), rosuvastatin (HR 1.18 [95% CI 1.10–1.26]), and simvastatin (HR 1.10 [95% CI 1.04–1.17]); the absolute risk for incident diabetes was ~31 and ~34 events per 1,000 person-years for atorvastatin and rosuvastatin, respectively.[80] There was no significantly increased risk with fluvastatin (HR 0.95 [95% CI 0.81–1.11]) or lovastatin (HR 0.99 [95% CI 0.86–1.14]).

A meta-analysis of 13 randomized statin trials with 91,140 participants showed an odds ratio of 1.09 for a new diagnosis of diabetes so that (on average) treatment of 255 patients with statins for 4 years resulted in one additional case of diabetes while simultaneously preventing 5.4 vascular events among those 255 patients.[81]

Younger patients (age <40 years) and/or type 1 diabetes. There is very little evidence of CV benefit of lipid treatment for primary prevention in younger patients (<40 years of age) with diabetes or those with type 1 diabetes of any age. Even though patients age <40 years either with diabetes type 1 or type 2 have a lower risk of developing CV events over a 10-year period, their lifetime ASCVD risk is higher than for patients without diabetes. In the presence of established ASCVD or additional ASCVD risk factors, similar statin therapy approaches can be used for patients with type 1 or type diabetes. According to the 2018 ACC/AHA guideline, younger adults (age 20–39 years) with diabetes that is either of long duration (≥10 years of type 2, ≥20 years of type 1), albuminuria (≥30, cg of albumin/mg creatinine) eGFR <60ml/min/1.73m^2, retinopathy, neuropathy, or ankle-brachial index (ABI <0.9), it may be reasonable to initiate statin therapy.[82]

Statins are contraindicated in pregnancy, and caution should be used when prescribing statins to any woman with childbearing potential. Statins should be stopped 1–2 months before the pregnancy is attempted, or as soon as the pregnancy is discovered.[82]

Dose and intensity of statin. The intensity of statin therapy is divided into three categories: high intensity, moderate intensity, and low intensity. High-intensity statin therapy typically lowers LDL-C levels by ~50%, moderate intensity statin therapy by 30%–49%, and low-intensity statin therapy by <30% (see Table 5.3). Low-dose statin therapy is generally not recommended in patients with diabetes due to the high ASCVD risk from diabetes but is sometimes the only dose of statin that a patient can tolerate due to side effects such as myalgia; for such patients, a less potent statin can be used.

HYPERTRIGLYCERIDEMIA

Low levels of HDL-C, together with elevated triglyceride levels, are the most prevalent pattern of lipid abnormality in individuals with type 2 diabetes. The strength of the evidence of CV benefit for treating these lipid fraction (low HDL-C and high triglyceride) is substantially less robust than that for lowering LDL-C by statin therapy.[83]

In the FIELD study, which consisted of 9,795 patients with type 2 diabetes (age 50–75 years) who were not taking statin at the initiation of study, showed that use of fenofibrate did not reduce overall CV outcome.[78]

Mild hypertriglyceridemia (fasting or nonfasting triglyceride 175–499 mg/dL), more commonly seen in patients with diabetes, and in many instances mild hypertriglyceridemia, can be satisfactorily managed by lifestyle and dietary modification such as weight loss, abstinence from alcohol, low-fat diet, and better glycemic control. Nutrition recommendations for these patients include a moderate increase in monounsaturated fat intake, with <10% of calories from saturated and polyunsaturated fats, and a more moderate intake of carbohydrate. Secondary risk factors for hypertriglyceridemia such as diabetes, chronic liver or kidney disease and/or nephrotic syndrome, hypothyroidism, and medications that raise triglycerides should also be identified and addressed. Severe hypertriglyceridemia (fasting triglycerides ≥500 mg/dL and especially ≥1,000 mg/dL) may be a risk factor for pancreatitis. In such patients with severe hypertriglyceridemia, fibric acid derivatives and/or fish oil [2–4 g/daily] can be used to reduce the risk of pancreatitis.

According to the REDUCE-IT trial, for patients with ASCVD or additional CV risk factors, on a statin with controlled LDL-C but elevated triglycerides (135–499 mg/dL), the addition of icosapent ethyl can be considered to reduce CV risk.[84]

Fish Oil and Statin Combination

The REDUCED-IT trial studied 8,179 patients who were ≥45 years of age with established CVD or were ≥50 years of age, had diabetes together with at least one additional CV risk factor, had been taking statin, and had a fasting triglyceride level of 135–499 mg/dL and an LDL-C level of 41–100 mg/d. They were followed for a median of 4.9 years. More than 50% of the studied population had type 2 diabetes (~58%). Compared with a placebo, addition of 2 g of icosapent ethyl twice daily to statin resulted in lower CV outcome (17.2% in subjects in the treatment group vs. 22.0% in subjects in the placebo group). Therefore, for patients with ASCVD or other cardiac risk factors on statin with controlled LDL-C (<100 mg/dL) but high triglyceride (135–499mg/dL), icosapent ethyl can be added to reduce CV risk.[84]

Earlier trials like ASCEND and ORIGIN failed to show CV benefits. The ASCEND study,[85] which studied 1,548 patients with diabetes without evidence of ASCVD, and the ORIGIN trial,[86] which studied high CV risk patients with diabetes or prediabetes, did not reduce CV outcome. The mechanism of icosapent ethyl for reduction of a CV event is still unknown, and the underlying reason the REDUCE-IT trial showed different outcomes from earlier trials is still unelucidated. Some experts attributed the difference in study design, studied population, underlying ASCVD risks, formula, and dosage of fish oil to the discrepancy in the results among these trials.

Combination Lipid-Lowering Therapy

The 2018 AHA/American College of Cardiology guideline on the management of blood cholesterol recommends considering the addition of nonstatin therapy for very high-risk ASCVD patients when LDL-C ≥ 70 mg/dL (≥1.8 mmol/L). Very high-risk ASCVD patients include patients with a history of multiple major ASCVD events or one major ASCVD event and multiple high-risk conditions. In these patients, ezetimibe can be added to maximally tolerated statin therapy when the LDL-C level remains ≥70 mg/dL (≥1.8 mmol/L). If the LDL-C level remains ≥70 mg/dL (≥1.8 mmol/L) on maximally tolerated statin and ezetimibe therapy, adding a PCSK9 inhibitor is reasonable, although long-term safety (>3 years) is uncertain.[82]

Statin and Ezetimibe Combination

The IMProved Reduction of Outcomes: Vytorin Efficacy International Trial (IMPROVE-IT) was a randomized controlled trial in 18,144 patients comparing the addition of 10 mg of ezetimibe to 40 mg of simvastatin therapy versus simvastatin alone; subjects were ≥50 years old with a history of a recent ACS.[87] Combination treatment with ezetimibe and simvastatin resulted in a 2% absolute reduction in major adverse CV events (HR 0.936 [95% CI 0.89–0.99]; $P = 0.016$). End-of-trial mean LDL-C was 70 mg/dL (≥1.8 mmol/L) in the statin group and 54 mg/dL (1.39 mmol/L) in the combination group. In this trial, absolute CV risk reduction was more pronounced in patients with diabetes (27% of studied population), with the combination therapy reducing major adverse CV events by 5% (40% vs. 45% cumulative incidence at 7 years), with a relative risk reduction of 14% (HR 0.86 [95% CI 0.78–0.94]) over monotherapy with simvastatin.[88]

Statin and PCSK9 Inhibitor Combination

PSCK 9 inhibitors (evolocumab and alirocumab) represent a new class of cholesterol-lowering medication. They are the monoclonal antibodies that inhibit PCSK9 and can lower LCL-C ~60%. PCSK9 binds to LDL receptors, causing their degradation; inhibiting PCSK9 with a monoclonal inhibitor means more LDL receptors are recycled to the surface of hepatocytes, resulting in increased clearance of LDL-C from the circulation.[89] PCSK9 inhibitors are approved as adjunctive therapy for patients with ASCVD or familial hypercholesterolemia who are receiving maximally tolerated statin therapy but require additional lowering of LDL-C. The ODDYSSEY OUTCOMES trial with alirocumab[90] and the FOURIER trial with evolocumab[91] are placebo-controlled trials evaluating the addition of PCSK9 inhibitors to maximally tolerated doses of statin therapy in participants at high risk for ASCVD or previous history of ACS. They demonstrated a significant reduction in LDL-C, ranging from 36% to 59%.

In the FOURIER trial, evolocumab significantly reduced the risk of the primary composite end point of CV death, MI, stroke, hospitalization for unstable angina, or coronary revascularization compared with the placebo (11.3% vs. 9.8%), representing a 15% relative risk reduction ($P < 0.001$) during the median follow-up of 2.2 years; the combined end point of CV death, MI, or stroke was reduced by 20%, from 7.4% to 5.9% ($P < 0.001$).[91] Importantly, similar benefits were seen in a prespecified subgroup of patients with diabetes, which represented 40% of the studied subjects. Evolocumab in this trial did not increase the risk of new-onset diabetes or result in worsening of glycemic control in subjects with diabetes.[92]

In the ODDYSSEY OUTCOMES trial (N = 18,924; ~29% with diabetes) during the median follow-up of 2.8 years, a composite primary end point event (composite of death from coronary heart disease, nonfatal MI, fatal or nonfatal ischemic stroke, or unstable angina requiring hospitalization) occurred in 903 patients (9.5%) in the alirocumab group and in 1,052 patients (11.1%) in the placebo group.[90] Alirocumab reduced total nonfatal CV events (HR 0.87 [95% CI 0.82–0.93]) and death (HR 0.83 [95% CI 0.71–0.97]). There were 190 fewer first and 385 fewer total nonfatal CV events or deaths observed with alirocumab compared with the placebo.[93]

Statin and Fibrate Combination

Adding a fibrate to statin therapy failed to reduce CV outcomes (fatal CV events, nonfatal MI, or nonfatal stroke) in the ACCORD-Lipid study, when compared with simvastatin alone, among patients with type 2 diabetes who were at high risk for CVD. However, subgroup analyses showed some differences in treatment effects; for example, men tended to benefit more than women from the combination, and so did participants with both elevated triglycerides (≥204 mg/dl [2.3 mmol/L]) and low a HDL-C level (≤34 mg/dl [0.88 mmol/L]).[94] Combining fibrates with statins can increase the risk for abnormal transaminase levels, myositis, and rhabdomyolysis. The risk of rhabdomyolysis is more common when combining a statin with gemfibrozil than fenofibrate, especially in patients with underlying renal insufficiency.[95]

Statin and Niacin Combination

Combination therapy with a statin and niacin is not recommended due to the lack of efficacy on major ASCVD outcomes and increased side effects. The AIM-HIGH Clinical Trial randomized >3,000 patients with established ASCVD (about one-third of subjects have diabetes), LDL-C levels (<180 mg/dL [<4.7 mmol/L]), low HDL-C levels (men <40 mg/dL [<1.0 mmol/L] and women <50 mg/dL [<1.3 mmol/L]), and elevated triglyceride levels of 150–400 mg/dL (1.7–4.5 mmol/L) to statin therapy plus extended-release niacin (1,500–2,000 mg per day) or placebo. This trial was stopped prematurely due to lack of efficacy on primary ASCVD outcomes (first event of the composite of death from CHD, nonfatal MI, ischemic stroke, hospitalization for an ACS, or symptom-driven coronary or cerebral revascularization) and a possible increase in the risk of stroke.[96] In addition, 81% of study subjects were followed up for an additional mean 1.1 year after the trial was halted; at that time, 95% of subjects remained on statin, but only 4% were still taking extended-released niacin. At a mean total follow-up of 4.1 years, there were 343 primary CV end points in the niacin arm and 305 CV end points in placebo participants (HR 1.11 [95% CI 0.96–1.30]). Ischemic stroke was also not significantly different after extended follow-up in the two groups (2.2% vs 1.5%, $P = 0.13$).[97]

The Heart Protection Study 2–Treatment of HDL to Reduce the Incidence of Vascular Events (HPS2-THRIVE) trial, which studied 25,673 patients with CVD (32% with diabetes) for a median follow-up of 3.9 years, also failed to show a benefit in adding 2 g of extended-release niacin and 40 mg of laropiprant (an antagonist of the prostaglandin D2 receptor DP1 that has been shown to improve adherence to niacin therapy) to background statin therapy. Niacin–laropiprant was associated with an increased incidence of new-onset diabetes (absolute excess, 1.3%; $P < 0.001$) and worsening hyperglycemia among those with diabetes. In addition, there was an increase in adverse effects of the gastrointestinal system, musculoskeletal system, skin, and, unexpectedly, infection and bleeding.[98]

SMOKING CESSATION

It is recommended by the American Diabetes Association to advise all patients with diabetes not to use cigarettes and other tobacco products or Electronic Nicotine Delivery Systems (ENDS).[99]

Cigarette smoking remains a strong and independent risk factor for ASCVD and premature death,[100] which is even higher among individuals with diabetes.[101] Not only the active smoker but also patients with diabetes who are exposed to second-hand smoke have a high risk of CVD, premature death, microvascular complications, and worse glycemic control when compared with nonsmokers.[102] Smoking is also associated with the development/ the mechanism of diabetes, but the mechanism remains unclear.[103]

Smoking cessation, even among older adults, is beneficial in reducing excess CV risk.[104] Quitting tobacco 15 years or longer reduces the risk of heart failure and death to the risk level of people who never smoked.[105] Tobacco dependence is a chronic disease that requires highly skilled chronic disease management. Ongoing efforts should be made by the practitioner to assist the patient in discontinuing cigarette smoking, including enrollment in formal smoking cessation programs, behavioral modification, and use of nicotine patches. Some individuals may benefit from a trial of bupropion HCl or varenicline to relieve some withdrawal symptoms.

ENDS, often called e-cigarettes, are a new class of tobacco product that emits aerosol containing fine and ultrafine particulates, nicotine, and toxic gases that may increase the risk of CV and pulmonary disease.[106] There is increased public popularity of e-cigarettes due to perceptions that e-cigarettes are less harmful than regular cigarette smoking.[107,108]

Arrhythmias and hypertension with e-cigarette use have also been reported.[109] The evidence on the use of ENDS as a smoking-cessation tool in adults (including pregnant women) and adolescents is insufficient[110] or limited.[111] There are emerging evidences of side effects such as pulmonary immune homeostasis and antimicrobial immunity and concern for the long-term safety of ENDS.[112]

GLUCOSE-LOWERING THERAPIES AND CV OUTCOMES

Newer classes of antihyperglycemic agents, such as sodium–glucose cotransporter 2 (SGLT-2) inhibitors (e.g., empagliflozin) and glucagon-like peptide 1 (GLP-1) agonists (e.g., liraglutide), were introduced within the last decade and have demonstrated CV benefits and mortality reduction in high CV risk patients with diabetes. The American Diabetes Association/European Association for the Study of Diabetes guidelines currently recommend considering these two classes of medications in patients with type 2 diabetes and established ASCVD, heart failure, or chronic kidney disease who need intensification of therapy beyond metformin and lifestyle management, after considering drug-specific risk and individual patient factors.[59,59a]

GLP-1 Receptor Agonist Trials

In the LEADER trial, a randomized controlled trial of >9,000 participants with ~4-year follow-up, adding **liraglutide** to standard care improved survival and reduced CV outcomes.[113] All-cause mortality was lower in the liraglutide group (8.2%) than in the placebo group (9.6%) (HR 0.85 [95% CI 0.74–0.97]; $P=0.02$). The rate of composite of CV events (CV death, nonfatal MI, or nonfatal stroke) was also lower in the liraglutide group (13%) than in the placebo group (15%) (HR 0.87 [95% CI 0.78–0.97]; $P < 0.001$ for noninferiority; $P = 0.01$ for superiority). Deaths from CV causes were significantly reduced in the liraglutide group (4.7%) compared with the placebo group (6.0%) (HR 0.78 [95% CI 0.66–0.93]; $P = 0.007$).

On the other hand, the CV outcome trial with **lixisenatide,** a short-acting and less potent GLP-1 receptor agonist (GLP-1RA), did not significantly change the rate of major CV events in patients with type 2 diabetes who had experienced a recent ACS.[114]

The Evaluation of Lixisenatide in Acute Coronary Syndrome (ELIXA) trial studied the once-daily GLP-1RA lixisenatide on CV outcomes in patients with type 2 diabetes who had had a recent acute coronary event. Lixisenatide showed noninferiority ($P < 0.0001$) but did not showed superiority ($P = 0.81$) compared with placebo.[114]

The Exenatide Study of Cardiovascular Event Lowering (EXSCEL) trial studied 14,752 patients with type 2 diabetes (73.1% had previous CVD) for a median follow-up of 3.2 years. It reported that major CV events were numerically lower with use of **extended-release exenatide** compared with a placebo, although this difference was not statistically significant. However, all-cause mortality was lower in the exenatide group (HR 0.86 [95% CI 0.77–0.97]).[115]

The SUSTAIN-6 trial evaluated CV and other long-term outcomes with **Semaglutide** in subjects with type 2 diabetes and was the randomized trial powered to test noninferiority of semaglutide for the purpose of initial regulatory approval. In this study, 3,297 patients with type 2 diabetes were randomized to receive once-weekly semaglutide (0.5 mg or 1.0 mg) or a placebo for 2 years. The primary outcome (the first occurrence of CV death, nonfatal MI, or nonfatal stroke) occurred in 108 patients (6.6%) in the semaglutide group vs. 146 patients (8.9%) in the placebo group (HR 0.74 [95% CI 0.58–0.95]; $P < 0.001$). In this trial, the risk reduction of the primary outcome was driven by a significant decrease in the rate of nonfatal stroke and a nonsignificant decrease in the rate of nonfatal MI, with no difference in CV death.[116]

IPIONEER 6, a noninferior phase 3 trial which studied 3,297 patients with type 2 diabetes for a median follow-up of 15.9 months, proved that once-daily **oral semaglutide** was noninferior to the placebo for the primary composite outcome of CV death, nonfatal MI, or nonfatal stroke (HR 0.79 [95% CI 0.57–1.11]; $P < 0.001$ for noninferiority).[117] It became the first available oral GLP-1RA since U.S. Food and Drug Administration approval in September 2019.[118] The long-term CV effects of oral semaglutide will be further tested in a large, longer-term outcomes trial.

The REWIND trial studied ~9,990 patients with type 2 diabetes at risk for CV events or with a history of CVD. Study participants had a mean age of 66 years and a mean duration of diabetes of ~10 years. Approximately 32% of participants had a prior history of atherosclerotic CV events at baseline. After a medial follow-up of 5.4 years, the primary composite outcome of nonfatal MI, nonfatal stroke, or death from CV causes occurred in 12.0% and 13.4% of participants in the dulaglutide and placebo treatment groups, respectively (HR 0.88 [95% CI 0.79–0.99]; $P = 0.026$). **Dulaglutide** also did not showed statistically significant reduction in the incidence of all-cause mortality, revascularization, hospital admissions for heart failure, or unstable angina compared with the placebo.[119]

SGLT2 Inhibitor Trials

The EMPA-REG Outcome trial with **empagliflozin** (an SGLT2 inhibitor), which studied >7,000 participants (99% had established ASCVD) and a median follow-up of 3 years, showed a significant reduction in the composite end point of CV mortality, nonfatal MI, or nonfatal stroke by 14% (absolute rate 10.5% in the empagliflozin group vs. 12.1% in the placebo group; HR 0.86 [95% CI 0.74–0.99]; $P = 0.04$ for superiority), as well as a reduction in CV mortality by 38% (absolute rate 3.7% in the empagliflozin group vs. 5.9% in the placebo group; HR 0.62 [95% CI 0.49–0.77]; $P < 0.001$).[120] It is noteworthy that >20% of the study participants were not on a statin, raising questions about the magnitude of the treatment benefit attributable to empagliflozin per se. A meta-analysis of 81 trials (n = 37,195 participants) reported that SGLT-2 inhibitors appeared to reduce both all-cause and CV mortality, primarily due to reduction in the risk of heart failure in patients with diabetes.[121]

The CANVAS study consisted of 10,142 patients with type 2 diabetes and high CV risk (66% of subjects had established CVD). Patients treated with **canagliflozin** had a lower risk of CV events than those who received a placebo. The rate of the primary outcome was lower with canagliflozin than with a placebo (occurring in 26.9 vs. 31.5 participants per 1,000 patient-years; HR 0.86 [95% CI 0.75–0.97]; $P < 0.001$ for noninferiority = 0.02 for superiority).[122]

The initial finding of lower-limb amputation risk with canagliflozin that was noted in the CANVAS study (6.3 vs. 3.4 participants per 1,000 patient-years; HR 1.97 [95% CI 1.41–2.75]) was not reproduced in the CREDENCE study.[123]

Canagliflozin in the CREDENCE study was also found to have significant CV benefits; lower risk of the composite of CV death, MI, or stroke (HR 0.80 [95% CI 0.67–0.95]; $P = 0.01$); of hospitalizations for heart failure (HR 0.61 [95% CI 0.47–0.80]; $P < 0.001$); and of the composite of CV death or hospitalization for heart failure (HR 0.69 [95% CI 0.57–0.83]; $P < 0.001$). This trial also showed significant renal benefit with the use of canagliflozin. The relative risk of the renal-specific composite of end-stage kidney disease, a doubling of the creatinine level, or death from renal causes was lower by 34% (HR 0.66 [95% CI 0.53–0.81]; $P < 0.001$), and the relative risk of end-stage kidney disease was lower by 32% (HR 0.68 [95% CI 0.54–0.86]; $P = 0.002$). This trial was stopped early at interim analysis, a median follow-up of 2.62 years, due to conclusive evidence of efficacy and safety.[123]

In the DECLARE-TIMI 58 trial, **dapagliflozin** did not show a lower rate of MACE (Major Adverse Cardiovascular Event) compared with a placebo (8.8% in the dapagliflozin group and 9.4% in the placebo group; HR 0.93 [95% CI 0.84–1.03]; $P = 0.17$). A lower rate of CV death or hospitalization for heart failure was noted (4.9% vs. 5.8%; HR 0.83 [95% CI 0.73–0.95]; $P = 0.005$), which reflected a lower rate of hospitalization for heart failure (HR 0.7 [95% CI 0.61–0.88]). No difference was seen in CV death between groups. It is noteworthy that 59% of participants did not have established ASCVD.[124]

DIABETES AND HEART FAILURE

According to the Framingham study, ≤50% of patients with type 2 diabetes may develop heart failure.[125] Heart failure patients with diabetes have a higher mortality and worse prognosis compared with those without diabetes.[126]

SGLT-2 inhibitors such as empagliflozin in the EMPA-REG OUTCOME trial,[120] canagliflozin in the CANVAS trial[122] and CREDENCE trial,[123] and dapagliflozin in the DECLARE-TIMI 58 trial[124] showed significant reduction in heart failure hospitalization of 35%, 33%, 39%, and 27%, respectively, compared with a placebo. Since most of the patients in these trials did not have heart failure at the baseline, DAPA-HF (a study dedicated to heart failure patients) was conducted. The DAPA-HF trial, which studied 4,744 patients with heart failure, proved that dapagliflozin reduced the risk of worsening heart failure or death from CVD causes compared with a placebo. There is no difference in adverse events (renal dysfunction, hypoglycemia, and volume depletion) between dapagliflozin and a placebo. Approximately 42% of subjects had diabetes, and the benefit of dapagliflozin on heart failure and CV death was noted to be the same between patients with diabetes and without diabetes.[127] Therefore, SGLT-2 inhibitors should be strongly considered in patients with diabetes and heart failure.

Thiazolidinediones (rosiglitazone and pioglitazone) are associated with a 2%–3% increased risk of heart failure[128] and hence should be avoided in patients with symptomatic heart failure (NY heart failure classification class III and IV). In the PROactive Study (PROspective pioglitAzone Clinical Trial In macroVascular Events), 5,238 patients with type 2 diabetes and high CV risk were studied for an average duration of 34.5 months. While the reduction of the prespecified primary outcome (death, MI, stroke, ACS, leg amputation, or coronary or leg revascularization) failed to reach statistical significance for pioglitazone, there was a significant 16% reduction in the secondary composite end point of all-cause mortality, non-fatal MI, and stroke (HR 0.84 [95% CI 0.72–0.98]; $P = 0.027$). Although mortality rates from heart failure did not differ between groups, 6% of patients in the pioglitazone group and 4% in the placebo group were admitted to the hospital with heart failure.[129] The CV effect of pioglitazone was also studied in a meta-analysis of 19 clinical trials of people with diabetes (N = 16 390). Similar to the result from the PROactive trial, pioglitazone was associated with a significantly lower risk of death, MI, or stroke (HR, 0.82 [95% CI 0.72–0.94]; $P = 0.005$). Higher incidence of serious heart failure was noted in the pioglitazone group compared with the control subjects (2.3% vs. 1.8%) (HR 1.41 [95% CI 1.14–1.76]; $P = 0.002$).[130]

Concerning **incretin-based therapies,** clinical trials regarding DPP-4 inhibitors' effect on heart failure showed mixed results. The SAVOR-TIMI 53 study showed that patients treated with saxagliptin were more likely to be hospitalized for heart failure than those given a placebo (3.5% vs. 2.8%, respectively).[131] Other multicenter, randomized, double-blind noninferiority trials—the Cardiovascular and Renal Microvascular Outcome Study With Linagliptin (CARMELINA),[132] Examination of Cardiovascular Outcomes with Alogliptin versus Standard of Care (EXAMINE),[133] and Trial Evaluating Cardiovascular Outcomes with Sitagliptin (TECOS)[134]—all did not show any association between DPP-4 inhibitor use and heart failure. GLP-1RA, lixisenatide, liraglutide, semaglutide, exenatide QW, albiglutide, or dulaglutid have a neutral effect on hospitalization due to heart failure compared with a placebo.[37] A retrospective cohort analysis of 1,499,650 patients with diabetes (79,800 subjects with a history of heart failure) showed that neither DDP-4 inhibitors nor GLP-1RAs are associated with a risk of hospitalization due to heart failure, compared with other oral antidiabetic medications. The results were consistent among analyses specified for patients with or without a history of heart failure and for patients taking DPP-4 inhibitors or GLP-1RAs.[135]

Metformin can be used in patients with diabetes with stable well-compensated heart failure as long as renal function remains within the recommended range for use (eGFR >30 mL/minute/1.73 m^2) and the risk of lactic acidosis is extremely low (~0.03 cases per 1,000 patient-years, with ~0.015 fatal cases per 1,000 patient-years).[136]

CONCLUSION

In summary, patients with diabetes continue to have an increased risk for CV events, which can be reduced with recommended primary and secondary prevention approaches, such as healthy dietary habits and increased physical activity, lipid management, blood pressure control, tobacco cessation, and antiplatelet therapy, when indicated. Currently approved SGLT2 inhibitors or GLP-1RA appear to reduce CV risk. Therefore, individuals with diabetes at CV high risk or with established

ASCVD can benefit from use of SGLT2 inhibitors and certain GLP-1RA. Patients with chronic kidney disease and heart failure can additionally benefit from treatment with SGLT2 inhibitors.

REFERENCES

1. UK Prospective Diabetes Study (UKPDS) Group. Intensive blood-glucose control with sulphonylureas or insulin compared with conventional treatment and risk of complications in patients with type 2 diabetes (UKPDS 33). *Lancet* 1998;352(9131):837–853

2. Ohkubo Y, Kishikawa H, Araki E, Miyata T, Isami S, Motoyoshi S, et al. Intensive insulin therapy prevents the progression of diabetic microvascular complications in Japanese patients with non–insulin-dependent diabetes mellitus: a randomized prospective 6-year study. *Diabetes Research and Clinical Practice* 1995;28(2):103–117

3. Patel A, MacMahon S, Chalmers J, Neal B, Woodward M, Billot L, et al. Effects of a fixed combination of perindopril and indapamide on macrovascular and microvascular outcomes in patients with type 2 diabetes mellitus (the ADVANCE trial): a randomised controlled trial. *Lancet* 2007;370(9590):829–840

4. The ACCORD Study Group, Gerstein HC, Miller ME, Genuth S, Ismail-Beigi F, Buse JB, et al. Long-term effects of intensive glucose lowering on cardiovascular outcomes. *N Engl J Med* 2011;364(9):818–828

5. Vokonas PS, Kannel WB. Diabetes mellitus and coronary heart disease in the elderly. *Clin Geriatr Med* 1996;12(1):69–78

6. Garcia MJ, McNamara PM, Gordon T, Kannel WB. Morbidity and mortality in diabetics in the Framingham population. Sixteen year follow-up study. *Diabetes* 1974;23(2):105–111

7. Haffner SM, Lehto S, Ronnemaa T, Pyorala K, Laakso M. Mortality from coronary heart disease in subjects with type 2 diabetes and in nondiabetic subjects with and without prior myocardial infarction. *N Engl J Med* 1998;339(4):229–234

8. American Diabetes Association. Statistics about diabetes [article online], 2015. Available from http://www.diabetes.org/diabetes-basics/statistics/

9. Taylor KS, Heneghan CJ, Farmer AJ, Fuller AM, Adler AI, Aronson JK, et al. All-cause and cardiovascular mortality in middle-aged people with type 2 diabetes compared with people without diabetes in a large U.K. primary care database. *Diabetes Care* 2013;36(8):2366–2371

10. American Diabetes Association. Economic costs of diabetes in the U.S. in 2017. *Diabetes Care* 2018;41(5):917–928

11. United States Renal Data System. 2016 USRDS Annual Data Report: epidemiology of kidney disease in the United States [article online]. National Institutes of Health, National Institute of Diabetes and Digestive and Kidney Diseases, Bethesda, MD, 2018. Available from https://www.usrds.org/2018/view/Default.aspx

12. Centers for Disease Control and Prevention. National Diabetes Statistics Report, 2020: Estimates of Diabetes and Its Burden in the United States [Internet], 2020. Available from https://www.cdc.gov/diabetes/data/statistics/statistics-report.html

13. Gregg EW, Li Y, Wang J, Burrows NR, Ali MK, Rolka D, et al. Changes in diabetes-related complications in the United States, 1990–2010. *N Engl J Med* 2014;370(16):1514–1523

14. Rawshani A, Rawshani A, Franzen S, Eliasson B, Svensson AM, Miftaraj M, et al. Mortality and cardiovascular disease in type 1 and type 2 diabetes. *N Engl J Med* 2017;376(15):1407–1418

15. Gregg EW, Cheng YJ, Srinivasan M, Lin J, Geiss LS, Albright AL, et al. Trends in cause-specific mortality among adults with and without diagnosed diabetes in the USA: an epidemiological analysis of linked national survey and vital statistics data. *Lancet* 2018;391(10138):2430–2440

16. Holman RR, Paul SK, Bethel MA, Matthews DR, Neil HA. 10-year follow-up of intensive glucose control in type 2 diabetes. *N Engl J Med* 2008;359(15):1577–1589

17. Stratton IM, Adler AI, Neil HA, Matthews DR, Manley SE, Cull CA, et al. Association of glycaemia with macrovascular and microvascular complications of type 2 diabetes (UKPDS 35): prospective observational study. *BMJ* (clinical research ed) 2000;321(7258):405–412

18. Buse JB, Bigger JT, Byington RP, Cooper LS, Cushman WC, Friedewald WT, et al. Action to Control Cardiovascular Risk in Diabetes (ACCORD) trial: design and methods. *Am J Cardiol* 2007;99(12a):21i–33i

19. Gerstein HC, Miller ME, Genuth S, Ismail-Beigi F, Buse JB, Goff DC, Jr., et al. Long-term effects of intensive glucose lowering on cardiovascular outcomes. *N Engl J Med* 2011;364(9):818–828

20. The ACCORD Study Group. Nine-year effects of 3.7 years of intensive glycemic control on cardiovascular outcomes. *Diabetes Care* 2016;39(5):701–708

21. Ismail-Beigi F, Craven T, Banerji MA, Basile J, Calles J, Cohen RM, et al. Effect of intensive treatment of hyperglycaemia on microvascular outcomes in type 2 diabetes: an analysis of the ACCORD randomised trial. *Lancet* 2010;376(9739):419–430

22. Murray AM, Hsu FC, Williamson JD, Bryan RN, Gerstein HC, Sullivan MD, et al. ACCORDION MIND: results of the observational extension of the ACCORD MIND randomised trial. *Diabetologia* 2017;60(1):69–80

23. Duckworth W, Abraira C, Moritz T, Reda D, Emanuele N, Reaven PD, et al. Glucose control and vascular complications in veterans with type 2 diabetes. *N Engl J Med* 2009;360(2):129–139

23a. Control Group, Turnbull FM, Abraira C, et al. Intensive glucose control and macrovascular outcomes in type 2 diabetes [published correction appears in Diabetologia. 2009 Nov;52(1):2470. Control Group [added]]. Diabetologia. 2009;52(11):2288–2298. doi:10.1007/s00125-009-1470-0

24. Zoungas S, Chalmers J, Neal B, Billot L, Li Q, Hirakawa Y, et al. Follow-up of blood-pressure lowering and glucose control in type 2 diabetes. *N Engl J Med* 2014;371(15):1392–1406

25. Reaven PD, Emanuele NV, Wiitala WL, Bahn GD, Reda DJ, McCarren M, et al. Intensive glucose control in patients with type 2 diabetes—15-year follow-up. *N Engl J Med* 2019;380(23):2215–2224

26. Matheus AS, Tannus LR, Cobas RA, Palma CC, Negrato CA, Gomes MB. Impact of diabetes on cardiovascular disease: an update. *Int J Hypertens* 2013;2013:653789. doi: 10.1155/2013/653789. Epub 2013 Mar 4

27. Secrest AM, Becker DJ, Kelsey SF, Laporte RE, Orchard TJ. Cause-specific mortality trends in a large population-based cohort with long-standing childhood-onset type 1 diabetes. *Diabetes* 2010;59(12):3216–3222

28. Zhang ZM, Rautaharju PM, Prineas RJ, Rodriguez CJ, Loehr L, Rosamond WD, et al. Race and sex differences in the incidence and prognostic significance of silent myocardial infarction in the Atherosclerosis Risk in Communities (ARIC) Study. *Circulation* 2016;133(22):2141–2148

29. Upchurch CT, Barrett EJ. Clinical review: screening for coronary artery disease in type 2 diabetes. *J Clin Endocrinol Metab* 2012;97(5):1434–1442

30. Bax JJ, Young LH, Frye RL, Bonow RO, Steinberg HO, Barrett EJ. Screening for coronary artery disease in patients with diabetes. *Diabetes Care* 2007;30(10):2729–2736

31. Young LH, Wackers FJ, Chyun DA, Davey JA, Barrett EJ, Taillefer R, et al. Cardiac outcomes after screening for asymptomatic coronary artery disease in patients with type 2 diabetes: the DIAD study: a randomized controlled trial. *JAMA* 2009;301(15):1547–1555

32. Greenland P, Alpert JS, Beller GA, Benjamin EJ, Budoff MJ, Fayad ZA, et al. 2010 ACCF/AHA guideline for assessment of cardiovascular risk in asymptomatic adults: a report of the American College of Cardiology Foundation/American Heart Association Task Force on Practice Guidelines. *Circulation* 2010;122(25):e584–e636

33. Look AHEAD Research Group. Eight-year weight losses with an intensive lifestyle intervention: the look AHEAD study. *Obesity* 2014;22(1):5–13

34. Wing RR, Bolin P, Brancati FL, Bray GA, Clark JM, Coday M, et al. Cardiovascular effects of intensive lifestyle intervention in type 2 diabetes. *N Engl J Med* 2013;369(2):145–154

35. Gaede P, Vedel P, Larsen N, Jensen GV, Parving HH, Pedersen O. Multifactorial intervention and cardiovascular disease in patients with type 2 diabetes. *N Engl J Med* 2003;348(5):383–393

36. Gaede P, Lund-Andersen H, Parving HH, Pedersen O. Effect of a multifactorial intervention on mortality in type 2 diabetes. *N Engl J Med* 2008;358(6):580–591

37. American Diabetes Association. 10. Cardiovascular disease and risk management: standards of medical care in diabetes 2020. *Diabetes Care* 2020;43(Suppl. 1):S111–S134

38. Baigent C, Blackwell L, Collins R, Emberson J, Godwin J, Peto R, et al. Aspirin in the primary and secondary prevention of vascular disease: collaborative meta-analysis of individual participant data from randomised trials. *Lancet* 2009;373(9678):1849–1860

39. Bowman L, Mafham M, Wallendszus K, Stevens W, Buck G, Barton J, et al. Effects of aspirin for primary prevention in persons with diabetes mellitus. *N Engl J Med* 2018;379(16):1529–1539

40. Gaziano JM, Brotons C, Coppolecchia R, Cricelli C, Darius H, Gorelick PB, et al. Use of aspirin to reduce risk of initial vascular events in patients at moderate risk of cardiovascular disease (ARRIVE): a randomised, double-blind, placebo-controlled trial. *Lancet* 2018;392(10152):1036–1046

41. McNeil JJ, Wolfe R, Woods RL, Tonkin AM, Donnan GA, Nelson MR, et al. Effect of aspirin on cardiovascular events and bleeding in the healthy elderly. *N Engl J Med* 2018;379(16):1509–1518

42. Pignone M, Alberts MJ, Colwell JA, Cushman M, Inzucchi SE, Mukherjee D, et al. Aspirin for primary prevention of cardiovascular events in people with diabetes. *J Am Coll Cardiol* 2010;55(25):2878–2886

43. Campbell CL, Smyth S, Montalescot G, Steinhubl SR. Aspirin dose for the prevention of cardiovascular disease: a systematic review. *JAMA* 2007;297(18):2018–2024

44. Rothwell PM, Cook NR, Gaziano JM, Price JF, Belch JFF, Roncaglioni MC, et al. Effects of aspirin on risks of vascular events and cancer according to bodyweight and dose: analysis of individual patient data from randomised trials. *Lancet* 2018;392(10145):387–399

45. Vandvik PO, Lincoff AM, Gore JM, Gutterman DD, Sonnenberg FA, Alonso-Coello P, et al. Primary and secondary prevention of cardiovascular disease: antithrombotic therapy and prevention of thrombosis, 9th ed: American College of Chest Physicians evidence-based clinical practice guidelines. *Chest* 2012;141(Suppl. 2):e637S–e668S

46. Bhatt DL, Bonaca MP, Bansilal S, Angiolillo DJ, Cohen M, Storey RF, et al. Reduction in ischemic events with ticagrelor in diabetic patients with prior myocardial infarction in PEGASUS-TIMI 54. *J Am Coll Cardiol* 2016;67(23):2732–2740

47. de Boer IH, Bangalore S, Benetos A, Davis AM, Michos ED, Muntner P, et al. Diabetes and hypertension: a position statement by the American Diabetes Association. *Diabetes Care* 2017;40(9):1273–1284

48. UK Perspective Diabetes Study Group. Tight blood pressure control and risk of macrovascular and microvascular complications in type 2 diabetes: UKPDS 38. UK Prospective Diabetes Study Group. *BMJ* (Clinical research ed) 1998;317(7160):703–713

49. Hansson L, Zanchetti A, Carruthers SG, Dahlof B, Elmfeldt D, Julius S, et al. Effects of intensive blood-pressure lowering and low-dose aspirin in patients with hypertension: principal results of the Hypertension Optimal Treatment (HOT) randomised trial. HOT Study Group. *Lancet* 1998;351(9118):1755–1762

50. Heart Outcomes Prevention Evaluation (HOPE) Study Investigators. Effects of ramipril on cardiovascular and microvascular outcomes in people with diabetes mellitus: results of the HOPE study and MICRO-HOPE substudy. Heart Outcomes Prevention Evaluation Study Investigators. *Lancet* 2000;355(9200):253–259

51. Cushman WC, Evans GW, Byington RP, Goff DC, Jr., Grimm RH, Jr., Cutler JA, et al. Effects of intensive blood-pressure control in type 2 diabetes mellitus. *N Engl J Med* 2010;362(17):1575–1585

52. Pepine CJ, Handberg EM, Cooper-DeHoff RM, Marks RG, Kowey P, Messerli FH, et al. A calcium antagonist vs a non–calcium antagonist hypertension treatment strategy for patients with coronary artery disease: The International Verapamil-Trandolapril Study (INVEST): a randomized controlled trial. *JAMA* 2003;290(21):2805–2816

53. Wright JT, Jr., Williamson JD, Whelton PK, Snyder JK, Sink KM, Rocco MV, et al. A randomized trial of intensive versus standard blood-pressure control. *N Engl J Med* 2015;373(22):2103–2016

54. Whelton PK, Carey RM, Aronow WS, Casey DE, Jr., Collins KJ, Dennison Himmelfarb C, et al. 2017 ACC/AHA/AAPA/ABC/ACPM/AGS/APhA/ASH/ASPC/NMA/PCNA guideline for the prevention, detection, evaluation, and management of high blood pressure in adults: executive summary: a report of the American College of Cardiology/American Heart Association Task Force on Clinical Practice Guidelines. *J Am Coll Cardiol* 2018;71(19):2199–2269

55. Magee LA, von Dadelszen P, Rey E, Ross S, Asztalos E, Murphy KE, et al. Less-tight versus tight control of hypertension in pregnancy. *N Engl J Med* 2015;372(5):407–417

56. Brown MA, Magee LA, Kenny LC, Karumanchi SA, McCarthy FP, Saito S, et al. Hypertensive disorders of pregnancy: ISSHP classification, diagnosis, and management recommendations for international practice. *Hypertension* 2018;72(1):24–43

57. Hypertension in pregnancy. Report of the American College of Obstetricians and Gynecologists' Task Force on Hypertension in Pregnancy. *Obstet Gynecol* 2013;122(5):1122–1131

58. Appel LJ, Moore TJ, Obarzanek E, Vollmer WM, Svetkey LP, Sacks FM, et al. A clinical trial of the effects of dietary patterns on blood pressure. *N Engl J Med* 1997;336(16):1117–1124

59. American Diabetes Association. 10. Cardiovascular disease and risk management: standards of medical care in diabetes 2019. *Diabetes Care* 2019;42(Suppl. 1):S103–S123

59a. Cosentino F, Grant PJ, Aboyans V, et al. 2019 ESC Guidelines on diabetes, pre-diabetes, and cardiovascular diseases developed in collaboration with the EASD. Eur Heart J. 2020;41(2):255–323. doi:10.1093/eurheartj/ehz486

60. Braunwald E, Domanski MJ, Fowler SE, Geller NL, Gersh BJ, Hsia J, et al. Angiotensin-converting-enzyme inhibition in stable coronary artery disease. *N Engl J Med* 2004;351(20):2058–2068

61. Yusuf S, Teo K, Anderson C, Pogue J, Dyal L, Copland I, et al. Effects of the angiotensin-receptor blocker telmisartan on cardiovascular events in high-risk patients intolerant to angiotensin-converting enzyme inhibitors: a randomised controlled trial. *Lancet* 2008;372(9644):1174–1183

62. Bangalore S, Fakheri R, Toklu B, Messerli FH. Diabetes mellitus as a compelling indication for use of renin angiotensin system blockers: systematic review and meta-analysis of randomized trials. *BMJ* (Clinical research ed) 2016;352:i438

63. Ettehad D, Emdin CA, Kiran A, Anderson SG, Callender T, Emberson J, et al. Blood pressure lowering for prevention of cardiovascular disease and death: a systematic review and meta-analysis. *Lancet* 2016;387(10022):957–967

64. Kezerashvili A, Marzo K, De Leon J. Beta blocker use after acute myocardial infarction in the patient with normal systolic function: when is it "ok" to discontinue? *Curr Cardiol Rev* 2012;8(1):77–84

65. Carlberg B, Samuelsson O, Lindholm LH. Atenolol in hypertension: is it a wise choice? *Lancet* 2004;364(9446):1684–1689

66. Weber MA, Bakris GL, Jamerson K, Weir M, Kjeldsen SE, Devereux RB, et al. Cardiovascular events during differing hypertension therapies in patients with diabetes. *J Am Coll Cardiol* 2010;56(1):77–85

67. Williams B, MacDonald TM, Morant S, Webb DJ, Sever P, McInnes G, et al. Spironolactone versus placebo, bisoprolol, and doxazosin to determine the optimal treatment for drug-resistant hypertension (PATHWAY-2): a randomised, double-blind, crossover trial. *Lancet* 2015;386(10008):2059–2068

68. Bakris GL, Agarwal R, Chan JC, Cooper ME, Gansevoort RT, Haller H, et al. Effect of finerenone on albuminuria in patients with diabetic nephropathy: a randomized clinical trial. *JAMA* 2015;314(9):884–894

69. Bomback AS, Klemmer PJ. Mineralocorticoid receptor blockade in chronic kidney disease. *Blood Purif* 2012;33(1-3):119–124

70. Gheorghiade M, Bohm M, Greene SJ, Fonarow GC, Lewis EF, Zannad F, et al. Effect of aliskiren on postdischarge mortality and heart failure readmissions among patients hospitalized for heart failure: the ASTRONAUT randomized trial. *JAMA* 2013;309(11):1125–1135

71. Shaw JE, Punjabi NM, Naughton MT, Willes L, Bergenstal RM, Cistulli PA, et al. The effect of treatment of obstructive sleep apnea on glycemic control in type 2 diabetes. *Am J Respir Crit Care Med* 2016;194(4):486–492

72. Estruch R, Ros E, Salas-Salvado J, Covas MI, Corella D, Aros F, et al. Primary prevention of cardiovascular disease with a Mediterranean diet supplemented with extra-virgin olive oil or nuts. *N Engl J Med* 2018;378(25):e34

73. Eckel RH, Jakicic JM, Ard JD, de Jesus JM, Houston Miller N, Hubbard VS, et al. 2013 AHA/ACC guideline on lifestyle management to reduce cardiovascular risk: a report of the American College of Cardiology/American Heart Association Task Force on Practice Guidelines. *J Am Coll Cardiol* 2014;63(25 Pt B):2960–2984

74. Collins R, Armitage J, Parish S, Sleigh P, Peto R, Heart Protection Study Collaborative G. MRC/BHF Heart Protection Study of cholesterol-lowering with simvastatin in 5963 people with diabetes: a randomised placebo-controlled trial. *Lancet* 2003;361(9374):2005–2016

75. Colhoun HM, Betteridge DJ, Durrington PN, Hitman GA, Neil HA, Livingstone SJ, et al. Primary prevention of cardiovascular disease with atorvastatin in type 2 diabetes in the Collaborative Atorvastatin Diabetes Study (CARDS): multicentre randomised placebo-controlled trial. *Lancet* 2004;364(9435):685–696

76. Mihaylova B, Emberson J, Blackwell L, Keech A, Simes J, Barnes EH, et al. The effects of lowering LDL cholesterol with statin therapy in people at low risk of vascular disease: meta-analysis of individual data from 27 randomised trials. *Lancet* 2012;380(9841):581–590

77. Baigent C, Keech A, Kearney PM, Blackwell L, Buck G, Pollicino C, et al. Efficacy and safety of cholesterol-lowering treatment: prospective meta-analysis of data from 90,056 participants in 14 randomised trials of statins. *Lancet* 2005;366(9493):1267–1278

78. Keech A, Simes RJ, Barter P, Best J, Scott R, Taskinen MR, et al. Effects of long-term fenofibrate therapy on cardiovascular events in 9795 people with type 2 diabetes mellitus (the FIELD study): randomised controlled trial. *Lancet* 2005;366(9500):1849–1861

79. Taylor F, Huffman MD, Macedo AF, Moore TH, Burke M, Davey Smith G, et al. Statins for the primary prevention of cardiovascular disease. *Cochrane Database Syst Rev* 2013(1):Cd004816

80. Carter AA, Gomes T, Camacho X, Juurlink DN, Shah BR, Mamdani MM. Risk of incident diabetes among patients treated with statins: population based study. *BMJ* (Clinical research ed) 2013;346:f2610

81. Sattar N, Preiss D, Murray HM, Welsh P, Buckley BM, de Craen AJ, et al. Statins and risk of incident diabetes: a collaborative meta-analysis of randomised statin trials. *Lancet* 2010;375(9716):735–742

82. Grundy SM, Stone NJ, Bailey AL, Beam C, Birtcher KK, Blumenthal RS, et al. 2018 AHA/ACC/AACVPR/AAPA/ABC/ACPM/ADA/AGS/APhA/ASPC/NLA/PCNA guideline on the management of blood cholesterol. *Circulation* 2018:Cir0000000000000625

83. Singh IM, Shishehbor MH, Ansell BJ. High-density lipoprotein as a therapeutic target: a systematic review. *JAMA* 2007;298(7):786–798

84. Bhatt DL, Steg PG, Miller M, Brinton EA, Jacobson TA, Ketchum SB, et al. Cardiovascular risk reduction with icosapent ethyl for hypertriglyceridemia. *N Engl J Med* 2019;380(1):11–22

85. Bowman L, Mafham M, Wallendszus K, Stevens W, Buck G, Barton J, et al. Effects of n-3 fatty acid supplements in diabetes mellitus. *N Engl J Med* 2018;379(16):1540–1550

86. Bosch J, Gerstein HC, Dagenais GR, Diaz R, Dyal L, Jung H, et al. N-3 fatty acids and cardiovascular outcomes in patients with dysglycemia. *N Engl J Med* 2012;367(4):309–18

87. Cannon CP, Blazing MA, Giugliano RP, McCagg A, White JA, Theroux P, et al. Ezetimibe added to statin therapy after acute coronary syndromes. *N Engl J Med* 2015;372(25):2387–2397

88. Giugliano RP, Cannon CP, Blazing MA, Nicolau JC, Corbalan R, Spinar J, et al. Benefit of adding ezetimibe to statin therapy on cardiovascular outcomes and safety in patients with versus without diabetes mellitus: results from IMPROVE-IT (Improved Reduction of Outcomes: Vytorin Efficacy International Trial). *Circulation* 2018;137(15):1571–1582

89. Cohen JC, Boerwinkle E, Mosley TH, Jr., Hobbs HH. Sequence variations in PCSK9, low LDL, and protection against coronary heart disease. *N Engl J Med* 2006;354(12):1264–1272

90. Schwartz GG, Steg PG, Szarek M, Bhatt DL, Bittner VA, Diaz R, et al. Alirocumab and cardiovascular outcomes after acute coronary syndrome. *N Engl J Med* 2018;379(22):2097–2107

91. Sabatine MS, Giugliano RP, Keech AC, Honarpour N, Wiviott SD, Murphy SA, et al. Evolocumab and clinical outcomes in patients with cardiovascular disease. *N Engl J Med* 2017;376(18):1713–1722

92. Sabatine MS, Leiter LA, Wiviott SD, Giugliano RP, Deedwania P, De Ferrari GM, et al. Cardiovascular safety and efficacy of the PCSK9 inhibitor evolocumab in patients with and without diabetes and the effect of evolocumab on glycaemia and risk of new-onset diabetes: a prespecified analysis of the FOURIER randomised controlled trial. *Lancet Diabetes Endocrinol* 2017;5(12):941–950

93. Szarek M, White HD, Schwartz GG, Alings M, Bhatt DL, Bittner VA, et al. Alirocumab reduces total nonfatal cardiovascular and fatal events: the ODYSSEY OUTCOMES trial. *J Am Coll Cardiol* 2019;73(4):387–396

94. Ginsberg HN, Elam MB, Lovato LC, Crouse JR, 3rd, Leiter LA, Linz P, et al. Effects of combination lipid therapy in type 2 diabetes mellitus. *N Engl J Med* 2010;362(17):1563–1574

95. Jones PH, Davidson MH. Reporting rate of rhabdomyolysis with fenofibrate + statin versus gemfibrozil + any statin. *Am J Cardiol* 2005;95(1):120–122

96. Boden WE, Probstfield JL, Anderson T, Chaitman BR, Desvignes-Nickens P, Koprowicz K, et al. Niacin in patients with low HDL cholesterol levels receiving intensive statin therapy. *N Engl J Med* 2011;365(24):2255–2267

97. Probstfield JL, Boden WE, Anderson T, Branch K, Kashyap M, Fleg JL, et al. Cardiovascular outcomes during extended follow-up of the AIM-HIGH trial cohort. *J Clin Lipidol* 2018;12(6):1413–1419

98. Landray MJ, Haynes R, Hopewell JC, Parish S, Aung T, Tomson J, et al. Effects of extended-release niacin with laropiprant in high-risk patients. *N Engl J Med* 2014;371(3):203–212

99. American Diabetes Association. 5. Facilitating behavior change and well-being to improve health outcomes: standards of medical care in diabetes 2020. *Diabetes Care* 2020;43(Suppl. 1):S48–S65

100. Pan A, Wang Y, Talaei M, Hu FB. Relation of smoking with total mortality and cardiovascular events among patients with diabetes mellitus: a meta-analysis and systematic review. *Circulation* 2015;132(19):1795–1804

101. Jha P, Ramasundarahettige C, Landsman V, Rostron B, Thun M, Anderson RN, et al. 21st-Century hazards of smoking and benefits of cessation in the United States. *N Engl J Med* 2013;368(4):341–350

102. Kar D, Gillies C, Zaccardi F, Webb D, Seidu S, Tesfaye S, et al. Relationship of cardiometabolic parameters in non-smokers, current smokers, and quitters in diabetes: a systematic review and meta-analysis. *Cardiovasc Diabetol* 2016;15(1):158

103. Sliwinska-Mosson M, Milnerowicz H. The impact of smoking on the development of diabetes and its complications. *Diab Vasc Dis Res* 2017;14(4):265–276

104. Mons U, Muezzinler A, Gellert C, Schottker B, Abnet CC, Bobak M, et al. Impact of smoking and smoking cessation on cardiovascular events and mortality among older adults: meta-analysis of individual participant data from prospective cohort studies of the CHANCES consortium. *BMJ* (Clinical research ed) 2015;350:h1551

105. Ahmed AA, Patel K, Nyaku MA, Kheirbek RE, Bittner V, Fonarow GC, et al. Risk of heart failure and death after prolonged smoking cessation: role of amount and duration of prior smoking. *Circ Heart Fail* 2015;8(4):694–701

106. Bhatnagar A. Cardiovascular perspective of the promises and perils of e-cigarettes. *Circ Res* 2016;118(12):1872–1875

107. Huerta TR, Walker DM, Mullen D, Johnson TJ, Ford EW. Trends in e-cigarette awareness and perceived harmfulness in the U.S. *Am J Prev Med* 2017;52(3):339–346

108. Pericot-Valverde I, Gaalema DE, Priest JS, Higgins ST. E-cigarette awareness, perceived harmfulness, and ever use among U.S. adults. *Prev Med* 2017;104:92–99

109. Lippi G, Favaloro EJ, Meschi T, Mattiuzzi C, Borghi L, Cervellin G. E-cigarettes and cardiovascular risk: beyond science and mysticism. *Semin Thromb Hemost* 2014;40(1):60–65

110. Force UPST. Final recommendation statement: tobacco smoking cessation in adults, including pregnant women: behavioral and pharmacotherapy interventions [Internet], 2015. [cited 7 Aug 2017]. Available from https://www.uspreventiveservicestaskforce.org/Page/Document/UpdateSummaryFinal/tobacco-use-in-adults-and-pregnant-women-counseling-and-interventions1?ds=1&s=tobacco

111. Livingston CJ, Freeman RJ, Costales VC, Westhoff JL, Caplan LS, Sherin KM, et al. Electronic nicotine delivery systems or e-cigarettes: American College of Preventive Medicine's Practice Statement. *Am J Prev Med* 2019;56(1):167–178

112. Madison MC, Landers CT, Gu BH, Chang CY, Tung HY, You R, et al. Electronic cigarettes disrupt lung lipid homeostasis and innate immunity independent of nicotine. *J Clin Invest* 2019;129(10):4290–4304

113. Marso SP, Daniels GH, Brown-Frandsen K, Kristensen P, Mann JF, Nauck MA, et al. Liraglutide and cardiovascular outcomes in type 2 diabetes. *N Engl J Med* 2016;375(4):311–322

114. Pfeffer MA, Claggett B, Diaz R, Dickstein K, Gerstein HC, Kober LV, et al. Lixisenatide in patients with type 2 diabetes and acute coronary syndrome. *N Engl J Med* 2015;373(23):2247–2257

115. Holman RR, Bethel MA, Mentz RJ, Thompson VP, Lokhnygina Y, Buse JB, et al. Effects of once-weekly exenatide on cardiovascular outcomes in type 2 diabetes. *N Engl J Med* 2017;377(13):1228–1239

116. Marso SP, Bain SC, Consoli A, Eliaschewitz FG, Jodar E, Leiter LA, et al. Semaglutide and cardiovascular outcomes in patients with type 2 diabetes. *N Engl J Med* 2016;375(19):1834–1844

117. Husain M, Birkenfeld AL, Donsmark M, Dungan K, Eliaschewitz FG, Franco DR, et al. Oral semaglutide and cardiovascular outcomes in patients with type 2 diabetes. *N Engl J Med* 2019;381(9):841–851

118. Food and Drug Administration. FDA approves first oral GLP-1 treatment for type 2 diabetes [article online], Sept 2019. [updated Feb 22nd 2020]. Available from https://www.fda.gov/news-events/press-announcements/fda-approves-first-oral-glp-1-treatment-type-2-diabetes

119. Gerstein HC, Colhoun HM, Dagenais GR, Diaz R, Lakshmanan M, Pais P, et al. Dulaglutide and cardiovascular outcomes in type 2 diabetes (REWIND): a double-blind, randomised placebo-controlled trial. *Lancet* 2019;394(10193):121–130

120. Zinman B, Wanner C, Lachin JM, Fitchett D, Bluhmki E, Hantel S, et al. Empagliflozin, cardiovascular outcomes, and mortality in type 2 diabetes. *N Engl J Med* 2015;373(22):2117–2128

121. Saad M, Mahmoud AN, Elgendy IY, Abuzaid A, Barakat AF, Elgendy AY, et al. Cardiovascular outcomes with sodium-glucose cotransporter-2 inhibitors in patients with type II diabetes mellitus: a meta-analysis of placebo-controlled randomized trials. *Int J Cardiol* 2017;228:352–358

122. Neal B, Perkovic V, Mahaffey KW, de Zeeuw D, Fulcher G, Erondu N, et al. Canagliflozin and cardiovascular and renal events in type 2 diabetes. *N Engl J Med* 2017;377(7):644–657

123. Perkovic V, Jardine MJ, Neal B, Bompoint S, Heerspink HJL, Charytan DM, et al. Canagliflozin and renal outcomes in type 2 diabetes and nephropathy. *N Engl J Med* 2019;380(24):2295–2306

124. Wiviott SD, Raz I, Bonaca MP, Mosenzon O, Kato ET, Cahn A, et al. Dapagliflozin and cardiovascular outcomes in type 2 diabetes. *N Engl J Med* 2019;380(4):347–357

125. Kannel WB, Hjortland M, Castelli WP. Role of diabetes in congestive heart failure: the Framingham study. *Am J Cardiol* 1974;34(1):29–34

126. Lehrke M, Marx N. Diabetes mellitus and heart failure. *Am J Med* 2017;130(6):S40–S50

127. McMurray JJV, Solomon SD, Inzucchi SE, Kober L, Kosiborod MN, Martinez FA, et al. Dapagliflozin in patients with heart failure and reduced ejection fraction. *N Engl J Med* 2019;381(21):1995–2008

128. Singh S, Loke YK, Furberg CD. Thiazolidinediones and heart failure: a teleo-analysis. *Diabetes Care* 2007;30(8):2148–2153

129. Dormandy JA, Charbonnel B, Eckland DJ, Erdmann E, Massi-Benedetti M, Moules IK, et al. Secondary prevention of macrovascular events in patients with type 2 diabetes in the PROactive Study (PROspective pioglitAzone Clinical Trial In macroVascular Events): a randomised controlled trial. *Lancet* 2005;366(9493):1279–1289

130. Lincoff AM, Wolski K, Nicholls SJ, Nissen SE. Pioglitazone and risk of cardiovascular events in patients with type 2 diabetes mellitus: a meta-analysis of randomized trials. *JAMA* 2007;298(10):1180–1188

131. Scirica BM, Bhatt DL, Braunwald E, Steg PG, Davidson J, Hirshberg B, et al. Saxagliptin and cardiovascular outcomes in patients with type 2 diabetes mellitus. *N Engl J Med* 2013;369(14):1317–1326

132. Rosenstock J, Perkovic V, Johansen OE, Cooper ME, Kahn SE, Marx N, et al. Effect of linagliptin vs placebo on major cardiovascular events in adults with type 2 diabetes and high cardiovascular and renal risk: The CARMELINA randomized clinical trial. *JAMA* 2019;321(1):69–79

133. Zannad F, Cannon CP, Cushman WC, Bakris GL, Menon V, Perez AT, et al. Heart failure and mortality outcomes in patients with type 2 diabetes taking alogliptin versus placebo in EXAMINE: a multicentre, randomised, double-blind trial. *Lancet* 2015;385(9982):2067–2076

134. Green JB, Bethel MA, Armstrong PW, Buse JB, Engel SS, Garg J, et al. Effect of sitagliptin on cardiovascular outcomes in type 2 diabetes. *N Engl J Med* 2015;373(3):232–242

135. Filion KB, Azoulay L, Platt RW, Dahl M, Dormuth CR, Clemens KK, et al. A multicenter observational study of incretin-based drugs and heart failure. *N Engl J Med* 2016;374(12):1145–1154

136. Crowley MJ DC, McDuffie JR, et al. Metformin use in patients with contraindications or precautions [Internet]. Washington, DC, U.S. Department of Veterans Affairs. Available from https://www.ncbi.nlm.nih.gov/books/NBK409379] Accessed 1 Sep 2016

MICROVASCULAR COMPLICATIONS

Uma Gunasekaran, MD

DIABETIC RETINOPATHY

Worldwide, there are ~93 million people with diabetic retinopathy (DR), 17 million with proliferative diabetic retinopathy (PDR), 21 million with diabetic macular edema (DME), and 28 million with vision-threatening DR. Longer diabetes duration and poor glycemic and blood pressure control have a strong association with DR.[1] Approximately 12,000–24,000 new cases of DR are diagnosed yearly in the U.S.[2]

As in type 1 diabetes, the development and progression of retinopathy in type 2 diabetes is duration dependent and associated with higher glycemic levels. DR is the most common cause of vision loss among people with diabetes and the leading cause of blindness among working-age adults in the U.S.[3] Glaucoma, cataracts, and other disorders of the eye occur earlier and more frequently in people with diabetes. Glycemic control prevents or delays the onset of retinopathy. Other risk factors that were shown to increase the risk of retinopathy include hypertension, nephropathy, and hyperlipidemia. Although relatively fewer people with type 2 diabetes, compared with type 1 diabetes, develop PDR, DME may be more common. In addition to retinopathy, patients with type 2 diabetes develop cataracts more frequently and at an earlier age than do people without diabetes.

The frequency of visual impairment related to diabetes makes effective patient education crucial. Table 5.4 presents patient teaching points concerning retinopathy.

Table 5.4–What Patients Need to Know—Retinopathy

- Inform patients newly diagnosed with type 2 diabetes that vision loss is a possibility and that routine screening begins at diagnosis, even if asymptomatic.
- Instruct patients regarding the relationship between hyperglycemia, hypertension, dyslipidemia, and diabetic retinopathy, focusing on risk factor control to preserve eyesight.
- Ensure that patients understand the importance of routine dilated eye examinations or retinal photography performed by or interpreted by an ophthalmologist or optometrist because retinopathy outcomes are better with early detection and treatment.
- Reassure patients concerning transient vision changes associated with casual glycemic fluctuations and temporary changes in retinopathy status due to changes in glycemic therapy or pregnancy.
- Inform patients of the sight-saving procedures, including photocoagulation and intraocular injections, that are available for severe nonproliferative, proliferative retinopathy, and DME.
- Suggest support programs and community services for patients with visual impairments or blindness.
- Counseling should be provided to women with preexisting diabetes prior to pregnancy about the risk of development and/or progression of diabetic retinopathy.

Source: Wong.[4]

Stages of Diabetic Retinopathy

The stages of DR are mild to moderate nonproliferative diabetic retinopathy (NPDR), severe NPDR, PDR, and DME.

Mild to moderate nonproliferative diabetic retinopathy. NPDR is the earliest stage and is characterized by microaneurysms (mild NPDR), dot and blot hemorrhages, hard exudates, and cotton wool spots (moderate NPDR) (Fig. 5.2).[4] Most individuals with long-term type 2 diabetes eventually develop NPDR, but in many cases, it does not progress and has no effect on visual acuity.

Severe nonproliferative retinopathy. Certain retinal lesions represent an advanced form of NPDR (Fig. 5.3). These lesions include intraretinal hemorrhage, beading" of the retinal veins, and intraretinal microvascular abnormalities, which are dilated, tortuous retinal capillaries, or perhaps newly formed vessels within the retina.[4] When these lesions are found together, the risk of progression to the proliferative stage is increased, and the presence of any of these signs should prompt referral to an ophthalmologist who is knowledgeable and experienced in the management of DR.

Proliferative diabetic retinopathy. PDR (Fig. 5.4) is the most vision-threatening stage of DR and is characterized by neovascularization (new vessel formation) on the surface of the retina, sometimes extending into the posterior vitreous in response to ischemia.[4] PDR threatens vision because the new vessels are prone to bleed, especially if they are stretched by contraction of the vitreous. If bleeding into the preretinal space or vitreous occurs, the patient is likely to report "floaters" or "cobwebs" in the field of vision. The patient who has a major retinal hemorrhage will experience a sudden, painless loss of vision. The proliferation of fibrous tissue that often follows can lead to retinal detachment as fibrous tissue contracts.

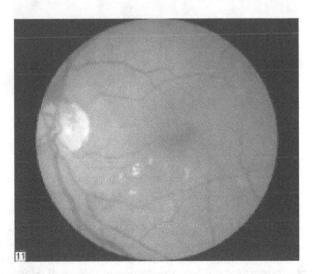

Figure 5.2 Moderate nonproliferative diabetic retinopathy. This image presents scattered exudates, microaneurysms, and dot and blot hemorrhages. *Source*: LeBlond, R. *DeGowin's Diagnostic Examination*. 10th Edition.

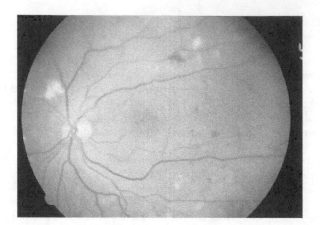

Figure 5.3 Severe nonproliferative retinopathy. This image shows a large number of hemorrhages along with mild diabetic macular edema. *Source*: American Academy of Ophthalmology Basic and Clinical Science Series. Section 12. Retina and Vitreous, 2008–2009. 109–132.

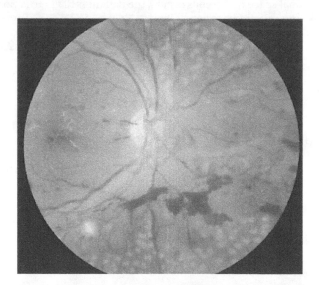

Figure 5.4 Proliferative diabetic retinopathy. This image shows neovascular vessels, retinal and vitreous hemorrhage, cotton wool spots, and macular exudate. Peripheral round spots signify recent panretinal photocoagulation. *Source*: Jameson, AS, et al. Harrison's Principles of Internal Medicine. 20th Edition.

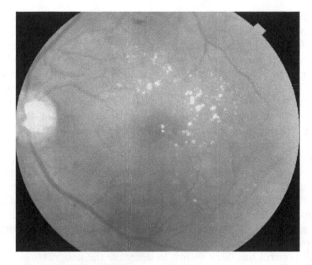

Figure 5.5 Diabetic macular edema. This image shows exudates in the macula indicative of macular edema. *Source*: Lenier S. *Deep learning predicts OCT measures of diabetic macular thickening*. Ophthalmology Times. May 21, 2019.

Diabetic macular edema. The macula is responsible for central vision. DME (Fig. 5.5) can be present in either nonproliferative or proliferative retinopathy and can result in vision loss. The breakdown of the blood retinal barrier by various metabolic factors causes vascular permeability and the leakage of plasma proteins such as albumin. The plasma proteins increase the oncotic pressure in the neural interstitium, resulting in DME.[5] The presence of DME is suspected if there are hard exudates in close proximity to the macula. Circinate hard exudates near the macula are especially suspicious. Any of these findings should prompt referral to an ophthalmologist with expertise in treating DR.[4] Chronic hyperglycemia, hypertension,[6] and hyperlipidemia[7] cholesterol are known to increase the risk of developing DME.

Prevention of Vision Loss from Retinopathy

Large, prospective clinical trials such as Diabetes Control and Complications Trial (DCCT)[8] and the U.K. Prospective Diabetes Study (UKPDS)[9] demonstrated that intensive treatment of hyperglycemia to near-normal levels prevents or ameliorates DR. Furthermore, the EDIC follow-up trial demonstrated that patients with early, intensive diabetes control in the DCCT had a lower incidence of progression of DR during long-term follow-up, a concept known as metabolic memory.[10] Additionally, the small Kumamoto study in Japan demonstrated the benefit of improved glycemic control in patients with type 2 diabetes,[11] and the Wisconsin Epidemiologic Study of Diabetic Retinopathy found a strong association between baseline glycated hemoglobin and the incidence and progression of retinopathy in patients with type 2 diabetes, independent of treatment.[12] The FIELD study has demonstrated that the rate of first laser treatments for DR is reduced in patients on fenofibrate therapy, especially in patients with pre-identified retinopathy.[13] More recently, the ACCORD trial demonstrated the benefits of both intensive glycemia treatment and lipid management (with a combination of statin and fenofibrate) in preventing retinopathy progression in patients with type 2 diabetes at high risk of a CVD event.[14] Also, two large prospective studies, the Diabetic Retinopathy Study[15] and the Early Treatment of Diabetic Retinopathy Study,[16] provided strong support for the benefits of photocoagulation therapy (laser therapy), which decreases the risk of vision loss in patients with PDR or DME. Therefore, timely identification of patients at risk is a major means of preventing vision loss.

The UKPDS also provided evidence that blood pressure control prevents the appearance and progression of retinopathy,[17] although the Appropriate Blood Pressure Control in Diabetes Trial did not confirm a difference in retinopathy between intensive and moderate blood pressure control.[18] Furthermore, the ACCORD trial also found no benefit in retinopathy rates with further lowering of blood pressure levels <120 mmHg.[14,19] ACE inhibitors and angiotensin receptor blockers (ARBs) have also shown benefit in patients with DR.[20]

Glycemic control has been shown to decrease the progression of retinopathy and should therefore be at the forefront of treatment in patients with DR. Consideration should also be given to the addition of fenofibrate therapy with individuals with mild NPDR and proper management of hypertension with the use of ACE inhibitors or ARBs.

Evaluation and Referral

Because patients may be asymptomatic, or the changes involved in DR may be subtle and can escape detection by direct ophthalmoscopy, all patients with type 2 diabetes should have an initial examination with a complete visual history, visual acuity examination, and careful dilated pupil ophthalmoscopic examination by an ophthalmologist or optometrist. The evaluations should begin at diabetes diagnosis, because the duration of hyperglycemia before diagnosis of type 2 diabetes is uncertain, and many patients already have retinopathy at diagnosis. Subsequent evaluations should occur every 1–2 years if no retinopathy was previously identified.[7] These evaluations can be performed with a dilated pupil ophthalmoscopic examination by an ophthalmologist or optometrist or via retinal photography with remote reading by experts, especially in areas without eye care professionals. Retinal photography is not a substitute for comprehensive exams, and their frequency should be directed by an eye care professional.[7] The recommended timing intervals for rescreening and referral are listed in Table 5.5. Note that 25%–50% of patients with any high-risk characteristic may sustain severe visual loss within 2 years unless photocoagulation or intravitreal anti-vascular endothelial growth factor treatment is performed.[21]

Note also that visual acuity changes are frequently related to fluctuating glycemic levels and corresponding changes in the hydration of the crystalline lens. Thus, a presenting symptom of diabetes in a patient with severe hyperglycemia may be a change in vision (commonly blurring of vision). Likewise, a patient whose glycemic levels are decreased in response to appropriate treatment may experience acute, but temporary, visual changes and should be forewarned as well as reassured that these will resolve over time.

Table 5.5–Timing Intervals for Rescreening or Referral of Patients with Type 2 Diabetes to Ophthalmologist or Optometrist

Classification	Rescreening interval (low–intermediate resource country)	Rescreening interval (high resource country)	Referral to ophthalmologist or optometrist
No apparent DR, mild NPDR, and no DME	1–2 years	Rescreen in 1–2 years	Referral not required
Mild NPDR	1–2 years	6–12 months	Referral not required
Moderate NPDR	6–12 months	3–6 months	Referral required
Severe NPDR	<3 months	<3 months	Referral required
PDR	<1 month	<1 month	Referral required
Noncenter involving DME	3 months	3 months	Referral required
Center involving DME	1 month	1 month	Referral required

DME, diabetic macular edema; DR, diabetic retinopathy; NPDR, nonproliferative diabetic retinopathy; PDR, proliferative diabetic retinopathy.

Source: Adapted from original tables in Wong.[4]

Pregnancy is associated with an increased risk for the development or progression of DR, and all women should be counseled on this. Pregnant women should be screened prior to pregnancy or in the first trimester and monitored every trimester as well as 1 year postpartum based on the degree of retinopathy present.[7] Rapid improvement and intensive glycemic control in the presence of retinopathy is often associated with worsening of retinopathy.[22] Approximately 50%–70% of patients with known DR have progression during pregnancy.[23,24] Women with gestational diabetes are not at risk of developing retinopathy during their pregnancy and do not need retinal screening.[25]

Treatment of Retinopathy

The ophthalmologic treatment of DR depends on the stage of disease. There is no commonly accepted therapy for NPDR other than improved glycemic, blood pressure, and lipid control. Panretinal photocoagulation is considered the treatment of choice for patients who have PDR with high-risk characteristics as it reduces the risk of severe visual loss by ~60%.[15] Photocoagulation slows progressive visual loss in patients with DME by 50%.[16]

Photocoagulation is used to stop neovascularization before recurrent hemorrhages into the vitreous cause irreparable damage. Sometimes photocoagulation is used to treat eyes with NPDR before high-risk characteristics have developed. However, the risks of photocoagulation are such that usually only one eye is treated; treatment of the other eye is deferred unless high-risk characteristics develop. If retinal detachment and massive vitreous hemorrhage occur, closed vitrectomy can be used to remove bloody vitreous and bands of fibrous tissue. During the procedure, clear fluid is infused to replace vitreous, and traction on the retina is relieved. Depending upon other comorbid ophthalmic conditions, vitrectomy can restore some vision.[26,27]

The use of intravitreal antivascular endothelial growth factor (anti-VEGF) drugs such as aflibercept, ranibizumab, and bevacizumab is the treatment of choice for DME.[4] Additionally, these drugs have been shown to be noninferior treatments for PDR compared with photocoagulation for the first 2 years.[28] Bevacizumab has also been an effective treatment against neovascularization.[29]

Intravitreal corticosteroids can be used in the treatment of DME but are more commonly used in the treatment of glaucoma and cataracts.

DIABETIC KIDNEY DISEASE

Diabetic kidney disease, manifested as persistent albuminuria, impaired glomerular filtration rate (GFR), or both, occurs in 20%–40% of individuals with diabetes and is the leading cause of end-stage renal disease (ESRD).[30] Patients with type 1 diabetes more commonly progress to ESRD than patients with type 2 diabetes.[31] The prevalence of diabetic kidney disease is 36% among the four cohorts of National Health and Nutrition Examination Survey participants in 2016, a decline from 44% previously.[32] Diabetic kidney disease is less common if the duration of diabetes is >10 years. The highest incidence rate, 3%, is seen 10–20 years after diabetes diagnosis. Native Americans, Hispanic individuals, Asians, and African Americans have a higher risk of developing diabetic kidney disease compared with non-Hispanic Caucasians.[33] The high morbidity of kidney disease related to diabetes makes effective patient education crucial. Table 5.6 presents patient teaching points concerning nephropathy.

Clinical Presentation of Nephropathy

The development of diabetic nephropathy is asymptomatic, and its detection relies on laboratory screening. The usual course of diabetic nephropathy in type 2 diabetes is not as stereotypical as in type 1 diabetes, but nephropathy tends to progress through several defined stages. The first sign of developing nephropathy is the occurrence of elevated albumin excretion (>30 mg albumin/24 h or spot albumin/creatinine >30 mg/g). Whether persistent albuminuria carries the same risk for the eventual development of clinical nephropathy in type 2 diabetes as seems to be the case in type 1 diabetes is unclear. As nephropathy progresses, "clinical" (dipstick positive, ≥300 mg albuminuria/24 h)

Table 5.6–What Patients Need to Know—Nephropathy

- Optimizing glycemic control prevents or delays nephropathy.
- Annual urine and blood tests are the only way to detect the "silent" onset of diabetic kidney disease.
- Regular blood pressure checks are vital because untreated hypertension damages the kidney, precipitating the onset of renal disease, and accelerates its progression.
- Effectively treating hypertension with medication, weight loss, and/or sodium restriction will help prevent or slow the progression of diabetic kidney disease.
- Consider newer anti-glycemic agents (sodium–glucose cotransporter 2 inhibitors [SGLT2i]), which delay the progression of established diabetic kidney disease.
- If there are signs of progressive nephropathy, explain the course of the disease and the options for treatment with dialysis and renal transplantation.

proteinuria occurs. In contrast to type 1 diabetes, hypertension usually is present before the development of clinical proteinuria. In addition, a significant proportion of patients with type 2 diabetes can develop renal insufficiency without significant albuminuria.[34] Eventually, nephrotic-range proteinuria develops, followed by decreasing GFR with rising serum creatinine, until ESRD occurs.

The importance of early identification is emphasized by evidence that intervention can lead to regression or remission of UACR of 30–299 mg/g,[35] whereas overt proteinuria (UACR >300 mg/day) is far more difficult to reverse. Nevertheless, specific interventions when overt proteinuria exists have been proven to slow the decline in GFR and reduce the incidence of kidney failure. Future approaches for early identification may include genetic screening for susceptibility loci and evaluation for early urinary biomarkers of diabetic renal disease.

Conditions That Influence Renal Function

Despite efforts at prevention, ~20%–40% of all patients with diabetes will develop some degree of nephropathy by 10 years after diagnosis.[7] In patients with diabetes, risk factors can be separated into those that increase susceptibility to damage, initiate damage, or cause progression of disease. These are summarized in Table 5.7.

Similar to DR, early intensive glycemic control delays the progression of diabetic kidney disease in patients with type 1 and type 2 diabetes.[37,38] In patients with type 2 diabetes enrolled in the UKPDS, there was a 24% reduction in microvascular complications, including diabetic kidney disease, in patients with early intensive glycemic control 10 years following the conclusion of the study, exemplifying the persistence of metabolic memory.[39] Intensive glycemic treatment in the ACCORD trial delayed the onset of albuminuria (UACR ≥300 mg/g).[40] Intensive glucose control in the ADVANCE trial was associated with a reduced risk of new or worsening nephropathy, new onset of albuminuria (UACR ≥300 mg/g).[41]

Hypertension may precipitate the onset or further accelerate the process of diabetic kidney disease. Systolic blood pressures >140 mmHg have been shown to increase the risk for ESRD and death by 38%.[42] In a recent meta-analysis, systolic blood pressure lowering <140 mmHg was associated with an absolute risk reduction of 9% in albuminuria in addition to a significantly lower risk of mortality.[43] Virtually all patients with diabetes who develop nephropathy develop hypertension.

Prevention and Treatment of Diabetic Renal Disease

Two methods can be used for albuminuria screening: measurement of the albumin-to-creatinine ratio in a random spot collection or a 24-h collection with creatinine, allowing the simultaneous measurement of creatinine clearance.[7] The spot measurement of the albumin-to-creatinine ratio is the easiest to perform and has a good predictive value. A value of >30 mg/g creatinine or an albumin excretion of >30 mg/24 h is considered abnormal. Due to the variability of urinary albumin excretion, two different specimens should be collected within 3–6 months of confirming the diagnosis. Elevated urine albumin not necessarily associated with nephropathy can be seen with exercise, infection, fever, congestive heart failure, marked hyperglycemia, menstruation, and marked hypertension around the time of the urine collection.[7] For screening purposes, serum creatinine with estimation

Table 5.7–Risk Factors for Diabetic Kidney Disease

Risk factor	Susceptibility	Initiation	Progression
Demographic			
Older age	+		
Sex (men)	+		
Race/ethnicity (black, American Indian, Hispanic, Asian/Pacific Islanders)	+		+
Hereditary			
Family history of diabetic kidney disease	+		
Genetic kidney disease		+	
Systemic conditions			
Hyperglycemia	+	+	+
Obesity	+	+	+
Hypertension	+	+	+
Kidney injuries			
Acute kidney injury		+	+
Toxins		+	+
Smoking	+		+
Dietary factors			
High protein intake	+		+

Source: Alicic.[36]

of GFR and urine albuminuria assessment should be done at diagnosis of type 2 diabetes and repeated at least twice annually in the presence of albuminuria.[7]

The presence of persistent albuminuria may be the first indication of incident nephropathy and, if present, should prompt aggressive treatment of even modestly elevated blood pressure, as studies have shown that improved blood pressure control can reduce hypertension-exacerbated albuminuria and delay progression of kidney disease.[44] ACE inhibitors and ARBs are particularly beneficial as they have been shown to slow the progression of UACR of 30–299 mg/g to clinical proteinuria and the development of ESRD.[45,46] ACE inhibitors and ARBs appear to provide equivalent benefit in diabetic kidney disease and can be used in patients with persistent albuminuria.[47] For this reason, guidelines advocate for the use of ACE inhibitors/ARBs, even in nonhypertensive patients with a UACR of 30–299 mg/g. However, there is no preventive role for ACE inhibitors or ARBs in patients with diabetes who have normal blood pressure and normal urine albumin levels.[7]

Combining ACE inhibitors with ARBs might further reduce albuminuria, but it does not appear to provide any benefit to renal function; the combination is associated with an increased risk of hyperkalemia and acute kidney injury, and it should be avoided.[48,49] In patients with diabetes with aldosterone escape (the return of protein excretion to pretreatment values after months or years), mineralocorticoid receptor antagonists (aldosterone antagonists) such as spironolactone, eplerenone, or finerenone have been shown to reduce proteinuria and can be used to treat resistant hypertension.[50-52] An additional intervention is the renin blocker aliskiren, which when given in addition to ARBs—as reported in the Aliskiren in the Evaluation of Proteinuria in Diabetes (AVOID) study—caused further reduction of albuminuria in patients with type 2 diabetes.[53] Longer-term studies are needed to better understand if these additional interventions can impact the progression of diabetic nephropathy.

In the past few years, multiple Food and Drug Administration (FDA)-mandated cardiovascular outcome trials have been conducted on some of the newer antidiabetic drug classes, including dipeptidyl peptidase-4 inhibitors (DDP4i), glucagon-like peptide 1 (GLP-1) receptor agonists, and sodium–glucose cotransporter-2 inhibitors (SGLT2i). In many of these trials, which enrolled individuals with type 2 diabetes with or at high risk for CVD, renal effects were examined as secondary outcomes, with one trial (CREDENCE) looking at kidney function as a primary end point.

The renal outcomes of patients taking DPP-4i have been examined only as a secondary end point in most trials to date. These are summarized in Table 5.8. Most of the DPP-4i currently approved have no significant impact on improving renal function; in the SAVOR-TIMI 53 trial saxagliptin showed improvement in subjects with UACR of 30–299 mg/g compared with a placebo. More information about DPP-4i may be found in Chapter 3.

Table 5.8–Summary of Renal Outcomes with the Use of Dipeptidyl Peptidase-4 Inhibitors*

Medication	Urinary albumin excretion (mg/g creatinine)	Progression to ESRD	Death due to renal failure	Sustained decrease of ≥40% in eGFR from baseline	Summary
Alogliptin[54]	Reduced by 1 mg/g creatinine at 78 weeks			Reduced by 1 ml/min/1.73 m² at 26 weeks	No clinical impact on diabetic renal disease
Linagliptin[55]	No difference	No difference	No difference	No difference	
Sitagliptin[56]	Not measured	Not measured	Not measured	Reduced by 1.34 ml/min/1.73 m² at 26 weeks	
Saxagliptin[57]	Improvement	Not measured	Not measured	Not measured	Improvement in UACR of 30–299 mg/g

eGFR, estimated glomerular filtration rate; ESRD, end-stage renal disease.

*All measured as secondary outcomes after primary end point of trial met; treatment comparison is to placebo.

Table 5.9—Summary of Renal Outcomes with the Use of Glucagon-like Peptide 1 Receptor Agonists*

Medication	Urinary albumin excretion (mg/g creatinine)	Progression to ESRD	Death due to renal failure	Sustained decrease of ≥40% in eGFR from baseline	Summary
Dulaglutide[58]	Not measured	Not measured	Not measured		No clinical impact on diabetic kidney disease
Exenatide[59]	Less progression of UACR ≥ 300 mg/g				Unclear impact on diabetic kidney disease
Liraglutide[60]	Less progression to UACR 30–299 mg/g	No significant change	No significant change		Less progression of disease
Lixisenatide[61]	Less incidence of UACR 30–299 mg/g and progression to UACR ≥ 300 mg/			No significant change	Less incidence and progression of disease
Semaglutide[62]	Less persistence of UACR ≥ 300 mg/		Not measured		Less progression of disease

GFR, estimated glomerular filtration rate; ESRD, end-stage renal disease.

*All measured as secondary outcomes after primary end point of trial met.

The renal outcomes of patients taking GLP-1 receptor agonists has also been examined as a secondary end point. These are summarized in Table 5.9. Most of the GLP-1 receptor agonists currently approved have an impact on the incidence and/or progression of albuminuria (UACR of 30–299 mg/g) with the exception of dulaglutide, which did not assess albuminuria. In general, GLP-1 receptor agonists are beneficial in patients with diabetic nephropathy. More information about GLP-1 receptor agonists may be found in Chapter 3.

The renal outcomes of patients taking SGLT2i have been examined as a primary end point in the CREDENCE trial using canagliflozin and as a secondary end point in trials for empagliflozin and dapagliflozin. These are summarized in Table 5.10. All of the SGLT2i show improvement in various aspects of diabetic kidney disease, but only dapagliflozin shows this improvement with patients who have an eGFR of 60 ml/min/1.73 m^2 or greater. Given their class effect, SGLT2i should be strongly considered in patients with diabetic nephropathy. More information about SGLT2i may be found in Chapter 3.

With regards to blood pressure management in patients with diabetic nephropathy, the American College of Cardiology and the American Heart Association recommend initiation or titration of antihypertensive medications to a target blood pressure of <130/80 mmHg,[67] while the American Diabetes Association[68] and the Eighth Joint National Commission on High Blood Pressure (JNC 8)[69] recommend a target of <140/90 mmHg or <130/80 mmHg based on individual characteristics. All agree that diuretics, ACE inhibitors, ARBs, and calcium channel blockers may all be used as first-line therapy for treatment of hypertension. ACE inhibitors and ARBs should be considered in the presence of persistent albuminuria even when blood pressure is not elevated.[67-69]

In patients with chronic kidney disease not requiring dialysis, dietary protein intake should be ~0.8 g/kg/day, which is the usual daily recommended allowance.[30] In addition, sodium intake should be limited to <2,300 mg daily to facilitate blood pressure control and reduce CVD risk.[70] In patients with reduced eGFR, potassium levels should be monitored and potassium intake restricted in the setting of hyperkalemia.[68]

Consultation with a nephrologist is suggested in specific circumstances: (a) uncertainty about the etiology of kidney disease (e.g., in a patient with nephropathy and no retinopathy), (b) rapid decline in GFR, (c) GFR <30 ml/min requiring discussion of renal replacement options, (d) management of chronic kidney disease complications.[7] Nephrologists assist with patient education regarding renal disease, monitoring of renal disease progression, and blood pressure control. With further progression in renal insufficiency, the nephrologist's role expands to include managing the secondary complications such as anemia and secondary hyperparathyroidism, which typically develop in late stage 3 chronic kidney disease (estimated GFR <40 ml/min). In addition, the role of the dietitian becomes increasingly important in assisting with management of sodium and protein intake, hyperphosphatemia, hyperkalemia, and overall nutrition.[7]

As patients with diabetes approach end-stage renal failure, the nephrologist assumes a more central role in the coordination of care. The primary goals of management at this stage are transplantation evaluation and preparation for dialysis, usually in parallel. Early referral to a nephrologist (i.e., >4 months before initiation of dialysis) has been associated with lower risk of death.[71] Because preemptive renal transplantation occurs in ~17% of cases,[72] dialysis preparation remains imperative. This practice involves patient education and training, coordination of Medicare and

Table 5.10—Summary of Renal Outcomes with the Use of Sodium–Glucose Cotransporter 2 Inhibitors

Medication	Urinary albumin excretion (mg/g creatinine)	Progression to ESRD	Death due to renal failure	Sustained decrease of ≥40% in eGFR from baseline	Summary
Canagliflozin[63,64]	Reduction regardless of prior renal status		Fewer deaths	No significant change	Improvement in incidence and progression of albuminuria, ESRD, death due to renal failure
Empagliflozin[65*]	Reduction in patients with UACR of 30–299 mg/g or eGFR <60 ml/min/1.73 m²	Less progression	No significant change	Reduction of serum creatinine doubling by 44%	Improvement in progression of albuminuria, ESRD, and doubling of eGFR
Dapagliflozin[66*]	Not measured				Improvement in ESRD, death due to renal failure, and sustained decrease of ≥40% in eGFR from baseline in patients with eGFR >60 ml/min/1.73 m² only

eGFR, estimated glomerular filtration rate.

*Measured as secondary outcomes after primary end point of trial met.

insurance coverage, and choosing a dialysis center. Renal nurses and social workers play prominent roles in this process. Another key aspect of dialysis preparation is vascular access planning, which requires cooperation among nephrologists, radiologists, and surgeons to determine the best approach for each individual patient.

In summary, diabetic kidney disease is a complication with significant morbidity and mortality. Optimal management requires cooperation and coordination among several specialties, with the roles of each specialty evolving as disease progression occurs.

DIABETIC FOOT PROBLEMS

Foot ulcers develop in 9.1–26.1 million people with diabetes annually worldwide, with 15%–25% of patients with diabetes developing a foot ulcer sometime during their lives.[73] Approximately 20% of moderate to severe diabetic infections lead to amputations.[74] Therefore, the clinician and patient who are conscientious about prevention, early detection, and prompt treatment of diabetic foot problems can make a significant impact on this complication.

Causes of Diabetic Foot Problems

Foot lesions in individuals with diabetes are the result of polyneuropathy, peripheral arterial disease, superimposed infection, foot deformity, or, most often, a combination of these complications.[75] A common pathway for the formation of diabetic foot ulcers is shown in Fig. 5.5. Damage from diabetic neuropathy can lead to foot deformity and callus formation, which can be followed by subcutaneous hemorrhage and ulcer formation. Neuropathic ulcers in the patient with diabetes often go undetected because they are usually painless.

In most patients with diabetes who have foot lesions, the primary pathophysiological event is the development of an insensitive foot secondary to polyneuropathy. Loss of foot sensation is often, but not always, accompanied by decreased vibratory sense and loss of ankle deep tendon reflexes. In addition to insensitivity, neuropathy may ultimately lead to a deformed foot secondary to tendon shortening (contractures), which leads to decreased mobility of the toes, abnormality in weight-bearing, calluses, and development of classic "hammer toe" deformities. The combination of foot insensitivity and foot deformities that shift weight distribution promotes the development of foot ulcers. Neuropathy also causes decreased sweating and dry skin. If left untreated, cracked and thickened skin can lead to infections and ulcerations. Diabetic neuropathy is also associated with an increased risk of foot fractures, which is possibly increased by the use of thiazolidinediones.

Neuroarthropathy (Charcot arthropathy) is an underrecognized complication of diabetic neuropathy that can result in disabling foot deformities. It usually occurs in the presence of adequate circulation. It is characterized by disintegration and disorganization of the bones in the lower leg and foot and can be precipitated by minimal trauma. Early recognition and appropriate treatment (offloading and possibly bisphosphonates) can substantially reduce permanent deformities.

The sudden development of a painful distal foot lesion, usually secondary to trauma, may signify underlying peripheral arterial disease (PAD), which is associated with findings of decreased or absent pulses, dependent rubor, and pallor on elevation. Additionally, the patient's history may include decreased walking speed, leg fatigue, or claudication. Testing should include at least one of the following in patients with a diabetic foot ulcer and PAD: skin perfusion pressure (≥40 mmHg), toe pressure (≥30 mmHg), or transcutaneous oxygen pressure (TcPO₂ ≥25mmHg). Urgent intervention should be considered in patients with ankle-brachial index <50mm Hg, toe pressure <30 mmHg, or TcPO₂ <25 mmHg.[7] The extent of the vascular disease and its potential for treatment by surgical intervention can be determined by Doppler noninvasive techniques and arteriography. Revascularization procedures, such as angioplasty and bypass, are often helpful in treating patients with severe, disabling claudication (at rest) or nonhealing ulcers or to aid healing of an amputation incision. Unfortunately, surgical intervention is not always effective in individuals with diabetes because many have diffuse vascular disease.

Infection is a frequent complication of both vascular and neuropathic ulcers (Fig. 5.6). Studies indicate that these infections are often mixed and that gram-positive organisms predominate.

Prevention of Foot Problems

There are five key components to foot care management:[76]

1. Regular inspection and examination of the at-risk foot.
2. Identification of the at-risk foot.
3. Education of patient, family, and healthcare providers.
4. Appropriate footwear.
5. Treatment of nonulcerative pathology.

Regular inspection should be performed at least annually and at every visit[7] for patients with risk factors. Patients' feet should be examined while the patient is supine and standing. Shoes and socks should also be inspected. Lack of patient symptoms does not denote a lack of foot pathology, and a full history and examination should be performed. Elements of a comprehensive foot exam are summarized in Table 5.11.[76]

To test for sensory loss, all of the following examinations should be performed:[76]

1. Assess pressure perception using the 10-g Semmes-Weinstein monofilament. First, apply the monofilament on the patient's hands to teach him or her what to feel. Ask the patient to close his or her eyes. Test three sites on each foot: the big toe pulp and the first and fifth metatarsus heads (Fig. 5.7). Apply the filament perpendicular to test the skin surface with sufficient force to cause the filament to bend ~45° (Fig. 5.7) and ask the patient *if* and *where* he or she felt pressure applied. Repeat the measurement twice at each site per foot in random order. Report the result separately for each foot in a ratio (e.g., 4/6 means the patient felt 4 touches of 6; 6/6 means the patient felt each application). During the procedure also ensure the patient is not automatically answering positively by assessing whether the patient perceives the monofilament when no filament is applied; if this is the case, further explain this procedure and its importance, and repeat the entire procedure.
2. Assess vibratory sensation using a 128 Hz tuning fork. The exam is performed by placing the tuning fork perpendicular to the bony part on the dorsal side of the distal phalanx of the first toe. Apply this at least twice and

also perform a "mock" test where the tuning fork is not vibrating to assess for accuracy (Fig. 5.8).

3. Assess discrimination. Test pinprick sensation on the dorsum of the foot without penetrating the skin.
4. Assess tactile sensation. Use cotton wool on the dorsum of the foot.
5. Assess reflexes. Specifically examine the Achilles tendon reflexes.
6. Assess proprioception in the toes and if absent in the ankle joint.

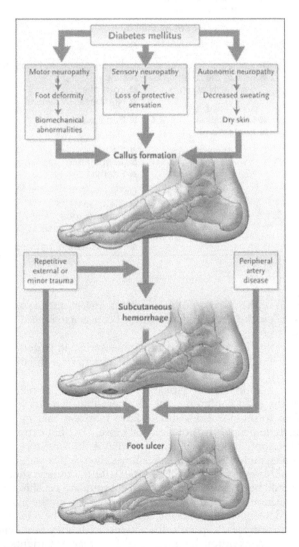

Figure 5.6 Common pathway of diabetic foot ulcer formation. *Source*: Armstrong.[74]

Table 5.11–History and Examination of Foot

History	History components
History	■ Previous ulcer/amputation ■ Previous foot education ■ Social isolation ■ Poor access to healthcare ■ Barefoot walking

	Foot examination	
	Symptoms	Signs
Neuropathy	■ Tingling in lower limb ■ Pain in the lower limb, especially at night	Using sensation and proprioception testing: ■ Loss of sensation ■ Numbness in general
Vascular status	■ Claudication ■ Rest pain	■ Pedal pulses
Skin		■ Color ■ Temperature ■ Edema
Bone/joint		Deformities: ■ Claw toes ■ Hammer toes ■ Bony prominences
Footwear/socks		■ Assessment of both inside and outside

Source: Bakker.[76]

Identification of the at-risk foot is critical for risk stratification. Fig. 5.9 presents examples of at-risk deformities and areas of concern in regard to callus formation as well.

Patient education is a critical preventive measure, and patient understanding of the education should be assessed. Table 5.12 summarizes the major points that should be covered.

Though foot examination is critical to the prevention of ulcers, inappropriate footwear is the most common cause of ulceration. Patients with neuropathy, ischemia, and/or foot deformities should have footwear that meets certain criteria. These include proper fit (not tight or loose), 1–2 cm extra length beyond the length of the foot, and ensuring the internal width of the shoe is as wide as the metatarsal phalangeal joints.[76] Furthermore, the toe box should be broad and square, laces should have three or four eyes per side, the tongue should be padded, and the shoe should be of a sufficient size to accommodate a cushioned insole. This allows for the cushioning and redistribution of pressure on the plantar surface of the foot.[7] If foot deformities are present, the patient should be referred for possible custom insoles or orthoses.[76] Specifically, patients with bony foot deformities that do not conform to conventional, commercial footwear or patients with Charcot foot will need custom-molded shoes.

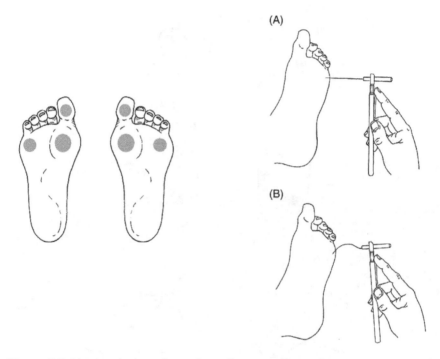

Figure 5.7 How and where to perform the monofilament exam.
Source: Bakker.[76]

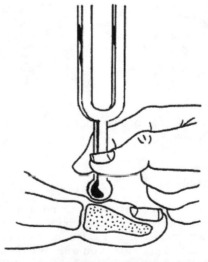

Figure 5.8 Application of the tuning fork for vibratory sensation testing.
Source: Bakker.[76]

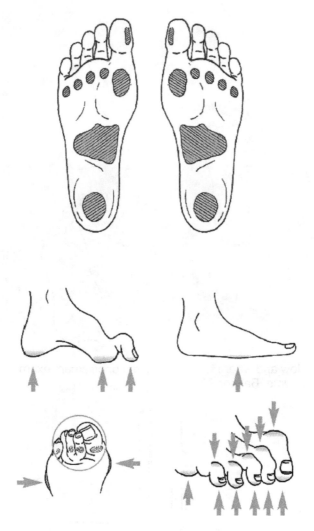

Figure 5.9 Examples and areas of increased risk of ulceration in the foot. *Source*: Bakker.[76]

Treatment of Foot Problems

Minor noninfected wounds can be treated with nonirritating antiseptic solution, daily dressing changes, and foot rest; use of antibiotics in noninfected wounds should be avoided.[77] More serious problems, such as foot deformities, infected lesions, and osteomyelitis, are best handled in consultation with specialists in diabetic foot care. Once an ulceration occurs, the likelihood for a poor and prolonged healing process is increased. Factors contributing to poor wound healing include male gender, duration

Table 5.12–What Patients Need to Know—Foot Care

- The patient, or family member in the case of a patient who is impaired by morbid obesity or blindness, has the major responsibility for prevention of foot problems.
- Cut toenails straight across and inspect the feet daily for cuts, abrasions, blisters, and corns.
- Regularly washing with warm water and mild soap, followed by thoroughly drying, is essential, especially between toes.
- Use moistening agents, such as lanolin, as needed but not between toes.
- Avoid prolonged soaking, strong chemicals such as Epsom salts or iodine, and "home surgery."
- Potential hazards that must be emphasized to all patients, especially those with peripheral neuropathy, are heat, cold, new shoes, constricting or mended socks, and, perhaps most important, going barefoot.
- Regular comprehensive foot exams should be completed by a healthcare provider.

Source: Bakker.[76]

of diabetes >10 years, older age, obesity, the presence of diabetic microvascular complications, peripheral vascular disease, elevated A1C, foot deformity, high plantar pressure, infections, and inappropriate foot self-care habits.[78] Infected foot ulcers usually require intravenous antibiotics, bedrest with foot elevation, and surgical debridement. Infection is a frequent complication of both vascular and neuropathic ulcers. Studies indicate that these infections are often mixed and that gram-positive organisms predominate.[77] Reducing plantar pressure using contact casts/specialized footwear accelerates healing. The utilization of shoes, insoles, and other modalities to offload plantar pressure sites is still the gold standard of care and maintenance, while total contact casting continues to be a more effective offloading device in the setting of healing ulcers.[79]

Charcot Foot

Charcot foot (neuropathic osteoarthropathy) is an underrecognized complication of diabetic peripheral neuropathy and is characterized by disintegration and disorganization of the bones in the foot and/or ankle. In the setting of sensory loss, repeated minor trauma triggers, via inflammation, various signaling pathways that result in bone destruction(3)(3).[80] It often presents as painless swelling of the ankle(s) associated with warmth, occasionally erythema and bounding peripheral pulses. The diagnosis is made based on clinical history, physical examination of the foot, and imaging.[81] Radiographic hallmarks of the disease include bony destruction, fragmentation, joint subluxation, and bony remodeling, which can be evident on X-rays, magnetic resonance imaging, or ultrasound. The proper treatment is immobilization of the limb with a total contact cast. Early recognition and appropriate treatment (offloading and total contact casting) can substantially reduce permanent deformities.

Acute Charcot foot usually presents as a red, swollen foot and should be immediately referred to a foot specialist. Promising therapies for acute Charcot foot are being investigated, including the use of bisphosphonates[82] and RANK-ligand monoclonal antibodies (denosumab).[83,84] Surgical intervention in acute or chronic Charcot foot are variable and are often used after the failure of conservative treatments or when surgical realignment is needed for severely deformed feet which predispose to foot ulceration.

DIABETIC NEUROPATHIES

The diabetic neuropathies are among the most common complications of diabetes. Neuropathy has a wide variety of manifestations in people with diabetes, and classification varies. An accepted classification is presented in Table 5.13.

Early recognition and appropriate management of neuropathy in patients with diabetes is important for a number of reasons: *1)* nondiabetic neuropathies may be present in patients with diabetes and may be treatable; *2)* a number of

Table 5.13–Classification of Diabetic Neuropathies

Diffuse neuropathy

	DSPN (Distal symmetric poly-neuropathy)	■ Primarily small-fiber neuropathy ■ Primarily large-fiber neuropathy ■ Mixed small- and large-fiber neuropathy (most common)
	Autonomic	■ Cardiovascular (reduced heart rate variability, resting tachycardia, orthostatic hypotension, sudden death from malignant arrhythmia) ■ Gastrointestinal (diabetic gastroparesis, enteropathy, colonic hypomotility) ■ Urogenital (diabetic cystopathy, erectile dysfunction, female sexual dysfunction) ■ Sudomotor dysfunction (distal hypohydrosis/anhidrosis, gustatory sweating) ■ Hypoglycemia unawareness [see section 4c, Special Therapeutic Situations: Major Acute Complications] ■ Abnormal pupillary function

Mononeuropathy (mononeuritis multiplex)

	Isolated cranial or peripheral nerve	
	Mononeuritis multiples	If confluent, can resemble polyneuropathy

Radiculopathy or polyradiculopathy

	Radiculoplexus neuropathy	Examples include lumbosacral polyra-diculopathy, proximal motor amytrophy
	Thoracic radiculopathy	

Common nondiabetic neuropathies

	Pressure palsies
	Chronic inflammatory demy-elinating polyneuropathy
	Radiculoplexus neuropathy

(continued)

Table 5.13 *(continued)*

Acute painful small-fiber neuropathies	Treatment induced
Hypothyroidism	
Folic acid/ Cyanobalamin deficiency	
Uremia	
Chronic alcoholism	
Chemotherapy	
Malignancy	
Infections	
Vasculitis	
Inherited neuropathies	
Syphilis	

Source: Pop-Busui.[85]

treatment options exist for symptomatic diabetic neuropathy; *3)* ≤50% of diabetic neuropathies may be asymptomatic, and patients are at risk of insensate injury to their feet.[85] Prevention of diabetic neuropathy by intensive glycemic control has been well shown in type 1 diabetes but less clearly in type 2 diabetes.[86]

Screening consists of assessment for distal symmetric polyneuropathy starting at diagnosis for patients with type 2 diabetes and after 5 years of diagnosis for patients with type 1 diabetes and annually thereafter.[7] Assessment should include a history and either temperature or pinprick sensation along with vibration sensation using a 128-Hz tuning fork. Annual 10-g monofilament testing in the feet should also be performed, as detailed earlier. Electrophysiological testing and referral to a neurologist for additional evaluation is rarely needed and should be done in patients with atypical neurologic symptoms such as motor greater than sensory neuropathy.[85]

The presence and severity of the neuropathy generally relates to the duration of diabetes and degree of hyperglycemia. In people with type 2 diabetes, neuropathy may be present at diagnosis. Painful neuropathy has also been identified in subjects with impaired glucose tolerance. Diabetic neuropathy is often associated with retinopathy and nephropathy. Both symptoms and deficits may have an adverse effect on quality of life in patients with neuropathy.

Symptoms and Diagnosis of Neuropathy

Based upon the type of nerve fibers affected, symptoms of neuropathy can vary (see Table 5.14). Assessment should follow the typical pattern of diabetic sensory neuropathy, which usually begins distally and moves proximally.

Because there are no distinguishing features unique to diabetic neuropathy, which should be considered a diagnosis of exclusion, all other possible causes of the neuropathy must be ruled out by careful history, physical exam, and laboratory testing.[87]

Table 5.14–Assessment for Diabetic Neuropathy

	Large myelinated nerve fibers	Small myelinated nerve fibers
Function	Pressure, balance	Nociception, protective sensation
Symptoms	Numbness, tingling, poor balance	Pain: burning, electric shocks, stabbing
Examination	Reduced or absent: ■ Ankle reflexes ■ Vibration perception ■ 10-g monofilament ■ Proprioception	Reduced or absent: ■ Hot/cold discrimination ■ Pinprick sensation

Source: Pop-Busui.[85]

These include hypothyroidism, folic acid/cyanocobalamin deficiency, uremia, chronic alcoholism, chemotherapy, renal disease, malignancy, infections, vasculitis, inherited neuropathies, syphilis, and chronic inflammatory demyelinating neuropathy.

The most common early symptom of diabetic neuropathy is from small fiber damage, which presents as pain and dysesthesias. Pain is also the most common cause for patients with diabetes to seek evaluation of neuropathy.[85]

Peripheral neuropathy commonly manifests as decreased tactile sensation, lack of temperature discrimination, sensory loss, and muscle weakness. Inability to walk on the heels is a sign of more severe neuropathy. The muscular weakness may lead to foot deformity, such as hammertoes and abnormal weight-bearing. The insensitivity leads to neglect of discomfort and injury, and contributes to the generation of foot ulcers (neurotrophic ulcers) and Charcot joints. Although polyneuropathy can affect the hands, most often hand symptoms are caused by carpal tunnel syndrome or ulnar neuropathy.

Treatment of Neuropathy

While tight glycemic control may prevent neuropathy,[86,88] it has not been shown to be an effective treatment of neuropathy.[88] Lifestyle modifications including aerobic exercise or resistance training as well as diet modification have shown some benefit in treatment in some studies.[89,90]

Painful peripheral neuropathy can be severe and debilitating and can impact quality of life, mobility, mood, and social interactions.[91] Treatment of painful neuropathy is limited to pharmacologic intervention,[92] is usually only partially effective, and is associated with frequent side effects. As such, pharmacologic treatment should be reserved for symptoms that interfere with quality of life or activities of daily living. While there are three FDA-approved treatments for painful neuropathy in the U.S. (pregabalin, duloxetine, and tapentadol), other options have been used for relief of painful symptomatology. Table 5.15 summarizes the most common pharmacologic interventions for neuropathic pain.

Autonomic Neuropathy

Diminished autonomic nerve function can cause a variety of signs and symptoms. Autonomic polyneuropathy, which usually occurs in concert with peripheral

Table 5.15–Pharmacologic Interventions for Neuropathic Pain

Medication	Most effective dose	Effect on neuropathic pain	Common side effects
Calcium channel α2-δ subunit ligands			
Gabapentin[93]*	1,200–3,600 mg daily	10%–20% reduction in pain	Dizziness, somnolence, water retention, and gait disturbance
Pregabalin[94]*	457–555 mg bid	48%–52% reduction in pain, seen as early as 1 week into treatment	Dizziness, nausea, vertigo, and somnolence
Selective norepinephrine and serotonin reuptake inhibitor			
Duloxetine[95]*	50 mg daily	<50% reduction in pain	Usually minor
Venlafaxine[96]	75–225 mg daily	Limited information about efficacy, not a first-line agent	Somnolence, dizziness, mild gastrointestinal symptoms
Opioid and atypical opioid analgesics: In general, the opioid analgesic class of medications offers very limited therapeutic benefit to patients with diabetic neuropathy. They should not be considered as first- or second-line therapy.			
Tapendatol extended release[97]*	100–250 mg bid	<30% reduction in pain	Nausea, anxiety, diarrhea, and dizziness, tolerance and addiction (less than others in this class)
Tramadol[98]*	100–400 mg daily	20% reduction in pain	
Extended release oxycodone[99]*	Poor evidence for efficacy		Withdrawal symptoms
Tricyclic antidepressants			
Amitryptiline[100]	Poor evidence for efficacy but anecdotal evidence shows benefit in a limited number of patients		
Nortryptiline[101]	Poor evidence for efficacy due to small trial size. Use pregabalin and/or duloxetine first.	Can be useful in patients with more nighttime symptoms	Contraindicated in patients with urinary retention and prolonged QT interval
Desipramine[102]	Poor evidence for efficacy due to trial design and bias. Do not use as first-line agent.		

*FDA-approved for treatment of neuropathic pain.

sensorimotor neuropathy, includes gastroparesis, diabetic diarrhea, constipation, fecal incontinence, neurogenic bladder, gustatory sweating, impaired cardiovascular reflexes and orthostatic hypotension, sexual dysfunction in men, dyspareunia in women, hypoglycemia unawareness, resting tachycardia, and sudomotor dysfunction, including both excessive and reduced sweating.[7] Clinically, autonomic neuropathy can develop as early as within a year of diagnosis of type 2 diabetes.[103]

Cardiovascular Autonomic Neuropathy

Cardiovascular autonomic neuropathy (CAN) represents the impairment of cardiovascular autonomic control in the setting of diabetes after the exclusion of other causes.[104] The prevalence of CAN is estimated to be between 20% and 73% in patients with type 2 diabetes.[105] CAN can be associated with coronary vessel ischemia, arrhythmias, silent myocardial infarctions, severe orthostatic hypotension, and sudden death syndrome.[106]

Risk factors and progression of disease. Established risk factors for developing CAN and disease progression include level of glycemic control, diabetes disease duration, hypertension, UACR of 30–299 mg/g, and dyslipidemia.[107] Predictors of CAN development include being female,[108] older age, and the presence of microvascular disease.[107]

Fig. 5.10 summarizes the natural progression of CAN. Subclinical CAN has a very subtle presentation and is often missed.

Screening, clinical manifestations, and diagnosis. Screening for CAN should be done at the time of diagnosis with patients with type 2 diabetes and particularly

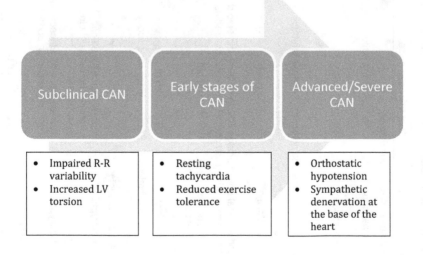

Figure 5.10 Natural progression of CAN. *Source:* Dimitropoulos.[105]

in patients with other macro-/microvascular complications[104] and a history of poor glycemic control.[109]

The most common manifestation of CAN is resting tachycardia with a heart rate of 90–130 bpm,[110] while a fixed heart rate lacking variation with sleep, stress, or exercise is often a sign of complete cardiac denervation.[111] Other clinical manifestations include exercise intolerance, orthostatic hypotension, silent ischemia, diabetic cardiomyopathy with subsequent left ventrical dysfunction, sudden cardiac death, perioperative and intraoperative complications, cerebrovascular disease, diabetic nephropathy, and lower limb vascular and neurologic complications.[105]

Assessment for CAN is described in Table 5.16.

Table 5.16–Testing for CAN

Test	How to perform test	Normal result
Heart response to deep breathing	■ Have patient perform paced deep breathing (expiration 5 sec, inspiration 5 sec) for a total of 6 cycles over 5 min. ■ Test heart rate using an electrocardiogram (ECG) over 120 consecutive beats (recording R-R interval).	■ Expect large accelerations during inspiration. ■ Expect large decelerations during expiration. ■ Average of either should not be lower than 10–15 beats/min.
Response to standing	Have patient lay down. ■ Test heart rate using an ECG from laying down to 45 sec after standing (recording R-R interval). ■ Note when patient stands.	1. Calculate the longest R-R interval between heart beats 20–40 after standing. 2. Calculate the shortest R-R interval between heart beats 5–25 after standing. 3. Calculate the ratio of 1 and 2; it should be at least 1.04.
Response to Valsalva maneuver	■ Have patient sit at rest for 15–20 min. ■ Have patient blow into specialized tube to maintain 40 mmHg for 15 sec. ■ Clamp nose and release after 15 sec. ■ Record R-R interval starting at rest through 40 beats after clamp release. ■ Perform three times and calculate the mean value.	1. Calculate the longest R-R interval after the clamp is removed. 2. Calculate the shortest R-R interval while the clamp is on. 3. Calculate the ratio of 1 and 2; it should be above 1.21.
Blood pressure response to standing	■ Have patient rest supine. ■ Measure blood pressure. ■ Have patient stand and remeasure blood pressure after 3 min.	■ Systolic blood pressure should not decline >20 mmHg. ■ Diastolic blood pressure should not decline >10 mmHg.

Source: Zygmunt.[112]

Criteria for CAN diagnosis and staging are (1) one abnormal cardio-vagal test identifies possible or early CAN; (2) at least two abnormal cardio-vagal tests are required for definite or confirmed CAN; and (3) the presence of orthostatic hypotension, in addition to heart rate test abnormalities, identifies severe or advanced CAN. Progressive stages of CAN are associated with an increasingly worse prognosis.[113]

The presence of CAN may identify patients with diabetes who are more prone to the dangerous effects of hypoglycemia, in particular among the group with cardiac disease.[114] Thus, CAN testing may serve to define the target of glycemic control according to the patient's risk profile and also to balance the advantage of aggressive diabetes treatment against the risk. However, it is still unproven that the presence of CAN should be a contraindication for intensive glycemic control.

Management of CAN. Unlike in type 1 diabetes, where intensive insulin treatment can improve CAN,[115] an intensive multifactorial cardiovascular risk intervention is required to reduce the progression or development of CAN among patients with type 2 diabetes and UACR of 30–299 mg/g. Multifactorial cardiovascular risk reduction was accomplished with a stepwise program of behavior modification and pharmacotherapy targeting hyperglycemia, hypertension, dyslipidemia, and UACR of 30–299 mg/g in addition to aspirin for secondary prevention of cardiovascular disease.[107]

There have been no particular lifestyle modifications that have been shown to prevent or treat CAN. Patients with autonomic neuropathy have an increased risk of exercise-induced injury through decreased cardiac responsiveness to exercise; they also experience impaired thermoregulation, orthostatic hypotension, impaired night vision, and greater susceptibility to hypoglycemia.[113] Patients with CAN should avoid high-intensity exercise without clearance from a physician and should be counseled about possible hypotension after vigorous activity. They should avoid physical exertion in hot or cold environments due to impaired thermoregulation. Recumbent cycling or water aerobics may be safer than standard exercise recommendations in patients with diabetes and in patients with orthostatic hypotension.[106]

Patients with orthostatic hypotension may find relief by nonpharmacological treatments such as (1) avoiding sudden changes in body posture to the head-up position; (2) avoiding medications that aggravate hypotension, such as tricyclic antidepressants and phenothiazines; (3) eating small, frequent meals to avoid the postprandial hypotension that may occur after a large carbohydrate-containing meal; (4) avoiding activities that involve straining; (5) elevating the head of the bed; and (6) wearing compression stockings.[116]

Physical activity and exercise should be encouraged to prevent deconditioning with repletion of fluid and salt as well.[7]

Pharmacologic agents for the treatment of orthostatic hypotension are summarized in Table 5.17. It is important to weigh the risks and benefits of using these medications in the context of preexisting comorbidities as these could be exacerbated. These patients tend to have supine hypertension requiring the use of short-acting medications such as guanfacine or clonidine (affect baroreceptor activity), isradipine (shorter-acting calcium blocker), or atenolol or metoprolol tartrate (shorter-acting beta blockers). Enalapril can be used as an alternative if other agents are not tolerated.[7]

Table 5.17–Pharmacologic Therapies for the Treatment of Orthostatic Hypotension

Medication	Dosage	Side effects
Midodrine	2.5 mg–10 mg tid	Piloerection, paresthesias, urinary retention, supine hypertension
Droxidopa	300 mg–1,800 mg/day	Headache, hypertension, dizziness, nausea
Fludrocortisone	0.05 mg–0.2 mg daily	Supine hypertension, hypokalemia, hypomagnesemia; doses >0.3mg/daily associated with fluid retention, hypertension, congestive heart failure
Erythropoietin	25–75 units/kg three times weekly	Hypertension, headache, thrombosis
Nonselective β-blockers	No clear evidence for efficacy in treating CAN	
Clonidine	0.1–0.6 mg/day	Limited use due to inconsistent hypertensive effect and serious side effects
Somatostatin analogs	25–200 µg/day	Use with caution as cases of severe hypertension have been reported
Pyridostigmine bromide[117]	60 mg daily	Nausea, diarrhea, abdominal cramps

Source: Pop-Busui.[116]

Gastroparesis

Autonomic neuropathic disorders of the gastrointestinal tract include esophageal dysmotility, gastroparesis, and diabetic enteropathies (i.e., small bowel dysmotility syndromes, diabetic diarrhea, and fecal incontinence).[118] Up to 30% of patients with type 2 diabetes are thought to have gastroparesis.[119]

Clinical manifestations and diagnosis. The diagnosis of diabetic gastroparesis is made by a combination of symptoms and signs along with delayed gastric emptying in the absence of mechanical obstruction. Prior to undergoing specialized testing, organic causes of gastric outlet obstruction or peptic ulcer disease must be ruled out using a either esophagogastroduodenoscopy or barium stomach study.[7] Symptoms and signs include early satiety, postprandial fullness, nausea, vomiting, bloating, and upper abdominal pain. A gastric emptying study should be performed, with the most conventional method being scintigraphy. Patients eat a meal of sulfur colloid–labeled egg with jam, toast, and water as recommended by the Society of Nuclear Medicine and the American Neurogastroenterology and Motility Society.[120] Measurements should be taken every 15 min over 4 h. Alternatively, breath tests using ^{13}C-octanoate or -spirulina have been shown to be effective in assessing gastric emptying but still require further validation prior to being recommended as a true alternative to scintigraphy.[121] It is important to note that significant hyperglycemia (>275mg/dL) can delay gastric emptying, so the fasting blood glucose should be less than this value at the time of testing.[122,123]

Treatment of gastroparesis. Patients with gastroparesis are at risk for nutritional deficiencies due to poor oral intake/tolerance, and nutritional support should be offered as needed. Meals should be smaller (and more frequent) and contain low-fat and low-residue/fiber. Increasing the liquid component of the meal can also be beneficial.[121]

While the short- and long-term effect of glycemic control in treating gastroparesis is unclear, acute hyperglycemia can further slow gastric emptying and exacerbate symptomatology. It is important to note that while GLP-1 receptor agonists can delay gastric emptying and are relatively contraindicated in gastroparesis, DPP-4 inhibitors do not.[121] Other therapies that might slow gastric emptying should be reviewed and possibly modified or discontinued (i.e., opioids, trichloroacetic acids, pramlintide).

Table 5.18 summarizes the pharmacologic therapies for diabetic gastroparesis. Close monitoring for side effects and drug-drug interactions is warranted.

The benefits of surgical treatments, including venting gastrostomy, gastrojejunostomy, pyloroplasty, and gastrectomy, have shown some possible benefit, but further larger studies are needed.[121] Gastric pacing (electrical stimulation) is FDA approved for treatment of severe and refractory gastroparesis, although its efficacy is variable.[124]

Diabetic Enteropathy

Constipation alternating with diarrhea is the most common manifestation of diabetic enteropathy. Though diabetic enteropathy is most commonly seen in poorly controlled patients with diabetes who have autonomic neuropathy, other causes include pancreatic insufficiency, bile salt malabsorption, steatorrhea, and medications such as metformin. Treatment is based on symptom relief, correction of fluid and electrolyte deficits, improvement of nutrition and glycemic control, and management of the underlying condition. Caution should be used with antidiarrheal agents due to the risk of toxic megacolon. Rifaximin is ≤84% effective in

Table 5.18–Pharmacologic Therapies for Diabetic Gastroparesis

Medication	Dosage	Side effects
Metoclopramide	5 mg tid as starting dose	Tardive dyskinesia (can be reversed with antihistamines and benzodiazepines), use lowest therapeutic dose
Domperidone	10 mg tid as starting dose	QT prolongation, hyperprolactinemia, drug-drug interactions
Erythromycin	Tachyphylaxis with long-term treatment	QT prolongation, drug-drug interactions
Gastric electrical stimulation	Studies show improvement, but further studies are still needed before the therapy can be universally recommended	
Intrapyloric botulinum injection	Not recommended as an efficacious treatment for diabetic gastroparesis	

Source: Camilleri.[121]

treating bacterial overgrowth as are amoxicillin-clavulanic acid, doxycycline, ciprofloxacin, metronidazole, neomycin, and norfloxacin. Constipation can be treated with hydration, exercise, and increased fiber intake and in severe cases lactulose or osmotic laxatives. Prucalopride improves constipation but has not been specifically studied in diabetic enteropathy.[125]

Urologic Dysfunction

Over 50% of patients with diabetes have a urologic dysfunction, which includes diabetic bladder dysfunction, sexual dysfunction, and urinary tract infections.[126]

Bladder dysfunction (Neurogenic bladder). Long-standing diabetes causes dysfunction of the detrusor muscle leading to voiding difficulties, principally weak stream, postvoid residual volume, and impairment of bladder sensation. Neurogenic bladder is characterized by a pattern of frequent, small voiding and incontinence and may progress to urinary retention. There is no evidence to show that improved glycemic control prevents the development of diabetic bladder dysfunction. Treatment should be targeted at eliminating symptoms. Because the major symptom is urinary retention, cholinergic agents could be used in addition to scheduling voiding at regular intervals and massaging the lower abdomen to aid in fully emptying the bladder. Treatment for urinary leakage can include cholinergic agents, scheduled voiding, Kegel exercises to strengthen pelvic floor muscles, and surgical procedures such as the pelvic sling or bladder neck suspension in females and artificial urinary sphincter in males.[127]

Male sexual dysfunction. Erectile dysfunction (ED), the persistent inability to achieve or maintain penile erection for successful sexual intercourse, is a cause of decreased quality of life in men.[128] Men with diabetes have a threefold increase in probability of developing ED compared with those without.[129] ED is a well-recognized index of cardiovascular risk and an independent predictor of coronary artery disease and CVD mortality.[130]

The ED pathogenesis in diabetes is multifactorial, related to neuropathy, accelerated atherosclerosis, and endothelial cell dysfunction. The decreased availability of nitric oxide from endothelial cells causes insufficient relaxation of the vascular smooth muscle of the corpora cavernosa.[131]

Key diagnostic procedures of ED include a comprehensive history (sexual, medical, drug use, risk factor assessment, and psychosocial factors) and routine laboratory tests (A1C, fasting blood glucose, lipid profile, and total testosterone [if available: bio-available or free testosterone instead of total]). Use of a validated questionnaire, such as the Sexual Health Inventory for Men (SHIM), can aid in the characterization of frequency and severity of ED symptoms.[132] It is important to establish the nature of the erectile problem and to distinguish it from other forms of sexual difficulty, such as penile curvature or premature ejaculation. Drugs associated with ED include antipsychotic medications, antidepressants (tricyclics, selective serotonin reuptake inhibitors, monoamine oxidase inhibitors), and antihypertensives (β-blockers, calcium channel blockers, thiazide diuretics, and ACE inhibitors).[133]

When psychological and endocrine causes of impotence have been ruled out, treatment should begin with lifestyle modification. There is no clear data that improving glycemic control improves ED in patients with type 2 diabetes.

Lifestyle modification, including weight loss, low intake of saturated fat, high consumption of monounsaturated fat and fiber, and moderate physical activity, are strongly correlated with improvement in ED.[134] Alcohol consumption has been associated with erectile dysfunction, though the evidence is not definitive[135] and therefore should also be considered with lifestyle modification.

Phosphodiesterase-5 inhibitors (i.e., sildanafil, vardenafil, and tadalafil) are the first-line pharmacologic treatment for ED. They are effective in the treatment of ED but not as effective as in men without diabetes. Caution should be used in patients with unstable or severe angina, recent myocardial infarction, certain arrhythmias, poorly controlled hypertension, and concomitant use of nitrates. Intracavernosal injection of papaverine, phentolamine, and prostaglandin E1 and intra-urethral administration of prostaglandin E1 are good alternatives for patients who do not respond adequately to phosphodiesterase-5 inhibitors.[131]

Female sexual dysfunction. Female sexual dysfunction can encompass disorders of sexual desire, arousal, orgasm, and pain.[136] Women with diabetes have a higher frequency of female sexual dysfunction than women without diabetes.[137] Women with longer duration of diabetes, older age, higher BMI, presence of cardiovascular disease, and presence of diabetic complications more commonly have sexual dysfunction,[138] with metabolic syndrome, atherogenic dyslipidemia, marital status, and depression being independent predictors.[139]

The pathogenesis of female sexual dysfunction is also multifactorial, similar to male sexual dysfunction. Regulation of blood flow to the clitoris is governed by nitric oxide, as it is in men, and therefore, hyperglycemia can also cause the same endothelial dysfunction and reduction in nitric oxide. Hyperglycemia also reduced the hydration of vaginal mucus membranes.

Treatment begins with lifestyle changes, psychotherapy, and optimal glycemic control. Lifestyle changes mainly include engaging in physical activity and adopting diet modifications for the prevention of cardiovascular risk factors. Studies have shown that these changes have a positive association with improving sexual dysfunction. Treatment of concomitant depression and possibly hormone replacement therapy in postmenopausal women can be considered.[131] Flibanserin is the only medication approved for the treatment of female sexual interest/arousal disorder but is not indicated for women who may have this disorder secondary to a comorbid medical condition such as diabetes.[140]

Other Varieties of Diabetic Neuropathy

In addition to symmetric polyneuropathy, people with diabetes are subject to a variety of other neuropathic syndromes. These syndromes include lumbosacral plexus neuropathies (also called femoral neuropathy or diabetic amyotrophy), truncal radiculopathy, upper-limb mononeuropathies (the entrapment neuropathies—carpal tunnel syndrome and ulnar neuropathy, which are more common in people with diabetes), and cranial neuropathy. These varieties of neuropathy are asymmetric and abrupt or subacute in onset, and they tend to follow a monophasic course with improvement over time. Nerve entrapments may require surgical intervention.[85]

Lumbosacral plexus neuropathy begins with unilateral pain in the thigh or buttock, then typically spreads to other parts of the same limb and then to the opposite limb due to involvement of the lumbosacral roots, plexus, and peripheral nerves. Patients may present with asymmetric limb weakness with severe deep pain and possibly weight loss ≤20–30 kg. On examination, there will be asymmetric proximal muscle wasting and weakness, as well as loss of reflexes in the affected knee and ankle with minimal sensory loss. It is more common in men with type 2 diabetes. Diagnosis is made clinically as there is no definitive test to confirm the diagnosis. Treatment includes pain control (with possibly opiates at onset, amitriptyline 10–75mg at night for insomnia, nonsteroidal anti-inflammatory agents, gabapentin, and/or steroids), physiotherapy, and maintaining glycemic control. Recovery usually occurs in several months to a year.[141]

The most commonly affected cranial nerves in diabetes are 3, 4, and 6, which innervate the extraocular muscles. The presentation of cranial neuropathy is usually of an extraocular palsy with ptosis and possibly pupillary dysfunction. Deficits fade over days to months, with many individuals having complete resolution of symptoms.[142]

The diagnosis of a diabetic neuropathy is often easily made on clinical evaluation with little testing necessary. People with diabetes can have neuropathy unrelated to their diabetes. When the clinical features are not typical (i.e., unilateral, predominantly upper limb, rapidly progressive, mainly motor) or consistent with the duration of diabetes and presence of other complications, other causes of neuropathy should be excluded.

REFERENCES

1. Yau JW, Rogers SL, Kawasaki R, Lamoureux EL, Kowalski JW, Bek T, et al. Global prevalence and major risk factors of diabetic retinopathy. *Diabetes Care* 2012;35(3):556–564. doi: 10.2337/dc11-1909. Epub 2012 Feb 4. PubMed PMID: 22301125; PubMed Central PMCID: PMCPMC3322721

2. Centers for Disease Control and Prevention. Economic studies: Vision health initiative [Internet], 2019. Available from https://www.cdc.gov/visionhealth/projects/economic_studies.htm. Accessed 17 May 2019

3. Centers for Disease Control and Prevention. Facts about diabetic eye disease [Internet], 2019. Available from https://nei.nih.gov/health/diabetic/retinopathy. Accessed 16 April 2019

4. Wong TY, Sun J, Kawasaki R, Ruamviboonsuk P, Gupta N, Lansingh VC, et al. Guidelines on diabetic eye care: the International Council of Ophthalmology recommendations for screening, follow-up, referral, and treatment based on resource settings. *Ophthalmology* 2018;125(10): 1608–1622. doi: 10.1016/j.ophtha.2018.04.007. Epub 2018 May 20. PubMed PMID: 29776671

5. Zhang X, Zeng H, Bao S, Wang N, Gillies MC. Diabetic macular edema: new concepts in patho-physiology and treatment. *Cell Biosci* 2014;4:27. doi: 10.1186/2045-3701-4-27. Epub 2014 Jun 24. PubMed PMID: 24955234; PubMed Central PMCID: PMCPMC4046142

6. Bhagat N, Grigorian RA, Tutela A, Zarbin MA. Diabetic macular edema: pathogenesis and treatment. *Surv Ophthalmol* 2009;54(1):1–32.

doi: 10.1016/j.survophthal.2008.10.001. Epub 2009 Jan 28. PubMed PMID: 19171208

7. American Diabetes Association. 11. Microvascular complications and foot care: standards of medical care in diabetes 2020. *Diabetes Care* 2020;43(Suppl. 1):S135–S151. doi: 10.2337/dc20-S011. Epub 2019 Dec 22. PubMed PMID: 31862754

8. Diabetes Control Complications Trial Research Group, Nathan DM, Genuth S, Lachin J, Cleary P, et al. The effect of intensive treatment of diabetes on the development and progression of long-term complications in insulin-dependent diabetes mellitus. *N Engl J Med* 1993;329(14):977–986. doi: 10.1056/NEJM199309303291401. Epub 1993 Sep 30. PubMed PMID: 8366922

9. UK Prospective Diabetes Study (UKPDS) Group. Effect of intensive blood-glucose control with metformin on complications in overweight patients with type 2 diabetes (UKPDS 34). UK Prospective Diabetes Study (UKPDS) Group. *Lancet* 1998;352(9131):854–865. Epub 1998 Sep 22. PubMed PMID: 9742977

10. Aiello LP, Group DER. Diabetic retinopathy and other ocular findings in the diabetes control and complications trial/epidemiology of diabetes interventions and complications study. *Diabetes Care* 2014;37(1):17–23. doi: 10.2337/dc13-2251. Epub 2013 Dec 21. PubMed PMID: 24356593; PubMed Central PMCID: PMCPMC3867989

11. Ohkubo Y, Kishikawa H, Araki E, Miyata T, Isami S, Motoyoshi S, et al. Intensive insulin therapy prevents the progression of diabetic microvascular complications in Japanese patients with non-insulin-dependent diabetes mellitus: a randomized prospective 6-year study. *Diabetes Res Clin Pract* 1995;28(2):103–117. Epub 1995 May 1. PubMed PMID: 7587918

12. Klein R, Knudtson MD, Lee KE, Gangnon R, Klein BE. The Wisconsin Epidemiologic Study of Diabetic Retinopathy: XXII the twenty-five-year progression of retinopathy in persons with type 1 diabetes. *Ophthalmology* 2008;115(11):1859–1868. doi: 10.1016/j.ophtha.2008.08.023. Epub 2008 Dec 11. PubMed PMID: 19068374; PubMed Central PMCID: PMCPMC2761813

13. Keech AC, Mitchell P, Summanen PA, O'Day J, Davis TM, Moffitt MS, et al. Effect of fenofibrate on the need for laser treatment for diabetic retinopathy (FIELD study): a randomised controlled trial. *Lancet* 2007;370(9600):1687–1697. doi: 10.1016/S0140-6736(07)61607-9. Epub 2007 Nov 9. PubMed PMID: 17988728

14. The ACCORD Study Group, ACCORD Eye Study Group, Chew EY, Ambrosius WT, Davis MD, Danis RP, et al. Effects of medical therapies on retinopathy progression in type 2 diabetes. *N Engl J Med* 2010;363(3):233–244. doi: 10.1056/NEJMoa1001288. Epub 2010 Jul 1. PubMed PMID: 20587587; PubMed Central PMCID: PMCPMC4026164

15. The Diabetic Retinopathy Study Research Group. Preliminary report on effects of photocoagulation therapy. *Am J Ophthalmol* 1976;81(4):383–396. Epub 1976 Apr 1. PubMed PMID: 944535

16. Early Treatment Diabetic Retinopathy Study Research Group. Photocoagulation for diabetic macular edema. Early Treatment Diabetic Retinopathy Study report number 1. *Arch Ophthalmol* 1985;103(12):1796–1806. Epub 1985 Dec 1. PubMed PMID: 2866759

17. Stratton IM, Kohner EM, Aldington SJ, Turner RC, Holman RR, Manley SE, et al. UKPDS 50: risk factors for incidence and progression of retinopathy in type II diabetes over 6 years from diagnosis. *Diabetologia* 2001;44(2):156–163. doi: 10.1007/s001250051594. Epub 2001 Mar 29. PubMed PMID: 11270671

18. Estacio RO, Jeffers BW, Gifford N, Schrier RW. Effect of blood pressure control on diabetic microvascular complications in patients with hypertension and type 2 diabetes. *Diabetes Care* 2000;23(Suppl. 2):B54–B64. Epub 2000 Jun 22. PubMed PMID: 10860192

19. Chew EY, Ambrosius WT, Davis MD, Danis RP, Gangaputra S, Greven CM, et al. Effects of medical therapies on retinopathy progression in type 2 diabetes. *N Engl J Med* 2010;363(3):233–244. doi: 10.1056/NEJMoa1001288. Epub 2010 Jul 1. PubMed PMID: 20587587; PubMed Central PMCID: PMCPMC4026164

20. Shih CJ, Chen HT, Kuo SC, Li SY, Lai PH, Chen SC, et al. Comparative effectiveness of angiotensin-converting-enzyme inhibitors and angiotensin II receptor blockers in patients with type 2 diabetes and retinopathy. *CMAJ* 2016;188(8):E148–E157. doi: 10.1503/cmaj.150771. Epub 2016 Apr 24. PubMed PMID: 27001739; PubMed Central PMCID: PMCPMC4868622

21. Baker CW, Glassman AR, Beaulieu WT, Antoszyk AN, Browning DJ, Chalam KV, et al. Effect of initial management with aflibercept vs laser photocoagulation vs observation on vision loss among patients with diabetic macular edema involving the center of the macula and good visual acuity: a randomized clinical trial. *JAMA* 2019;321(19):1880–1894. doi: 10.1001/jama.2019.5790. Epub 2019 May 1. PubMed PMID: 31037289; PubMed Central PMCID: PMCPMC6537845

22. Diabetes Control and Complications Trial Research Group. Effect of pregnancy on microvascular complications in the diabetes control and complications trial. The Diabetes Control and Complications Trial Research Group. *Diabetes Care* 2000;23(8):1084–1091. Epub 2000 Aug 11. PubMed PMID: 10937502; PubMed Central PMCID: PMCPMC2631985

23. Mallika P, Tan A, S A, T A, Alwi SS, Intan G. Diabetic retinopathy and the effect of pregnancy. *Malays Fam Physician* 2010;5(1):2–5. Epub 2010 Jan 1. PubMed PMID: 25606177; PubMed Central PMCID: PMCPMC4170393

24. Klein BE, Klein R. Gravidity and diabetic retinopathy. *Am J Epidemiol* 1984;119(4):564–569. doi: 10.1093/oxfordjournals.aje.a113773. Epub 1984 Apr 1. PubMed PMID: 6711545

25. Gunderson EP, Lewis CE, Tsai AL, Chiang V, Carnethon M, Quesenberry CP, Jr., et al. A 20-year prospective study of childbearing and incidence of diabetes in young women, controlling for glycemia before conception: the

Coronary Artery Risk Development in Young Adults (CARDIA) Study. *Diabetes* 2007;56(12):2990–2996. doi: 10.2337/db07-1024. Epub 2007 Sep 28. PubMed PMID: 17898128; PubMed Central PMCID: PMCPMC2952440

26. Sokol JT, Schechet SA, Rosen DT, Ferenchak K, Dawood S, Skondra D. Outcomes of vitrectomy for diabetic tractional retinal detachment in Chicago's county health system. *PLoS One* 2019;14(8):e0220726. doi: 10.1371/journal.pone.0220726. Epub 2019 Aug 21. PubMed PMID: 31430299; PubMed Central PMCID: PMCPMC6701761

27. Ross WH. Visual recovery after macula-off retinal detachment. *Eye* 2002;16(4):440–446. doi: 10.1038/sj.eye.6700192. Epub 2002 Jul 9. PubMed PMID: 12101451

28. Writing Committee for the Diabetic Retinopathy Clinical Research Network, Gross JG, Glassman AR, Jampol LM, Inusah S, Aiello LP, et al. Panretinal photocoagulation vs intravitreous ranibizumab for proliferative diabetic retinopathy: a randomized clinical trial. *JAMA* 2015;314(20):2137–2146. doi: 10.1001/jama.2015.15217. Epub 2015 Nov 14. PubMed PMID: 26565927; PubMed Central PMCID: PMCPMC5567801

29. Sivaprasad S, Prevost AT, Vasconcelos JC, Riddell A, Murphy C, Kelly J, et al. Clinical efficacy of intravitreal aflibercept versus panretinal photocoagulation for best corrected visual acuity in patients with proliferative diabetic retinopathy at 52 weeks (CLARITY): a multicentre, single-blinded, randomised, controlled, phase 2b, non-inferiority trial. *Lancet* 2017;389(10085):2193–2203. doi: 10.1016/S0140-6736(17)31193-5. Epub 2017 May 13. PubMed PMID: 28494920

30. Tuttle KR, Bakris GL, Bilous RW, Chiang JL, de Boer IH, Goldstein-Fuchs J, et al. Diabetic kidney disease: a report from an ADA Consensus Conference. *Diabetes Care* 2014;37(10):2864–2883. doi: 10.2337/dc14-1296. Epub 2014 Sep 25. PubMed PMID: 25249672; PubMed Central PMCID: PMCPMC4170131

31. Gheith O, Farouk N, Nampoory N, Halim MA, Al-Otaibi T. Diabetic kidney disease: world wide difference of prevalence and risk factors. *J Nephropharmacol* 2016;5(1):49–56. Epub 2015 Oct 9. PubMed PMID: 28197499; PubMed Central PMCID: PMCPMC5297507

32. United States Renal Data System. 2019 USRDS Annual Data Report: Epidemiology of kidney disease in the United States [article online], 2019. National Institutes of Health, National Institute of Diabetes and Digestive and Kidney Diseases, Bethesda, MD, 2019.Available from https://www.usrds.org/2018/view/v1_01.aspx. Accessed 17 May 2019

33. Spanakis EK, Golden SH. Race/ethnic difference in diabetes and diabetic complications. *Curr Diab Rep* 2013;13(6):814–823. doi: 10.1007/s11892-013-0421-9. Epub 2013 Sep 17. PubMed PMID: 24037313; PubMed Central PMCID: PMCPMC3830901

34. Retnakaran R, Cull CA, Thorne KI, Adler AI, Holman RR, Group US. Risk factors for renal dysfunction in type 2 diabetes: U.K. Prospective Diabetes Study 74. *Diabetes* 2006;55(6):1832–1839. doi: 10.2337/db05-1620. Epub 2006 May 30. PubMed PMID: 16731850

35. Perkins BA, Ficociello LH, Silva KH, Finkelstein DM, Warram JH, Krolewski AS. Regression of microalbuminuria in type 1 diabetes. *N Engl J Med* 2003;348(23):2285–2293. doi: 10.1056/NEJMoa021835. Epub 2003 Jun 6. PubMed PMID: 12788992

36. Alicic RZ, Rooney MT, Tuttle KR. Diabetic kidney disease: challenges, progress, and possibilities. *Clin J Am Soc Nephrol* 2017;12(12):2032–2045. doi: 10.2215/CJN.11491116. Epub 2017 May 20. PubMed PMID: 28522654; PubMed Central PMCID: PMCPMC5718284

37. The Diabetes Control and Complications (DCCT) Research Group. Effect of intensive therapy on the development and progression of diabetic nephropathy in the Diabetes Control and Complications Trial. *Kidney Int* 1995;47(6):1703–1720. Epub 1995 Jun 1. PubMed PMID: 7643540

38. UK Prospective Diabetes Study (UKPDS) Group. Intensive blood-glucose control with sulphonylureas or insulin compared with conventional treatment and risk of complications in patients with type 2 diabetes (UKPDS 33). *Lancet* 1998;352(9131):837–853. PubMed PMID: 9742976

39. Holman RR, Paul SK, Bethel MA, Matthews DR, Neil HA. 10-Year follow-up of intensive glucose control in type 2 diabetes. *N Engl J Med* 2008;359(15): 1577–1589. doi: 10.1056/NEJMoa0806470. PubMed PMID: 18784090

40. Ismail-Beigi F, Craven TE, O'Connor PJ, Karl D, Calles-Escandon J, Hramiak I, et al. Combined intensive blood pressure and glycemic control does not produce an additive benefit on microvascular outcomes in type 2 diabetic patients. *Kidney Int* 2012;81(6):586–594. doi: 10.1038/ki.2011.415. Epub 2011 Dec 15. PubMed PMID: 22166848; PubMed Central PMCID: PMCPMC4641306

41. The ADVANCE Collaborative Group, Patel A, MacMahon S, Chalmers J, Neal B, Billot L, et al. Intensive blood glucose control and vascular outcomes in patients with type 2 diabetes. *N Engl J Med* 2008;358(24):2560–2572. doi: 10.1056/NEJMoa0802987. Epub 2008 Jun 10. PubMed PMID: 18539916

42. Bakris GL, Weir MR, Shanifar S, Zhang Z, Douglas J, van Dijk DJ, et al. Effects of blood pressure level on progression of diabetic nephropathy: results from the RENAAL study. *Arch Intern Med* 2003;163(13):1555–1565. doi: 10.1001/archinte.163.13.1555. Epub 2003 Jul 16. PubMed PMID: 12860578

43. Emdin CA, Rahimi K, Neal B, Callender T, Perkovic V, Patel A. Blood pressure lowering in type 2 diabetes: a systematic review and meta-analysis. *JAMA* 2015;313(6):603–615. doi: 10.1001/jama.2014.18574. Epub 2015 Feb 11. PubMed PMID: 25668264

44. Abraham PA, Mascioli SR, Launer CA, Flack JM, Liebson PR, Svendsen KH, et al. Urinary albumin and N-acetyl-beta-D-glucosaminidase excretions in mild hypertension. *Am J Hypertens* 1994;7(11):965–974. Epub 1994 Nov 1. PubMed PMID: 7848623

45. Sano T, Hotta N, Kawamura T, Matsumae H, Chaya S, Sasaki H, et al. Effects of long-term enalapril treatment on persistent microalbuminuria in normotensive type 2 diabetic patients: results of a 4-year, prospective, randomized study. *Diabet Med* 1996;13(2):120–124. doi: 10.1002/(SICI)1096-9136(199602)13:2<120::AID-DIA6>3.0.CO;2-F. Epub 1996 Feb 1. PubMed PMID: 8641115

46. Brenner BM, Cooper ME, de Zeeuw D, Keane WF, Mitch WE, Parving HH, et al. Effects of losartan on renal and cardiovascular outcomes in patients with type 2 diabetes and nephropathy. *N Engl J Med* 2001;345(12):861–869. doi: 10.1056/NEJMoa011161. Epub 2001 Sep 22. PubMed PMID: 11565518

47. Barnett A. Preventing renal complications in type 2 diabetes: results of the diabetics exposed to telmisartan and enalapril trial. *J Am Soc Nephrol* 2006;17(4 Suppl. 2):S132–S135. doi: 10.1681/ASN.2005121326. Epub 2006 Mar 28. PubMed PMID: 16565237

48. Fried LF, Emanuele N, Zhang JH, Brophy M, Conner TA, Duckworth W, et al. Combined angiotensin inhibition for the treatment of diabetic nephropathy. *N Engl J Med* 2013;369(20):1892–1903. doi: 10.1056/NEJMoa1303154. Epub 2013 Nov 12. PubMed PMID: 24206457

49. Liebson PR, Amsterdam EA. Ongoing Telmisartan Alone and in Combination With Ramipril Global Endpoint Trial (ONTARGET): implications for reduced cardiovascular risk. *Prev Cardiol* 2009;12(1):43–50. Epub 2009 Mar 24. PubMed PMID: 19301691

50. Bakris GL, Agarwal R, Chan JC, Cooper ME, Gansevoort RT, Haller H, et al. Effect of finerenone on albuminuria in patients with diabetic nephropathy: a randomized clinical trial. *JAMA* 2015;314(9):884–894. doi: 10.1001/jama.2015.10081. Epub 2015 Sep 2. PubMed PMID: 26325557

51. Williams B, MacDonald TM, Morant S, Webb DJ, Sever P, McInnes G, et al. Spironolactone versus placebo, bisoprolol, and doxazosin to determine the optimal treatment for drug-resistant hypertension (PATHWAY-2): a randomised, double-blind, crossover trial. *Lancet* 2015;386(10008):2059–2068. doi: 10.1016/S0140-6736(15)00257-3. Epub 2015 Sep 29. PubMed PMID: 26414968; PubMed Central PMCID: PMCPMC4655321

52. Sato A, Hayashi K, Naruse M, Saruta T. Effectiveness of aldosterone blockade in patients with diabetic nephropathy. *Hypertension* 2003;41(1):64–68. Epub 2003 Jan 4. PubMed PMID: 12511531

53. Persson F, Lewis JB, Lewis EJ, Rossing P, Hollenberg NK, Parving HH. Aliskiren in combination with losartan reduces albuminuria independent of baseline blood pressure in patients with type 2 diabetes and nephropathy. *Clin J Am Soc Nephrol* 2011;6(5):1025–31. doi: 10.2215/CJN.07590810. Epub 2011 Feb 26. PubMed PMID: 21350110; PubMed Central PMCID: PMCPMC3087767

54. Mita T, Katakami N, Yoshii H, Onuma T, Kaneto H, Osonoi T, et al. Alogliptin, a dipeptidyl peptidase 4 inhibitor, prevents the progression of carotid atherosclerosis in patients with type 2 diabetes: the Study of

Preventive Effects of Alogliptin on Diabetic Atherosclerosis (SPEAD-A). *Diabetes Care* 2016;39(1):139–148. doi: 10.2337/dc15-0781. Epub 2015 Dec 3. PubMed PMID: 26628419

55. Rosenstock J, Perkovic V, Johansen OE, Cooper ME, Kahn SE, Marx N, et al. Effect of linagliptin vs placebo on major cardiovascular events in adults with type 2 diabetes and high cardiovascular and renal risk: the CARMELINA randomized clinical trial. *JAMA* 2019;321(1):69–79. doi: 10.1001/jama.2018.18269. Epub 2018 Nov 13. PubMed PMID: 30418475

56. Green JB, Bethel MA, Armstrong PW, Buse JB, Engel SS, Garg J, et al. Effect of sitagliptin on cardiovascular outcomes in type 2 diabetes. *N Engl J Med* 2015;373(3):232–242. doi: 10.1056/NEJMoa1501352. Epub 2015 Jun 9. PubMed PMID: 26052984

57. Scirica BM, Bhatt DL, Braunwald E, Steg PG, Davidson J, Hirshberg B, et al. Saxagliptin and cardiovascular outcomes in patients with type 2 diabetes mellitus. *N Engl J Med* 2013;369(14):1317–1326. doi: 10.1056/NEJMoa1307684. Epub 2013 Sep 3. PubMed PMID: 23992601.

58. Tuttle KR, Lakshmanan MC, Rayner B, Busch RS, Zimmermann AG, Woodward DB, et al. Dulaglutide versus insulin glargine in patients with type 2 diabetes and moderate-to-severe chronic kidney disease (AWARD-7): a multicentre, open-label, randomised trial. *Lancet Diabetes Endocrinol* 2018;6(8):605–617. doi: 10.1016/S2213-8587(18)30104-9. Epub 2018 Jun 19. PubMed PMID: 29910024

59. Bethel MA, Mentz RJ, et al. Renal outcomes in the EXenatide Study of Cardiovascular Event Lowering (EXSCEL). *Diabetes* 2018;67 (Suppl. 1):522.

60. Mann JFE, Orsted DD, Brown-Frandsen K, Marso SP, Poulter NR, Rasmussen S, et al. Liraglutide and renal outcomes in type 2 diabetes. *N Engl J Med* 2017;377(9):839–848 doi: 10.1056/NEJMoa1616011. Epub 2017 Aug 31. PubMed PMID: 28854085

61. Muskiet MHA, Tonneijck L, Huang Y, Liu M, Saremi A, Heerspink HJL, et al. Lixisenatide and renal outcomes in patients with type 2 diabetes and acute coronary syndrome: an exploratory analysis of the ELIXA randomised, placebo-controlled trial. *Lancet Diabetes Endocrinol* 2018;6(11):859–869. doi: 10.1016/S2213-8587(18)30268-7. Epub 2018 Oct 8. PubMed PMID: 30292589

62. Marso SP, Bain SC, Consoli A, Eliaschewitz FG, Jodar E, Leiter LA, et al. Semaglutide and cardiovascular outcomes in patients with type 2 diabetes. *N Engl J Med* 2016;375(19):1834–1844. doi: 10.1056/NEJMoa1607141. Epub 2016 Sep 17. PubMed PMID: 27633186

63. Perkovic V, de Zeeuw D, Mahaffey KW, Fulcher G, Erondu N, Shaw W, et al. Canagliflozin and renal outcomes in type 2 diabetes: results from the CANVAS Program randomised clinical trials. *Lancet Diabetes Endocrinol* 2018;6(9):691–704. doi: 10.1016/S2213-8587(18)30141-30144. Epub 2018 Jun 26. PubMed PMID: 29937267

64. Perkovic V, Jardine MJ, Neal B, Bompoint S, Heerspink HJL, Charytan DM, et al. Canagliflozin and renal outcomes in type 2 diabetes and nephropathy. *N Engl J Med* 2019. doi: 10.1056/NEJMoa1811744. Epub 2019 Apr 17. PubMed PMID: 30990260

65. Wanner C, Inzucchi SE, Lachin JM, Fitchett D, von Eynatten M, Mattheus M, et al. Empagliflozin and progression of kidney disease in type 2 diabetes. *N Engl J Med* 2016;375(4):323–334. doi: 10.1056/NEJMoa1515920. Epub 2016 Jun 15. PubMed PMID: 27299675

66. Wiviott SD, Raz I, Bonaca MP, Mosenzon O, Kato ET, Cahn A, et al. Dapagliflozin and cardiovascular outcomes in type 2 diabetes. *N Engl J Med* 2019;380(4):347–357. doi: 10.1056/NEJMoa1812389. Epub 2018 Nov 13. PubMed PMID: 30415602

67. Whelton PK, Carey RM, Aronow WS, Casey DE, Jr., Collins KJ, Dennison Himmelfarb C, et al. 2017 ACC/AHA/AAPA/ABC/ACPM/AGS/APhA/ASH/ASPC/NMA/PCNA guideline for the prevention, detection, evaluation, and management of high blood pressure in adults: executive summary: a report of the American College of Cardiology/American Heart Association Task Force on clinical practice guidelines. *J Am Soc Hypertens* 2018;12(8):579, e1–e73. doi: 10.1016/j.jash.2018.06.010. Epub 2018 Sep 17. PubMed PMID: 30219548

68. American Diabetes Association. 10. Cardiovascular disease and risk management: standards of medical care in diabetes 2020. *Diabetes Care* 2020;43(Suppl. 1): S111–S134. doi: 10.2337/dc20-S010. Epub 2019 Dec 22. PubMed PMID: 31862753

69. James PA, Oparil S, Carter BL, Cushman WC, Dennison-Himmelfarb C, Handler J, et al. 2014 Evidence-based guideline for the management of high blood pressure in adults: report from the panel members appointed to the Eighth Joint National Committee (JNC 8). *JAMA* 2014;311(5): 507–520. doi: 10.1001/jama.2013.284427. Epub 2013 Dec 20. PubMed PMID: 24352797

70. Mills KT, Chen J, Yang W, Appel LJ, Kusek JW, Alper A, et al. Sodium excretion and the risk of cardiovascular disease in patients with chronic kidney disease. *JAMA* 2016;315(20):2200–2210. doi: 10.1001/jama.2016.4447. Epub 2016 May 25. PubMed PMID: 27218629; PubMed Central PMCID: PMCPMC5087595

71. Kazmi WH, Obrador GT, Khan SS, Pereira BJ, Kausz AT. Late nephrology referral and mortality among patients with end-stage renal disease: a propensity score analysis. *Nephrol Dial Transplant* 2004;19(7):1808–1814. doi: 10.1093/ndt/gfg573. Epub 2004 Jun 17. PubMed PMID: 15199194

72. Jay CL, Dean PG, Helmick RA, Stegall MD. Reassessing preemptive kidney transplantation in the United States: are we making progress? *Transplantation* 2016;100(5):1120–1127. doi: 10.1097/TP.0000000000000944. Epub 2015 Oct 20. PubMed PMID: 26479285; PubMed Central PMCID: PMCPMC4989865

73. Singh N, Armstrong DG, Lipsky BA. Preventing foot ulcers in patients with diabetes. *JAMA* 2005;293(2):217–228. doi: 10.1001/jama.293.2.217. Epub 2005 Jan 13. PubMed PMID: 15644549

74. Armstrong DG, Boulton AJM, Bus SA. Diabetic foot ulcers and their recurrence. *N Engl J Med* 2017;376(24):2367–2375. doi: 10.1056/NEJMra1615439. Epub 2017 Jun 15. PubMed PMID: 28614678

75. Boulton AJ. The diabetic foot: from art to science. The 18th Camillo Golgi lecture. *Diabetologia* 2004;47(8):1343–1353. doi: 10.1007/s00125-004-1463-y. Epub 2004 Aug 17. PubMed PMID: 15309286

76. Bakker K, Apelqvist J, Schaper NC, International Working Group on Diabetic Foot Editorial B. Practical guidelines on the management and prevention of the diabetic foot 2011. *Diabetes Metab Res Rev* 2012;28 (Suppl. 1):225–231. doi: 10.1002/dmrr.2253. Epub 2012 Mar 1. PubMed PMID: 22271742

77. Lipsky BA, Berendt AR, Deery HG, Embil JM, Joseph WS, Karchmer AW, et al. Diagnosis and treatment of diabetic foot infections. *Clin Infect Dis* 2004;39(7):885–910. doi: 10.1086/424846. Epub 2004 Oct 9. PubMed PMID: 15472838

78. Yazdanpanah L, Nasiri M, Adarvishi S. Literature review on the management of diabetic foot ulcer. *World J Diabetes* 2015;6(1):37–53. doi: 10.4239/wjd.v6.i1.37. Epub 2015 Feb 17. PubMed PMID: 25685277; PubMed Central PMCID: PMCPMC4317316

79. Kavitha KV, Tiwari S, Purandare VB, Khedkar S, Bhosale SS, Unnikrishnan AG. Choice of wound care in diabetic foot ulcer: a practical approach. *World J Diabetes* 2014;5(4):546–556. doi: 10.4239/wjd.v5.i4.546. Epub 2014 Aug 16. PubMed PMID: 25126400; PubMed Central PMCID: PMCPMC4127589

80. Rogers LC, Frykberg RG, Armstrong DG, Boulton AJ, Edmonds M, Van GH, et al. The Charcot foot in diabetes. *Diabetes Care* 2011;34(9):2123–2129. doi: 10.2337/dc11-0844. Epub 2011 Aug 27. PubMed PMID: 21868781; PubMed Central PMCID: PMCPMC3161273

81. Kucera T, Shaikh HH, Sponer P. Charcot neuropathic arthropathy of the foot: a literature review and single-center experience. *J Diabetes Res* 2016;2016:3207043. doi: 10.1155/2016/3207043. Epub 2016 Sep 23. PubMed PMID: 27656656; PubMed Central PMCID: PMCPMC5021483

82. Durgia H, Sahoo J, Kamalanathan S, Palui R, Sridharan K, Raj H. Role of bisphosphonates in the management of acute Charcot foot. *World J Diabetes* 2018;9(7):115–126. doi: 10.4239/wjd.v9.i7.115. Epub 2018 Aug 7. PubMed PMID: 30079147; PubMed Central PMCID: PMCPMC6068741

83. Investigating the use of Prolia (denosumab) in the treatment of acute charcot neuroarthropathy [Internet], 2019. Available from https://clinicaltrials.gov/ct2/show/NCT03174366

84. Busch-Westbroek TE, Delpeut K, Balm R, Bus SA, Schepers T, Peters EJ, et al. Effect of single dose of RANKL antibody treatment on acute Charcot neuro-osteoarthropathy of the foot. *Diabetes Care* 2018;41(3):e21–e22. doi: 10.2337/dc17-1517. Epub 2017 Dec 24. PubMed PMID: 29273577

85. Pop-Busui R, Boulton AJ, Feldman EL, Bril V, Freeman R, Malik RA, et al. Diabetic neuropathy: a position statement by the American Diabetes Association. *Diabetes Care* 2017;40(1):136–154. doi: 10.2337/dc16-2042. Epub 2016 Dec 22. PubMed PMID: 27999003

86. Ang L, Jaiswal M, Martin C, Pop-Busui R. Glucose control and diabetic neuropathy: lessons from recent large clinical trials. *Curr Diab Rep* 2014;14(9):528. doi: 10.1007/s11892-014-0528-7. Epub 2014 Aug 21. PubMed PMID: 25139473; PubMed Central PMCID: PMCPMC5084623

87. Misra UK, Kalita J, Nair PP. Diagnostic approach to peripheral neuropathy. *Ann Indian Acad Neurol* 2008;11(2):89–97. doi: 10.4103/0972-2327.41875. Epub 2008 Apr 1. PubMed PMID: 19893645; PubMed Central PMCID: PMCPMC2771953

88. Pop-Busui R, Lu J, Brooks MM, Albert S, Althouse AD, Escobedo J, et al. Impact of glycemic control strategies on the progression of diabetic peripheral neuropathy in the Bypass Angioplasty Revascularization Investigation 2 Diabetes (BARI 2D) Cohort. *Diabetes Care* 2013;36(10):3208–3215. doi: 10.2337/dc13-0012. Epub 2013 Jun 13. PubMed PMID: 23757426; PubMed Central PMCID: PMCPMC3781573

89. Balducci S, Iacobellis G, Parisi L, Di Biase N, Calandriello E, Leonetti F, et al. Exercise training can modify the natural history of diabetic peripheral neuropathy. *J Diabetes Complications* 2006;20(4):216–223. doi: 10.1016/j.jdiacomp.2005.07.005. Epub 2006 Jun 27. PubMed PMID: 16798472

90. Singleton JR, Marcus RL, Jackson JE, M KL, Graham TE, Smith AG. Exercise increases cutaneous nerve density in diabetic patients without neuropathy. *Ann Clin Transl Neurol* 2014;1(10):844–849. doi: 10.1002/acn3.125. Epub 2014 Dec 11. PubMed PMID: 25493275; PubMed Central PMCID: PMCPMC4241811

91. Sadosky A, Schaefer C, Mann R, Bergstrom F, Baik R, Parsons B, et al. Burden of illness associated with painful diabetic peripheral neuropathy among adults seeking treatment in the US: results from a retrospective chart review and cross-sectional survey. *Diabetes Metab Syndr Obes* 2013;6:79–92. doi: 10.2147/DMSO.S37415. Epub 2013 Feb 14. PubMed PMID: 23403729; PubMed Central PMCID: PMCPMC3569051

92. Waldfogel JM, Nesbit SA, Dy SM, Sharma R, Zhang A, Wilson LM, et al. Pharmacotherapy for diabetic peripheral neuropathy pain and quality of life: A systematic review. *Neurology* 2017;88(20):1958–1967. doi: 10.1212/WNL.0000000000003882. Epub 2017 Mar 28. PubMed PMID: 28341643

93. Wiffen PJ, Derry S, Bell RF, Rice AS, Tolle TR, Phillips T, et al. Gabapentin for chronic neuropathic pain in adults. *Cochrane Database of Syst Rev*

2017;6:CD007938. doi: 10.1002/14651858.CD007938.pub4. Epub 2017 Jun 10. PubMed PMID: 28597471; PubMed Central PMCID: PMCPMC6452908

94. Freynhagen R, Strojek K, Griesing T, Whalen E, Balkenohl M. Efficacy of pregabalin in neuropathic pain evaluated in a 12-week, randomised, double-blind, multicentre, placebo-controlled trial of flexible- and fixed-dose regimens. *Pain* 2005;115(3):254–263. doi: 10.1016/j.pain.2005.02.032. Epub 2005 May 25. PubMed PMID: 15911152

95. Lunn MP, Hughes RA, Wiffen PJ. Duloxetine for treating painful neuropathy, chronic pain or fibromyalgia. *Cochrane Database of Syst Rev* 2014(1): CD007115. doi: 10.1002/14651858.CD007115.pub3. Epub 2014 Jan 5. PubMed PMID: 24385423

96. Gallagher HC, Gallagher RM, Butler M, Buggy DJ, Henman MC. Venlafaxine for neuropathic pain in adults. *Cochrane Database of Syst Rev* 2015(8):CD011091. doi: 10.1002/14651858.CD011091.pub2. Epub 2015 Aug 25. PubMed PMID: 26298465; PubMed Central PMCID: PMCPMC6481532

97. Schwartz S, Etropolski M, Shapiro DY, Okamoto A, Lange R, Haeussler J, et al. Safety and efficacy of tapentadol ER in patients with painful diabetic peripheral neuropathy: results of a randomized-withdrawal, placebo-controlled trial. *Curr Med Res Opin* 2011;27(1):151–162. doi: 10.1185/03007995.2010.537589. Epub 2010 Dec 18. PubMed PMID: 21162697

98. Duehmke RM, Derry S, Wiffen PJ, Bell RF, Aldington D, Moore RA. Tramadol for neuropathic pain in adults. *Cochrane Database of Syst Rev* 2017;6:CD003726. doi: 10.1002/14651858.CD003726.pub4. Epub 2017 Jun 16. PubMed PMID: 28616956; PubMed Central PMCID: PMCPMC6481580

99. Gaskell H, Derry S, Stannard C, Moore RA. Oxycodone for neuropathic pain in adults. *Cochrane Database of Syst Rev* 2016;7:CD010692. doi: 10.1002/14651858.CD010692.pub3. Epub 2016 Jul 29. PubMed PMID: 27465317; PubMed Central PMCID: PMCPMC6457997

100. Moore RA, Derry S, Aldington D, Cole P, Wiffen PJ. Amitriptyline for neuropathic pain in adults. *Cochrane Database of Syst Rev* 2015(7):CD008242. doi: 10.1002/14651858.CD008242.pub3. Epub 2015 Jul 7. PubMed PMID: 26146793; PubMed Central PMCID: PMCPMC6447238

101. Derry S, Wiffen PJ, Aldington D, Moore RA. Nortriptyline for neuropathic pain in adults. *Cochrane Database of Syst Rev* 2015;1:CD011209. doi: 10.1002/14651858.CD011209.pub2. Epub 2015 Jan 9. PubMed PMID: 25569864; PubMed Central PMCID: PMCPMC6485407

102. Hearn L, Moore RA, Derry S, Wiffen PJ, Phillips T. Desipramine for neuropathic pain in adults. *Cochrane Database of Syst Rev* 2014(9):CD011003. doi: 10.1002/14651858.CD011003.pub2. Epub 2014 Sep 24. PubMed PMID: 25246131

103. Pfeifer MA, Weinberg CR, Cook DL, Reenan A, Halter JB, Ensinck JW, et al. Autonomic neural dysfunction in recently diagnosed diabetic subjects. *Diabetes Care* 1984;7(5):447–453. Epub 1984 Sep 1. PubMed PMID: 6499637

104. Tesfaye S, Boulton AJ, Dyck PJ, Freeman R, Horowitz M, Kempler P, et al. Diabetic neuropathies: update on definitions, diagnostic criteria, estimation of severity, and treatments. *Diabetes Care* 2010;33(10):2285–2293. doi: 10.2337/dc10-1303. Epub 2010 Sep 30. PubMed PMID: 20876709; PubMed Central PMCID: PMCPMC2945176

105. Dimitropoulos G, Tahrani AA, Stevens MJ. Cardiac autonomic neuropathy in patients with diabetes mellitus. *World J Diabetes* 2014;5(1):17–39. doi: 10.4239/wjd.v5.i1.17. Epub 2014 Feb 26. PubMed PMID: 24567799; PubMed Central PMCID: PMCPMC3932425

106. Serhiyenko VA, Serhiyenko AA. Cardiac autonomic neuropathy: Risk factors, diagnosis and treatment. *World J Diabetes* 2018;9(1):1–24. doi: 10.4239/wjd.v9.i1.1. Epub 2018 Jan 24. PubMed PMID: 29359025; PubMed Central PMCID: PMCPMC5763036

107. Gaede P, Vedel P, Parving HH, Pedersen O. Intensified multifactorial intervention in patients with type 2 diabetes mellitus and microalbuminuria: the Steno type 2 randomised study. *Lancet* 1999;353(9153):617–622. doi: 10.1016/S0140-6736(98)07368-1. Epub 1999 Feb 25. PubMed PMID: 10030326

108. Pop-Busui R, Evans GW, Gerstein HC, Fonseca V, Fleg JL, Hoogwerf BJ, et al. Effects of cardiac autonomic dysfunction on mortality risk in the Action to Control Cardiovascular Risk in Diabetes (ACCORD) trial. *Diabetes Care* 2010;33(7):1578–1584. Epub 2010 Mar 11. doi: 10.2337/dc10-0125. PubMed PMID: 20215456; PubMed Central PMCID: PMCPMC2890362

109. Vinik AI, Freeman R, Erbas T. Diabetic autonomic neuropathy. *Semin Neurol* 2003;23(4):365–372. doi: 10.1055/s-2004-817720. Epub 2004 Apr 17. PubMed PMID: 15088257

110. Pop-Busui R. What do we know and we do not know about cardiovascular autonomic neuropathy in diabetes. *J Cardiovasc Transl Res* 2012;5(4):463–478. Epub 2012 May 31. doi: 10.1007/s12265-012-9367-6. PubMed PMID: 22644723; PubMed Central PMCID: PMCPMC3634565

111. Vinik AI, Ziegler D. Diabetic cardiovascular autonomic neuropathy. *Circulation* 2007;115(3):387–397. doi: 10.1161/CIRCULATIONAHA.106.634949. Epub 2007 Jan 24. PubMed PMID: 17242296

112. Zygmunt A, Stanczyk J. Methods of evaluation of autonomic nervous system function. *Arch Med Sci* 2010;6(1):11–18. doi: 10.5114/aoms.2010.13500. Epub 2010 Mar 1. PubMed PMID: 22371714; PubMed Central PMCID: PMCPMC3278937

113. Spallone V, Ziegler D, Freeman R, Bernardi L, Frontoni S, Pop-Busui R, et al. Cardiovascular autonomic neuropathy in diabetes: clinical impact,

assessment, diagnosis, and management. *Diabetes Metab Res Rev* 2011;27(7):639–653. doi: 10.1002/dmrr.1239. Epub 2011 Jun 23. PubMed PMID: 21695768

114. Cryer PE. Hypoglycemia-associated autonomic failure in diabetes. *Am J Physiol Endocrinol Metab* 2001;281(6):E1115–E1121. doi: 10.1152/ ajpendo.2001.281.6.E1115. Epub 2001 Nov 10. PubMed PMID: 11701423

115. Pop-Busui R, Low PA, Waberski BH, Martin CL, Albers JW, Feldman EL, et al. Effects of prior intensive insulin therapy on cardiac autonomic nervous system function in type 1 diabetes mellitus: the Diabetes Control and Complications Trial/Epidemiology of Diabetes Interventions and Complications study (DCCT/EDIC). *Circulation* 2009;119(22):2886–2893. doi: 10.1161/CIRCULATIONAHA.108.837369. Epub 2009 May 28. PubMed PMID: 19470886; PubMed Central PMCID: PMCPMC2757005

116. Pop-Busui R. Cardiac autonomic neuropathy in diabetes: a clinical perspective. *Diabetes Care* 2010;33(2):434–441. doi: 10.2337/dc09-1294. Epub 2010 Jan 28. PubMed PMID: 20103559; PubMed Central PMCID: PMCPMC2809298

117. Singer W, Sandroni P, Opfer-Gehrking TL, Suarez GA, Klein CM, Hines S, et al. Pyridostigmine treatment trial in neurogenic orthostatic hypotension. *Arch Neurol* 2006;63(4):513–518. doi: 10.1001/ archneur.63.4.noc50340. Epub 2006 Feb 16. PubMed PMID: 16476804

118. Krishnasamy S, Abell TL. Diabetic gastroparesis: principles and current trends in management. *Diabetes Ther* 2018;9(Suppl. 1):1–42. doi: 10.1007/ s13300-018-0454-9. Epub 2018 Jun 24. PubMed PMID: 29934758; PubMed Central PMCID: PMCPMC6028327

119. Hasler WL. Gastroparesis—current concepts and considerations. *Medscape J Med* 2008;10(1):16. Epub 2008 Mar 8. PubMed PMID: 18324326; PubMed Central PMCID: PMCPMC2258461

120. Abell TL, Camilleri M, Donohoe K, Hasler WL, Lin HC, Maurer AH, et al. Consensus recommendations for gastric emptying scintigraphy: a joint report of the American Neurogastroenterology and Motility Society and the Society of Nuclear Medicine. *Am J Gastroenterol* 2008;103(3):753–763. doi: 10.1111/j.1572-0241.2007.01636.x. Epub 2007 Nov 22. PubMed PMID: 18028513

121. Camilleri M, Parkman HP, Shafi MA, Abell TL, Gerson L, American College of G. Clinical guideline: management of gastroparesis. *Am J Gastroenterol* 2013;108(1):18–37, quiz 8. doi: 10.1038/ajg.2012.373. Epub 2012 Nov 14. PubMed PMID: 23147521; PubMed Central PMCID: PMCPMC3722580

122. Tang DM, Friedenberg FK. Gastroparesis: approach, diagnostic evaluation, and management. *Dis Mon* 2011;57(2):74–101. doi: 10.1016/j.disamonth.2010.12.007. Epub 2011 Feb 19. PubMed PMID: 21329779

123. Mihai BM, Mihai C, Cijevschi-Prelipcean C, Grigorescu ED, Dranga M, Drug V, et al. Bidirectional relationship between gastric emptying and plasma glucose control in normoglycemic individuals and diabetic patients. *J Diabetes Res* 2018;2018:1736959. doi: 10.1155/2018/1736959. Epub 2018 Nov 08. PubMed PMID: 30402500; PubMed Central PMCID: PMCPMC6192082

124. McCallum RW, Snape W, Brody F, Wo J, Parkman HP, Nowak T. Gastric electrical stimulation with Enterra therapy improves symptoms from diabetic gastroparesis in a prospective study. *Clin Gastroenterol Hepatol* 2010;8(11):947–954, quiz e116. doi: 10.1016/j.cgh.2010.05.020. Epub 2010 Jun 12. PubMed PMID: 20538073

125. Krishnan B, Babu S, Walker J, Walker AB, Pappachan JM. Gastrointestinal complications of diabetes mellitus. *World J Diabetes* 2013;4(3):51–63. doi: 10.4239/wjd.v4.i3.51. Epub 2013 Jun 19. PubMed PMID: 23772273; PubMed Central PMCID: PMCPMC3680624

126. Brown JS, Wessells H, Chancellor MB, Howards SS, Stamm WE, Stapleton AE, et al. Urologic complications of diabetes. *Diabetes Care* 2005;28(1): 177–185. Epub 2004 Dec 24. PubMed PMID: 15616253

127. Liu G, Daneshgari F. Diabetic bladder dysfunction. *Chin Med J (Engl)* 2014;127(7):1357–1364. Epub 2014 Apr 09. PubMed PMID: 24709194; PubMed Central PMCID: PMCPMC4426965

128. De Berardis G, Franciosi M, Belfiglio M, Di Nardo B, Greenfield S, Kaplan SH, et al. Erectile dysfunction and quality of life in type 2 diabetic patients: a serious problem too often overlooked. *Diabetes Care* 2002;25(2):284–291. doi: 10.2337/diacare.25.2.284. Epub 2002 Jan 30. PubMed PMID: 11815497

129. Feldman HA, Goldstein I, Hatzichristou DG, Krane RJ, McKinlay JB. Impotence and its medical and psychosocial correlates: results of the Massachusetts Male Aging Study. *J Urol* 1994;151(1):54–61. Epub 1994 Jan 1. PubMed PMID: 8254833

130. Katsiki N, Wierzbicki AS, Mikhailidis DP. Erectile dysfunction and coronary heart disease. *Curr Opin Cardiol* 2015;30(4):416–421. doi: 10.1097/HCO.0000000000000174. Epub 2015 Jun 8. PubMed PMID: 26049392

131. Maiorino MI, Bellastella G, Esposito K. Diabetes and sexual dysfunction: current perspectives. *Diabetes Metab Syndr Obes* 2014;7:95–105. doi: 10.2147/DMSO.S36455. Epub 2014 Mar 14. PubMed PMID: 24623985; PubMed Central PMCID: PMCPMC3949699

132. Pastuszak AW. Current Diagnosis and Management of Erectile Dysfunction. *Curr Sex Health Rep* 2014;6(3):164–176. doi: 10.1007/s11930-014-0023-9. Epub 2015 Apr 17. PubMed PMID: 25878565; PubMed Central PMCID: PMCPMC4394737

133. Smith S. Drugs that cause sexual dysfunction. *Psychiatry* 2007;6(3):111–114

134. Esposito K, Ciotola M, Giugliano F, Maiorino MI, Autorino R, De Sio M, et al. Effects of intensive lifestyle changes on erectile dysfunction in men. *J Sex Med* 2009;6(1):243–250. doi: 10.1111/j.1743-6109.2008.01030.x. Epub 2009 Jan 28. PubMed PMID: 19170853

135. Cheng JY, Ng EM, Chen RY, Ko JS. Alcohol consumption and erectile dysfunction: meta-analysis of population-based studies. *Int J Impot Res* 2007;19(4):343–352. doi: 10.1038/sj.ijir.3901556. Epub 2007 Jun 1. PubMed PMID: 17538641

136. Basson R, Berman J, Burnett A, Derogatis L, Ferguson D, Fourcroy J, et al. Report of the international consensus development conference on female sexual dysfunction: definitions and classifications. *J Urol* 2000;163(3): 888–893. Epub 2000 Feb 25. PubMed PMID: 10688001

137. Pontiroli AE, Cortelazzi D, Morabito A. Female sexual dysfunction and diabetes: a systematic review and meta-analysis. *J Sex Med* 2013;10(4): 1044–1051. doi: 10.1111/jsm.12065. Epub 2013 Jan 26. PubMed PMID: 23347454

138. Abu Ali RM, Al Hajeri RM, Khader YS, Shegem NS, Ajlouni KM. Sexual dysfunction in Jordanian diabetic women. *Diabetes Care* 2008;31(8): 1580–1581. doi: 10.2337/dc08-0081. Epub 2008 May 7. PubMed PMID: 18458140; PubMed Central PMCID: PMCPMC2494660

139. Esposito K, Maiorino MI, Bellastella G, Giugliano F, Romano M, Giugliano D. Determinants of female sexual dysfunction in type 2 diabetes. *Int J Impot Res* 2010;22(3):179–184. doi: 10.1038/ijir.2010.6. Epub 2010 Apr 9. PubMed PMID: 20376056

140. English C, Muhleisen A, Rey JA. Flibanserin (Addyi): the first FDA-approved treatment for female sexual interest/arousal disorder in premenopausal women. *P T* 2017;42(4):237–241. Epub 2017 Apr 7. PubMed PMID: 28381915; PubMed Central PMCID: PMCPMC5358680

141. Llewelyn D, Llewelyn JG. Diabetic amyotrophy: a painful radiculoplexus neuropathy. *Pract Neurol* 2019;19(2):164–167. doi: 10.1136/practneurol-2018-002105. Epub 2018 Dec 12. PubMed PMID: 30530723

142. Smith BE. Focal and Entrapment Neuropathis. In *Diabetes and the Nervous System*. Eds. Zochodne DW and Malik RA. Amsterdam (Netherlands). Elsevier BV, 2014.

Diabetes Self-Management Education and Behavior Change

Highlights

Diabetes Self-Management Education and Support
  Information or Education
  Benefits of DSMES
  Diabetes Education Referral
  Who Are Diabetes Educators?
  Person-Centered Learning
  Summary

Behavior Change
  Person-Centric Language
  Challenges to Making Behavior Change
  Emotional Barriers and Factors Influencing Behavior Change
  Diabetes Distress
  Strategies for Behavior Change: Motivational Interviewing
  Strategies for Facilitating Goal Setting with Motivational Interviewing
  Strategies for Behavior Change: Empowerment Approach
  SMART Goal Setting
  Ongoing Diabetes Self-Management Support
  Summary

Highlights
Diabetes Education and Behavior Change

■ There is a critical need for person-centered diabetes care, rather than patient-centered diabetes care, with diabetes health assessment, decision making, and education.

■ Individuals with diabetes are required to implement and sustain multiple diabetes self-care behaviors in order to maintain glycemic control, prevent diabetes complications, and optimize their quality of life.

■ The demands of diabetes self-care require current knowledge, personal engagement, and empowerment in order to effectively assume this lifelong responsibility. Diabetes self-management education and support for the person with diabetes (and his or her family/caregiver) provides current knowledge, skills, and resources to facilitate sustainable, effective diabetes self-care behavior change.

■ Social, environmental, financial, and cultural influences may interfere with diabetes self-care, despite the person's most concerted efforts.

■ Diabetes Care and Education Specialists are excellent partners in diabetes care, both for the referring provider or care team, as well as for the person living with diabetes.

■ Using a multidisciplinary team approach in the ongoing process of diabetes education, shared decision making, and individualized goal setting increases the likelihood of success.

■ Individualized, collaborative decision making and goal setting enables more effective behavior change.

Diabetes Self-Management Education and Behavior Change

Kellie Rodriguez, RN, MSN, MBA, CDCES
Nancy Drobycki, RN, MSN, CDCES

D iabetes is a challenging and unrelenting disease, demanding daily self-care to achieve desired health outcomes. Given that most people with diabetes spend more than 99% of their time outside of the health system, we will specifically refer to "person with diabetes" rather than "patient with diabetes" throughout this chapter. This emphasizes the critical need for person-centered diabetes care and education within the realm of clinical assessment and decision making.

There have been significant advancements in diabetes clinical practice guidelines, available pharmacotherapies, insulin delivery, and glucose monitoring technology; yet the achievement of required glucose, blood pressure, and cholesterol goals for people with diabetes remains largely unattainable.[1] The contributions and value of these treatment approaches to health outcomes is closely impacted by the lived world of the person with diabetes and his or her ability to successfully implement daily self-care behaviors. Diabetes self-care requires the person with diabetes (and his or her family/support individuals) to effectively cope with the daily rigors of the disease and the recommended treatment regimen, which is at the very core of effective diabetes education and behavior-change strategies.

Diabetes Care and Education Specialists (DCESs), formerly known as Diabetes Educators, comprise a group of multidisciplinary clinicians working in the care and education of people living with diabetes. The title change to DCES was undertaken to more accurately reflect the broader role the specialty serves with people with diabetes. DCESs are therefore excellent partners and resources for primary care providers and people living with diabetes. DCESs support the needs of providers and the person with diabetes through informed decision making and development of effective self-care behavior strategies, use of diabetes technologies, cardiometabolic and behavioral healthcare, and collaboration with other members of the healthcare team. All of these functions are performed while keeping the person with diabetes at the center of care.

DIABETES SELF-MANAGEMENT EDUCATION AND SUPPORT

Diabetes self-management education and support (DSMES) is the ongoing process of facilitating the knowledge, skills, and tools required for people living with diabetes that assess for and incorporate the person's lived world.[2] The Association of Diabetes Care and Education Specialists (ADCES), formerly the American Association of Diabetes Educators (AADE), outlines seven diabetes self-care behavior categories, known as the AADE7 Self-Care Behaviors® (Table 6.1).[3] The AADE7 Self-Care Behaviors® provides a framework of key content for diabetes education assessment and provision.

DCESs have the knowledge, skills, and resources to assess each individual with diabetes across all seven behavior categories to identify areas for required education intervention and promote empowerment toward successful diabetes self-care. In providing diabetes education, DCESs should utilize a curriculum that embraces the latest evidence and practice guidelines.[2] The DCES will utilize those areas of the curriculum that are required, based on the individualized assessment and referral specifications.

Diabetes education is delivered to the person with diabetes by one or more members of the multidisciplinary education team in an individual, group, or

Table 6.1–AADE7 Self-Care Behaviors

AADE7 Self-Care Behaviors®	Key education content
Healthy eating	Understanding macronutrients, developing a practical meal plan, counting carbohydrates, reading food labels, measuring serving sizes, understanding the effects on blood glucose levels, setting goals for healthy eating
Being active	Benefits of exercise, types of exercise, frequency and duration recommendations, reducing risk, maintaining motivation, monitoring progress
Monitoring	Monitoring glucose levels, glucose targets and check times, factors that impact glucose levels, recommended behavior changes, keeping track of glucose levels
Taking medication	Understanding medication actions, side effects, dosage, administration timing and techniques, adherence strategies
Problem solving	High and low blood glucose levels, assessing and addressing factors that contribute to glucose changes, tracking and understanding glucose results, safety factors
Reducing risk	Understanding and reducing the risk for developing diabetes complications, importance of timely healthcare follow-up and self-care checks
Healthy coping	Reducing stress, diabetes distress and depression, maintaining life balance, seeking support, maintaining motivation, effective communication

Source: American Association of Diabetes Educators.[3]

combined individual and group format based on the learning needs of the person with diabetes, the capacity of the diabetes education service, and mandatory reimbursement criteria. Systematic review of the effect on glucose control for adults with type 2 diabetes participating in DSMES identified the greatest A1C reduction in those who attended combined individual and group-based education intervention. Understandably, those individuals with diabetes participating in ≥10 h of diabetes education obtained a greater proportion of A1C improvement.[4] The teaching approach to DSMES also requires consideration. Education research supports a dynamic and interactive process of bidirectional engagement, motivation, problem solving, and teach-back instead of didactic, unidirectional teaching approaches.

INFORMATION OR EDUCATION

At this juncture, it is important to differentiate the terms *health education* and *information*, which are terms often (and erroneously) used interchangeably. Information relates to facts provided or learned about something or someone, representing more of a one-directional interaction.[5] Information is often exchanged from the care team to the person with diabetes (and/or family and support) at healthcare visits, without active person-centered engagement or involvement in the process. Information provided is usually a verbal or written interaction that does not address the core areas of diabetes self-care that include skill building and behavior change. The World Health Organization defines health education as consciously constructed opportunities for individuals or groups to build knowledge and life skills that support promotion and maintenance of health and well-being.[6] Given the chronicity of diabetes and the daily expectations for self-management of the disease, person-centered education provides the best foundation for successful health outcomes.

BENEFITS OF DSMES

DSMES demonstrates multiple benefits to health and well-being for those people living with diabetes, as well as those at risk (Table 6.2).[7] The benefits go beyond reducing clinical risk and extend into improved self-belief and psychosocial well-being with the daily demands of disease management.

Table 6.2–Benefits of Diabetes Self-Management Education

- Improved knowledge and self-efficacy
- A1C reduction (as much as 1%)
- Cardiovascular risk factor reduction
- Reduced onset or advancement of complications
- Improved psychosocial outcomes
- Improved quality of life

Source: Chrvalaa.[7]

Table 6.3–Referral Recommendations

❶	❷	❸	❹
Upon diagnosis	Annual follow-up assessment	With new complicating factors	With care transitions
Upon new diagnosis of diabetes	Review knowledge, skills, and behaviors, especially when not meeting targets. Identify required support to maintain positive behavior change.	Health is compromised due to physical, mental, emotional, and/or social factors.	Changes with aging, living conditions, care team, and/or insurance coverage.

Source: Powers.[4]

DIABETES EDUCATION REFERRAL

Every person with diabetes, upon diagnosis and beyond, should be referred for diabetes education given the clear benefits and recognition that chronic disease success is embedded in self-care. A Joint Position Statement was developed identifying four key times when a person with diabetes should be referred for diabetes education (Table 6.3).[4] The intended goals of the referral recommendations were to improve the care experience and health outcomes of people and populations living with diabetes.

DCESs are valuable partners to referring providers through their skills in assisting with the following:

■ Time-consuming diabetes education, training, and support.
■ Referral follow-up and status updates.
■ Meeting provider and healthcare-center outcome goals.

The 2017 *National Standards for Diabetes Self-Management Education and Support* define the criteria for evidence-based quality diabetes education services. Education services can receive accreditation by the American Diabetes Association or the ADCES, formerly known as the American Association of Diabetes Educators. Accreditation denotes the service is adhering to quality standards across 10 core domains, with the ability to seek reimbursement for education services rendered. If treating providers do not have a connection to a recognized diabetes education program, they can identify available options on the American Diabetes Association's and ADCES's websites.[8,9] A referral is required from the treating provider for accredited DSMES services to address requirements for the national standards and billing purposes. Referrals will require key information to ensure they comply with expected standards and transmit key information to the educator or education team for effective education coordination (Table 6.4).[4]

A referral will denote an implied partnership between the referring provider, diabetes educator, or service and the person living with diabetes. Person-centered care practices will guide the assessment and education intervention provided by the diabetes educator or diabetes education service. Based on the reasons for referral and assessed needs, the diabetes education service will schedule the required individual or group-based sessions, or combination thereof, to meet the person's needs.

Table 6.4–Referral Elements

- Diabetes type
- Treatment plan
- Reason for referral
- Special needs/barriers to learning

Source: Powers.[4]

WHO ARE DIABETES CARE AND EDUCATION SPECIALISTS?

Diabetes Care and Education Specialists are typically health professionals such as nurses, dietitians, pharmacists, providers, and behavioral health specialists, whereas support for diabetes health maintenance is often provided in the community by paraprofessionals such as community health workers and peer leaders.

Utilization of Certified Diabetes Care and Education Specialists (CDCESs), formerly Certified Diabetes Educators (CDEs) or health professionals Board Certified in Advanced Diabetes Management (BC-ADMs), who have undergone a credentialing process to demonstrate core knowledge and expertise in diabetes education and management respectively, is preferred wherever available.[10,11] For practices without a recognized diabetes education service in their geographic location, partnering with one of the local multidisciplinary clinicians or DCESs to best address required education and support services may be an option. In addition, using available internal resources or evidence-based online resources may also be considered.

PERSON-CENTERED LEARNING

DCESs develop expertise to target education strategies in the best way that the person comprehends and learns in order to optimize understanding and motivation. One recommended approach is to use a combination of visual, auditory, reading, or kinesthetic learning principles, otherwise referred to as VARK (Table 6.5).[12,13]

Table 6.5–VARK Learning

VARK	Learning modality
Visual	Diagrams, charts, graphs, demonstration
Auditory	Lectures, group discussion, recordings, speaking, web chat, and talking things through
Reading	Books, pamphlets, lists, diaries
Kinesthetic	Demonstration, practice or simulation, videos, concrete personal experiences, doing something

Source: Fleming.[13]

VARK learning principles focus on an individual's preferred learning modalities. Despite most people having a preferred learning style, people generally benefit from using a combination of approaches. In office visits, information is often exchanged via auditory transaction, which as a sole modality is likely to positively impact >25%–30% of people. Providers should utilize as many available VARK approaches as possible with their teaching approach.

SUMMARY

Diabetes is a disease where health outcomes are largely dependent on the ability of the person with diabetes to implement the recommended treatment approach and self-care responsibilities. The person with diabetes is expected to make major lifestyle adjustments to include practicing healthy eating habits, being physically active, taking medications as prescribed, monitoring glucose, reducing the risk of both acute and chronic diabetes complications, using situational problem solving, and employing healthy coping strategies in order to prevent disease progression and promote an optimum quality of life.[4,14] DSMES provides the required framework for facilitating the knowledge, skills, and tools required for effective diabetes self-care and behavior change. Utilization of DSMES referral guidelines, multidisciplinary healthcare clinicians, and available accredited diabetes services provides a needed resource for both practicing providers and people living with diabetes and their families.

BEHAVIOR CHANGE

Historically, healthcare providers have attempted to convince the person to make behavior changes through persuasion, instilling fear, using judgmental language, and strongly emphasizing the negative health outcomes of current unhealthy behaviors. Not only have these methods been unsuccessful in motivating behavior change, but they have been associated with imparting diabetes-associated stigma, inflicting shame and guilt, causing the person to omit important health information, and even alienating the person from his or her provider.[15,16]

PERSON-CENTRIC LANGUAGE

The language healthcare professionals use has a very powerful impact on the perceptions and behavior of not only colleagues but most importantly people seeking care.[15] Many individuals struggle with a plethora of negative emotions, which can actually interfere with their ability to learn and make behavior change.[17] Language that is person centered, empowering, and strengths based has been shown to enhance communication, motivation, health, and well-being.[15] There are therefore important language considerations for the healthcare team when talking to people with diabetes and their families (Table 6.6).

CHALLENGES TO MAKING BEHAVIOR CHANGE

Changing behavior and sustaining these changes is burdensome for most individuals with diabetes, despite their innate desire to live healthfully and

Table 6.6–Person-centric Language

Language usage recommendations	Avoid saying	Consider saying
Neutral, nonjudgmental, and based on facts, actions, or physiology/biology	"You could reduce your dose of insulin if you would just eat the right foods."	"Research shows us that what and how much we eat can impact our bodies' demand for insulin at mealtime."
Strengths based, respectful, inclusive, and imparts hope	"You are a poorly controlled diabetic."	"You are trying hard to reach your blood glucose targets, and this seems challenging for you."
Free from stigma	"She is noncompliant with taking her insulin."	"Shelly takes her insulin every other day due to financial reasons."
Fosters collaboration between person and provider	"You must stop eating lunch at fast food restaurants."	"What are some other lunch options that might work for you besides fast food?"
Person centered	"She is a diabetic."	"Shelly has diabetes."

Source: Dickinson.[15]

independently. It is recommended that providers partner with the person with diabetes to assess his or her current health situation, identify treatment targets, and collaborate to create a diabetes plan of care that is facilitated by the provider but driven by the person.[14,17] With many competing responsibilities of daily living, multiple barriers may coexist that interfere with the person's best efforts at reaching his or her diabetes self-care goals. It is recommended that providers help the person with diabetes identify these barriers and begin to establish ways to overcome them (Table 6.7).[4,14–17]

EMOTIONAL BARRIERS AND FACTORS INFLUENCING BEHAVIOR CHANGE

It is especially important that providers recognize the impact of emotional barriers and factors influencing behavior change. Psychological comorbidities, including anxiety, depression, life stressors, disordered eating, cognitive impairment, and diabetes distress, often go unrecognized and unmanaged, which may contribute to poor health outcomes.[4,18]

Psychosocial assessment and care should be integrated into the diabetes care plan of all people with diabetes, using a collaborative, person-centered approach. Assessment and reassessment should occur at the time of the initial visit, when there is a change in disease treatment or life circumstances, and at periodic intervals using standardized, validated assessment tools. Appropriate referrals to professional mental health counseling and community resources should be offered to all individuals with diabetes needing psychosocial-related services.[18]

Table 6.7–Barriers to Behavior Change

Barriers: May have one or multiple coexisting barriers	Assessment factors
Socioeconomic: financial and social	Food affordability/availability Medication affordability/availability Complexity of medication regimen: frequency, mode Employment status: multiple jobs Healthcare coverage status
Cultural	Cultural beliefs about using Allopathic medicine versus cultural healthcare practices in the management of diabetes
Emotional	Emotional well-being Diabetes distress Depression or other mental health condition Motivation
Lack of a support system	Support system availability and need: individual or group
Physical	Side effects of current treatment Presence of comorbidities Clinical characteristics Ability to be physically active Hearing/vision/speech impairment
Cognitive	Ability to learn: literacy and health literacy, numeracy, native language, age, relevance of information Level of education, learning style preference
Spiritual	Spiritual practices and laws that impact health behaviors (i.e., dietary fasting, use of medications)

Source: Davies.[14]

DIABETES DISTRESS

Diabetes distress refers to the negative emotional responses and perceived diabetes disease burden for the person with diabetes. Diabetes distress is not a comorbidity or diabetes complication; it the result of living with the daily demands of diabetes self-management.[19] Diabetes distress has a prevalence rate of 18%–45%, and several studies suggest that it has a greater negative impact on both behavioral and metabolic outcomes than depression symptoms.[19,20,21] The unrelenting demands for behavior change (healthy eating, medication dosing/adjustment, being physically active), along with disease progression and the looming possibility of diabetes-related complications, can be overwhelming and exhausting for the person with diabetes. High levels of diabetes distress are connected to higher A1C, lower self-efficacy, medication nonadherence, and poor dietary and physical activity habits.[18,20,22]

The Diabetes Distress Scale 2 (Table 6.8) is a validated, two-item assessment tool that can be quickly administered to the person with diabetes. The Diabetes Distress Scale 17 (DDS-17) is a 17-item survey that provides a more detailed

Table 6.8–Diabetes Distress Scale 2

Diabetes Distress Screening Scale (DDS-2)	Not a problem	Slight problem	Moderate problem	Somewhat serious problem	Serious problem	Very serious problem
1. Feeling over-whelmed by the demands of living with diabetes.						
2. Feeling that I am often failing with my diabetes routine.						

Source: Jeong.[19]

assessment of the person's level of diabetes distress. It has been recommended that individuals with positive findings on the DDS-2 be further assessed using the DDS-17.[19,23]

STRATEGIES FOR BEHAVIOR CHANGE: MOTIVATIONAL INTERVIEWING

Once barriers and influential factors are identified, it is recommended that providers implement a shared decision-making process to facilitate the development of a person-centered diabetes management plan.[4,14] Creating this plan requires the provider to see the world through the eyes of the person with diabetes and respect his or her viewpoint, even if the person's ideas about diabetes self-care seem misguided and flawed.[24]

Individuals with diabetes make healthcare decisions based on what makes sense to them, not necessarily what may be best for their diabetes self-management. Our current society refers to individuals seeking healthcare as "patients"; yet, if we expect them to follow dictated treatment protocols and provider mandates to make behavior change, we are setting them up for failure. Instead, we are called to invite the person with diabetes to take an active role in his or her diabetes self-care.[25] Utilizing the motivational interviewing approach will help the provider to facilitate the establishment of the person-centered diabetes management plan with corresponding behavior-change recommendations.[4,14,18,24,25]

The spirit of motivational interviewing is caring for and respecting the *whole* person, who ultimately decides his or her plan of action for personal goal attainment. It optimizes the possibility that individuals with a chronic illness will consider and make behavior changes with the goal of positive health outcomes.[24]

Berger and Villaume indicate that both resistance and ambivalence to change exist in individuals with a chronic illness, which is a key consideration before implementing motivational interviewing strategies.[24] They also believe that providers are more likely to think of people as being resistant to making change versus ambivalent to making change. As a result, they have identified two types of resistance: issue resistance and relational resistance[24] (Table 6.9).

Table 6.9–Types of Resistance to Change

Types of resistance	Definition	Situation
Issue resistance (ambivalence)	The person's reasoning and making sense about a behavior	"I will take metformin, but I am not taking insulin."
Relational resistance	How the provider responds to the person's issue resistance (ambivalence)	Does the provider respect/disrespect the person's situational thoughts and concerns? Is there success or failure to build rapport?

Source: Berger.[24]

One of the major cornerstones of motivational interviewing is facilitating "change talk"; however, one must first understand the differences between change talk and "resistance talk" to enable more effective change talk (Table 6.10).

Millner and Rollnick recommend that providers use four skills when facilitating and eliciting change talk with the key objective of avoiding the creation of additional resistance talk.[14] These skills are summarized in Table 6.11. This process of eliciting change talk puts the person with diabetes at the center of his or her diabetes plan of care. To further enable the behavior-change process, providers should facilitate access to DSMES, educate and inform the person of various treatment options, and seek his or her preferences, thereby empowering him or her to set behavior-change goals.[14]

Table 6.10–Change Talk versus Resistance Talk

Change talk versus resistance talk	Definition	Example statements
Change talk	Any talk by the person that focuses on the rationale for making behavior change to achieve his or her goal. It may range from seeking information to making a commitment to change.	"Just how painful are those insulin injections?" "It sounds like taking insulin is not so painful. I can start taking it once a day in the evening."
Resistance talk	Any talk by the person that focuses on the rationale for why the person does not need to or does not want to change behavior	"I am not taking insulin because when they put my mom on insulin, she had her toes amputated 3 months later." "I hate needles because I had a bad experience as a child."

Source: Berger.[24]

Table 6.11–Change Talk—OARS

Skills of eliciting change talk (OARS)	Purpose	Recommendations	Caution
Open-ended questions starting with *how, what, why,* and *when*	Encourages the person to openly speak about prospective behavior change	Ask about the following: ■ Advantages of changing ■ Disadvantages of not changing ■ Being successful in changing ■ Intention to change	Only ask questions that invite change talk. Some open-ended questions may invite resistance talk.
Affirmations	Encourages the person to progress through the change process by using supportive statements with emphasis on the person's vision	Affirm things that will elicit further change talk through encouraging words and supportive nonverbal communication styles.	Avoid affirmations that may be perceived as insincere and those that may elicit further resistance talk.
Reflective listening	Provides immediate feedback to the person that his or her thoughts and concerns have been heard by the provider	Reflect back to the person what you just heard the person say. Emphasize the positive talk and place less emphasis on the negative talk.	Avoid using common responses like "Ok," "Uh-huh," and "I get it," as these lack proof that the provider has really heard the person's concerns.
Summaries	Gathers the thoughts, emotions, and concerns of change talk into a clear, concise account	Create a sense that something great has just transpired. Compose the summary with positivity that encourages behavior change.	Avoid treating this as a trivial step. It may reveal how much has been accomplished in the course of the encounter and may form a very personal basis for making change.

Source: Berger.[24]

STRATEGIES FOR FACILITATING GOAL SETTING WITH MOTIVATIONAL INTERVIEWING

Developing discrepancies and reinforcing change talk involves identifying the core values of the person with diabetes and what he or she most wants to accomplish to optimize his or her diabetes health. It also assists the person to see whether current healthcare behaviors mirror or contradict the person's core values. Providers can then facilitate behavior change by adding factual information to help the person with diabetes discern differences between current health behaviors and

Table 6.12–Questions That Facilitate Use of Motivational Interviewing

1. What reasons do you have for wanting to make this change?

2. How might you go about change in order to succeed?

3. What are some ways for you to change?

4. How important is it for you to make this change and why?

5. Out of the options we have discussed, what is the most appealing to you?

Source: Piatt.[26]

how they interact/interfere with core values and desired health outcomes. Ultimately, individuals with diabetes assume personal responsibility for identifying any discrepancies and then using these discrepancies as motivation to set behavior-change goals. Five questions have been identified that can be utilized to facilitate behavior change[26] (Table 6.12).

STRATEGIES FOR BEHAVIOR CHANGE: EMPOWERMENT APPROACH

The Empowerment Approach theorizes that the person with diabetes will make and sustain behavior change over a longer period of time if these changes are self-directed. Most individuals with diabetes will need assistance in learning to set meaningful, measurable, and realistic goals. Table 6.13 outlines a four-step process for goal setting that supports collaboration. When setting goals, it is helpful to encourage the person with diabetes to think of these as experiments rather than as absolutes that will result in a success or a failure. Beginning the visit by asking about his or her experiment and what he or she learned as a result sets the agenda for the rest of the visit and future goal setting.[26]

SMART GOAL SETTING

Facilitating behavior-change goal setting is simplified by using the SMART acronym as listed in Table 6.14.[27] Explaining the rationale for using this method gives the person with diabetes the necessary understanding of the importance of this process. Often, goals are set that are vague and without meaning. For example, a patient may set a goal to lose weight, but without planned, defined metrics that can be tracked, are achievable and realistic, and have a specific time line, a "goal" becomes just a mere wish.

ONGOING DIABETES SELF-MANAGEMENT SUPPORT

Most studies indicate that sustaining behavioral changes is more difficult than making an initial change. Many individuals with diabetes will need ongoing follow-up and support to maintain the gains made through DSMES and initial goal setting. This type of support includes following up on goals set previously; assisting with stress management, diabetes-related distress, and coping; collaborating

Table 6.13–Empowerment Approach to Behavior Change

Behavioral steps in the empowerment approach	Suggested questions	Rationale
Identify the problem.	What is the most difficult or frustrating part of caring for your diabetes at this time?	Helps the person explore the details of his or her current situation
Determine the person's feelings and his or her influence on behavior.	How do you feel about this issue? How are your feelings influencing your behavior?	Integrates clinical, behavioral, and psychosocial aspects into diabetes care Identifies barriers that may exist to making behavior change
Identify a short-term behavior-change experiment.	What are some steps that you can take now to get you closer to where you want to be? What is one thing that you will do when you leave here to improve your situation?	Facilitating the setting of a self-directed, I-SMART Goal activates the person as the following: ■ Problem-solver ■ Change agent ■ Expert in his or her learning needs and approaches that work best for him or her
Implement the plan and evaluate the plan at the next visit.	How did the plan we discussed at your last visit work out for you? What have you learned? What would you do differently next time? What will you do when you leave here today?	Provides an opportunity to reflect on the experience and outcome of implementing this goal. Serves as a foundation for setting new goals and making further behavior changes.

Source: Piatt.[26]

to solve problems and overcome barriers; providing information about new or different treatment options; and asking the person to set new goals or recommit to revising existing goals.[4,14,23]

SUMMARY

Behavior change is a critical aspect of diabetes care that greatly affects the person with diabetes in his or her immediate and future health outcomes and quality of life. Providers have a significant role to play in supporting the person with diabetes in achieving behavior change and sustaining these changes to optimize quality of life. We can give evidence-based diabetes information; refer individuals with diabetes for diabetes self-management education services; empower the person with diabetes in his or her role as problem-solver and change agent; facilitate col-

Table 6.14–I-SMART Goals

SMART Goal	Definition	Recommendations/rationale
Important	What is most important for the person to change first?	Having the person choose what is most important to him or her will increase the likelihood of changing behavior.
Specific	What? Why? When? How?	Encourage the person to identify the details of his or her planned experiment.
Measurable	Goal should be tracked and measured.	Accurate tracking is needed to identify progress toward goal achievement.
Achievable	Requires commitment and should challenge the person somewhat, but not be over-whelming	Success in goal achievement will set the foundation for developing confidence and a sense of self-efficacy.
Realistic	Doable (not necessarily easy)	Work with the person as to what he or she is willing and able to do to achieve his or her goal.
Time defined	Set a time frame for the goal	Providing a clear target to work toward prompts the person to put the goal into action. Shorter time frames may provide more immediate feedback.

Source: Schreiner.[27]

laborative goal setting, and reevaluate the diabetes plan of care on a regular basis.[14] Ultimately, the person with diabetes is responsible for putting this knowledge and support into action for positive behavior change for optimum health outcomes.

Using a team approach to diabetes self-management education and care, with the person with diabetes as the team leader, has proven to be a successful approach in changing diabetes self-care behaviors and improving diabetes health outcomes. Activating the expertise of the DCES, registered nurse, registered dietitian, pharmacist, exercise physiologist, mental health professional, and social worker provides individuals with diabetes a variety of resources to effectively manage their condition. In addition, connections with local community diabetes self-management support resources should be offered, and individuals with diabetes should be encouraged to utilize these resources.

REFERENCES

1.   Ali MK et al. Achievement of goals in U.S. diabetes care, 1999–2010. *N Engl J Med* 2013;368:1613–1624

2.   Beck J et al. 2017 National standards for diabetes self-management and support. *Diabetes Educator* 2017;43(5):449–464

3.   American Association of Diabetes Educators. The Art and Science of Diabetes Self-Management Education Desk Reference. 4th ed. Chicago, American Association of Diabetes Educators, 2017

4. Powers MA, et al. Diabetes self-management education and support in type 2 diabetes: a joint position statement of the American Diabetes Association, the American Association of Diabetes Educators, and the Academy of Nutrition and Dietetics. *Diabetes Educ* 2015;41(4):417–430

5. Stevenson A, et al. *Oxford American Dictionary*. 3rd ed. Oxford, Oxford University Press, 2019

6. World Health Organization. List of basic terms. In *Health Promotion Glossary*, 1998. Available from https://www.who.int/healthpromotion/about/HPR%20Glossary%201998.pdf. Accessed 23 April 2019

7. Chrvalaa CA, Sherr D, Lipman RD. Diabetes self-management education for adults with type 2 diabetes mellitus: a systematic review of the effect on glycemic control. *Patient Educ Couns* 2016;99(6):926–943

8. American Diabetes Association. ERP Listing [Internet]. Available from https://professional.diabetes.org/erp_list_zip. Accessed 14 April 2020

9. Association of Diabetes Care and Education Specialists. Find a Diabetes Education Program in Your Area [Internet] 2020. Available from: https://www.diabeteseducator.org/living-with-diabetes/find-an-education-program. Accessed 14 April 2020

10. National Certification Board for Diabetes Educators. What is a Certified Disabilities Educator? Available from https://www.ncbde.org/certification_info/what-is-a-cde/. Accessed 24 Apr 2019

11. Association of Diabetes Care and Education Specialists. Board Certified-Advanced Diabetes Management (BC-ADM®). Available from https://www.diabeteseducator.org/education/certification/bc_adm. Accessed 24 Apr 2019

12. Leite WL, Svinicki M, Shi Y. Attempted validation of the scores of the VARK: learning styles inventory with multitrait-multimethod confirmatory factor analysis models. *Educ Psychol Meas* 2010;70:323–339

13. Fleming ND. Facts, fallacies and myths: VARK and learning preferences, 2012. Available from http://vark-learn.com/wp-content/uploads/2014/08/Some-Facts-About-VARK.pdf. Accessed 9 May 2019

14. Davies MJ, D'Alessio DA, et al. Management of hyperglycemia in type 2 diabetes, 2018: a consensus report by the American Diabetes Association (ADA) and the European Association for the Study of Diabetes (EASD). *Diabetes Care* 2018;1–33.

15. Dickinson JK, et al. The use of language in diabetes care and education. *Diabetes Care* 2017;40(12):1790–1799

16. Greene J, et al. Supporting patient behavior change: approaches used by primary care clinicians whose patients have an increase in activation levels. *Annals of Family Medicine* 2016;14(2):148–154.

17. Storzo GA, Moore M, Scholtz M. Delivering change that lasts. *ACSM's Health & Fitness Journal* 2015;19(2):20–26

18. Young SA, et al. The influence of patient and provider communication on diabetes care delivery. *J Ambulatory Care Manag* 2016;39(3):272–278

19. Jeong M, Reifsnider E. Associations of diabetes-related distress and depressive symptoms with glycemic control in Korean Americans with type 2 diabetes. *Diabetes Educator* 2018;44(6):531–540

20. American Diabetes Association. 5. Facilitating behavior change and well-being to improve health outcomes: standards of medical care in diabetes 2020. *Diabetes Care* 2020;43(Suppl. 1):S48–S65

21. Fisher L, et al. Diabetes distress but not clinical depression or depressive symptoms is associated with glycemic control in both cross-sectional and longitudinal analyses. *Diabetes Care* 2010;33(1):23–28

22. Gonzalvo JD, et al. A practical approach to mental health for the diabetes educator—AADE Practice Paper. *AADE in Practice* 2019:29–44

23. Polonsky WH, Fisher L. Diabetes Distress Scale. Diabetes Distress Assessment & Resource Center. Available from https://diabetesdistress.org. Accessed 3 May 2019

24. Berger BA, Villaume WA. *Motivational Interviewing for Health Care Professionals: A Sensible Approach*. Washington, DC, American Pharmacist's Association, 2013.

25. Van Ommen B, Wopereis S, et al. From diabetes care to diabetes cure—the integration of systems biology, ehealth and behavioral change. *Frontiers in Endocrinol* 2018;8(381):1–19

26. Piatt GA, Anderson B, Funnell MM. Theoretical and behavioral approaches to the self-management of health. In Educators, American Association of Diabetes. *The Art and Science of Diabetes Self-Management Education Desk Reference*. 4th ed. Chicago, American Association of Diabetes Educators, 2017, p. 85–114

27. Schreiner B. The diabetes self-management education process. In Educators, American Association of Diabetes. *The Art and Science of Diabetes Self-Management Education Desk Reference*. 4th ed. Chicago, American Association of Diabetes Educators, 2017, p. 29–84.

Index

Note: Page numbers followed by an *f* refer to figures. Page numbers followed by a *t* refer to tables.

Printed in the USA
CPSIA information can be obtained
at www.ICGtesting.com
JSHW010813100824
67803JS00010B/8

9 781580 406314